Radiotracers
in
Drug
Development

Radiotracers
in
Drug
Development

Graham Lappin
Simon Temple

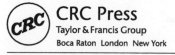

CRC Press
Taylor & Francis Group
Boca Raton London New York

CRC Press is an imprint of the
Taylor & Francis Group, an **informa** business
A TAYLOR & FRANCIS BOOK

First published 2006 by Taylor & Francis

Published in 2019 by
CRC Press
Taylor & Francis Group
6000 Broken Sound Parkway NW, Suite 300
Boca Raton, FL 33487-2742

© 2006 by Taylor & Francis Group, LLC
CRC Press is an imprint of Taylor & Francis Group, an Informa business

First issued in paperback 2019

No claim to original U.S. Government works

ISBN-13: 978-0-367-45372-5 (pbk)
ISBN-13: 978-0-8493-3347-7 (hbk)

Library of Congress Cataloging-in-Publication Data

Catalog record is available from the Library of Congress

**Visit the Taylor & Francis Web site at
http://www.taylorandfrancis.com**

**and the CRC Press Web site at
http://www.crcpress.com**

Preface

Synthetic pharmaceuticals are xenobiotics; they are compounds foreign to human metabolism and make no contribution to nutrition. Drugs, however, are not the only xenobiotics to which we are all exposed. Take the diet, for example. Countless xenobiotics have evolved in plants, animals and bacteria as chemical defense mechanisms. Other organisms that feed on them, such as humans, have coevolved biochemical systems that neutralize and remove these toxins. This chemical warfare extends well back in evolutionary time. Our detoxification mechanisms can be very efficient, evidenced by the fact that we do not experience toxic effects every time we ingest xenobiotics not previously encountered as we try some new foodstuff. Pharmaceuticals are xenobiotics that have been designed by humans to have targeted physiological effects in the never-ending battle against disease. To the body, however, pharmaceuticals are only another set of xenobiotics to be detoxified through metabolism and excretion. To the body, no distinction is made as to whether the xenobiotic is a drug, a synthetic chemical, or a natural compound. Indeed, this very fact goes some way to explode the modern myth of natural = good, unnatural = bad. There is irony in the fact that the body's detoxification systems will potentially eliminate drugs that might be lifesaving just as efficiently as other xenobiotics that might do harm.

Largely driven by the pharmaceutical industry, we now have a wide, yet still growing, understanding of the enzymology responsible for xenobiotic metabolism. Reflecting the influence of the pharmaceuticals industry, these enzymes are often referred to as drug metabolizing, although as discussed above, from an evolutionary perspective the presence of these enzymes has little to do with modern-day pharmaceuticals. An understanding of the way the body deals with foreign compounds is pivotal to developing effective new drugs. A drug might be exceedingly active in the test tube, but if the body breaks it down and excretes it so rapidly that the effect is not manifest in the patient, then the drug is of little use.

Not surprisingly, therefore, interest in the metabolism of xenobiotics grew significantly as the first pharmaceuticals were developed. To study the metabolic fate of a xenobiotic, it has to be followed through the body as it passes through the tissues and organs. Practically, this can be a very difficult process. The task demands that small amounts of compound be quantified within a vast and complex array of constitutive compounds. Moreover, as the xenobiotic is metabolized, its chemical structure is changed by metabolism, and therefore, in effect, it can hide from detection. These problems have been largely solved by the use of radiotracers, the subject of this book. By introducing a "tag" onto the xenobiotic, it effectively contains a radioactive homing signal, enabling the metabolic fate of the compound to be followed through the biological system. This approach has been used as a general research tool for many years. Indeed, as we shall see in Chapter 1, the photosynthetic pathway was elucidated back in the 1950s using just this technique.

If radiotracers are to be useful, they must be detected and quantified. There are many methods of detecting or imaging the label, and the choice very much depends upon the questions the experiments are designed to answer. Needless to say, there are many pitfalls of which the researcher must be aware. This book attempts to provide a general background to the use of radiotracers in the development of new pharmaceuticals and to place signposts over the pitfalls, in the hope that the researcher will not fall in. In recent times, new technologies have arisen for the detection and imaging of radiotracers, which have quietly revolutionized this science. Some of these technologies are not yet widely known, and so they are covered here in an attempt to spread the word.

The publishing of this book coincides with great angst in the pharmaceuticals industry. It is easy to forget, but modern drug therapy has developed over a remarkably short period. In the span of a single lifetime we have moved from the handful of drugs available at the end of the Second World War to the multi-billion dollar pharmaceutical industry that we see today. Many observers believe, however, that the pharmaceuticals industry today is in crisis. The number of new drugs approved each year is on the decline, while research and development costs are on the increase. If we have not already seen the last of the blockbuster drugs, many believe that their demise is not far away. There has been much debate on how to innovate the drug development process. No single technology will transform the pharmaceuticals industry; instead, each will play its own small yet important role. One of the many innovations has been to reevaluate the role that radiotracers play in drug development. Studies utilizing the unique properties of radiotracers are being conducted earlier in the development cycle, and greater use is being made of data derived from humans, as opposed to animal or *in vitro* models. Sizeable changes are afoot, although the conservatism of the pharmaceuticals industry should not be underestimated. There are few revolutions in this industry; it is more a matter of evolution and slow evolution at that.

Pharmaceutical development is a highly interdisciplinary field. This book touches upon only one aspect of drug development, but nevertheless, it crosses the boundaries of biology, chemistry, and physics. Researchers therefore have to be highly flexible and must be capable and willing to venture into fields where previously they had little knowledge or experience. For many, this is the joy of science, but it can also be frustrating, as the literature on the whole is written by experts for experts. This book is therefore aimed at both those new to metabolism research and those who are making the exciting journey to fresh pastures. It is not an in-depth review, but more an overview; nevertheless, it is hoped that even the most experienced metabolism scientist will find this a useful source of reference. This book attempts to place the use of radiotracer studies in context of the registration of drugs, and hence, it has a strong bias toward an industrial approach. Notwithstanding this, it is hoped that anyone researching into the metabolic fate of xenobiotics in general will find parts of the text useful.

Graham Lappin

Cross-References

Throughout the text there are cross-references to other sections by the section number: for example, 1.2.2, the first number (in this case 1) always indicating the chapter.

Authors

Graham Lappin

Dr. Graham Lappin, a veteran of 25 years in the business, started by researching into the metabolism of terpenoids in plants. He earned his bachelor's degree and Ph.D. from the University of Westminster, London, UK, followed by post-doctorial research at the University of Glasgow in Scotland. Graham then spent several years specializing in mammalian metabolism, and today he is dedicated to the study of drug metabolism in humans. Widely published in his field, Graham is a fellow of the UK's Institute of Biology and Royal Society of Chemistry, and is currently the head of research and development at Xceleron Ltd., a spin-out from the University of York, specializing in accelerator mass spectrometry. He would welcome any comments or question relating to this book via e-mail (glappin@glappin.com).

Simon Temple

After qualifying as a teacher in 1972, Simon Temple worked for two years in education. He left to pursue a career in sales with various companies in the scientific market place working on a range of different product types. In 1984 he joined Packard Instruments and in 1988 became responsible for the sales and marketing of the liquid scintillation consumable products. From this time he became closely involved with liquid scintillation products eventually becoming in 1995 the specialist responsible for both internal staff and customer training.

From 1995 until he left the company (by then PerkinElmer Life Sciences) he was closely involved in all aspects of liquid scintillation and gamma counting including flow scintillation analysis and microplate scintillation counting. A short while after leaving Perkin Elmer he formed DPM Solutions Ltd, a company dedicated to training in the theory and practice of liquid scintillation counting and gamma counting.

Simon runs training courses on liquid scintillation and gamma counting and acts as a consultant to various companies in the UK. He has recently become the managing director of raytest UK Ltd, concerned with the sales and service of radiochromatography, PET analysis and radiation protection instrumentation in the UK.

Contributors

Brian Whitby has more than 28 years of experience in the pharmaceutical contract industry. For the majority of this time he has specialized in carrying out whole-body autoradiography (WBA) experiments both at the qualitative and quantitative levels. He worked for 12 years at Huntingdon Life Sciences (formerly known as Huntingdon Research Centre) and for the past 16 years at Covance-Harrogate. As a senior scientist in the Drug Metabolism Department at Covance, he is a mentor for a group of experienced study directors and operational scientists who are dedicated to performing quantitative WBA studies. In addition to his duties at Covance, Brian is also the honorary chairman of the European Society for Autoradiography. In this role he is responsible for helping to organize major scientific meetings and training courses in Europe.

Barbara Koetz joined the Molecular Imaging Centre in Manchester, UK, in March 2005 as a PET oncology research fellow. She studied medicine in Münster, Germany, and, having spent most of her clinical training in the UK, became a member of the Royal College of Physicians, London in 1999. Prior to joining the imaging centre she worked as a specialist registrar in medical oncology at the University Hospital in Birmingham, where she obtained a master's degree in clinical oncology. She will be involved in developing response assessment tools for molecular targeted cancer treatments with a special interest in antiangiogenesis.

Pat Price studied at Cambridge and King's College Hospital Medical School, UK, qualifying in 1981. She trained in oncology at the Royal Marsden Hospital and took up a research position at the Institute of Cancer Research, London, winning the Cambridge University prize for best laboratory-based MD. While working at the Hammersmith Hospital, London as a senior lecturer, Pat developed a research interest in molecular imaging for oncology and headed the MRC and CRC PET Oncology Programmes. She moved to Manchester in 2000 to take up the Ralston Paterson Chair in radiation oncology and set up the new Manchester Molecular Imaging Centre, which she now directs.

Steve Newman is a scientific consultant based in Nottingham, UK. He has a Ph.D. from the Faculty of Medicine of the University of London. Steve was a principal physicist and honorary senior lecturer in the Department of Thoracic Medicine, Royal Free Hospital and School of Medicine from 1982 to 1991, and was a director of Pharmaceutical Profiles in Nottingham, from 1991 to 2004. He is a Fellow of the Institute of Physics and Engineering in Medicine, and also a Fellow of the Institute of Physics. He has given numerous lectures both at international conferences and within the pharmaceutical industry, and has published over 200 research papers, invited articles and book chapters.

Gary Pitcairn is currently head of development at Pharmaceutical Profiles, a company that specializes in evaluating drug delivery for the pharmaceutical industry.

Gary is responsible for all the scientific aspects of the laboratory and clinical studies undertaken with pulmonary and nasal inhalers. Prior to this post, Gary ran a small R&D group at the same company and successfully developed and patented a novel radiolabelling method applicable to a variety of different pharmaceutical dosage forms, thereby extending the role of scintigraphy in assessing drug delivery.

Contents

Contents

CHAPTER 1

Radiotracers and Drug Registration

Graham Lappin

CONTENTS

1.1 THE DRUG REGISTRATION PROCESS

There are three broad questions to answer in bringing a new drug to market: (1) Is it efficacious? (2) Is it safe? (3) What is the dose? These three questions are not independent from each other. At a given dose the drug will exhibit a certain efficacy and toxicity, while the ideal dose will optimize efficacy and minimize toxicity. The relationship among these three factors also differs between individual patients, depending upon the spread of response within a target population. At the outset, the relationship of efficacy, safety and dose within a patient population is unknown. It is the drug registration process that determines these relationships by means of an extensive range of scientific studies. Inappropriate properties in any one of these areas may lead to that particular drug being abandoned from the development process. To give an idea of the magnitude of the studies required to bring a new drug to market, at the time of writing (2005) the average development cost is around $800 million.[1]

The registration of new pharmaceuticals is heavily regulated by government agencies throughout the world. These agencies publish guidelines and regulations that set down data requirements for drug approval. The development of every new drug, however, raises questions peculiar to that compound. Each drug is in effect a hand-crafted, bespoke product. Drug registration is not merely a matter of blindly following a series of prescribed tests; on the contrary, it is highly science driven. The use of radiotracers (the subject of this book) is only one tool of many used by the pharmaceuticals industry in the science-driven drug registration process.

Before embarking on the subject of radiotracers, however, it is worth setting the scene with a general overview of the various stages of drug registration. How radiotracers are applied to this process can then be placed into context. Drug development can be divided into five general areas: discovery, preclinical, and three clinical phases (I to III). After the drug has been approved, there is then a period of postmarketing surveillance (phase IV). Each of these phases is outlined in Section 1.1.1 to Section 1.1.7. The process from drug discovery to market is often depicted as a development funnel, as shown in Figure 1.1. The majority of studies undertaken for the approval of a new drug are conducted using nonradiolabeled material. The efforts outlined in Section 1.1.1 to Section 1.1.7 are all in the nonradiolabeled category.

1.1.1 Discovery

Many thousands or millions of compounds are synthesized and then screened for pharmacological activity using *in vitro* techniques. While serendipity plays a role in the choice of synthesis, computer (*in silico*) models and a general understanding of drug metabolism also play an important part (Section 1.5.3). In a typical *in vitro* screen, compounds are assayed for their affinity for a receptor. A series of other screens then follow, to slowly whittle down the number of drug candidates, until a small number (perhaps only one) is selected for development. The screens are conducted using robotized, highly automated systems, in a process known as high-throughput screening. Drugs selected for development may not be those with the

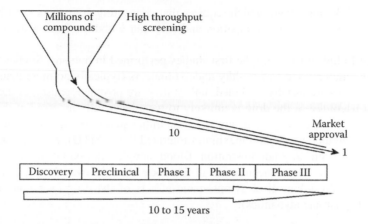

Figure 1.1 The drug development funnel. For every 10 candidate compounds that enter clinical trials, only one will make it to market.

highest binding affinities; instead, they will have a balance of predicted properties — a compromise among receptor affinity, water solubility, toxicity, and other parameters. At this early stage, the properties of the drug are estimated *in vitro* or *in silico*, typically using cell-based assays or enzyme kinetics, with perhaps some minimal animal data at the later stages of selection. Once the candidate drugs enter the development phase, costs begin to spiral, so there has been much debate on the effectiveness of the drug selection process.[2,3]

1.1.2 Preclinical Studies

Once it selects a drug for development, it is the usual objective of a pharmaceutical company to administer the drug candidate to human volunteers as quickly as possible. Before the drug can be administered to humans, however, a series of preclinical tests (pharmacology, safety pharmacology, short-term toxicity, and genotoxicity) must be performed, mainly using animals, to ensure the drug's safety. Such studies are sufficient to allow the drug to be tested on humans in phase I studies, but further testing is required with animals over longer periods to assess potential long-term toxicity, reproduction toxicity, and carcinogenicity of the drug candidate before it can be finally approved for medical use.

1.1.3 Phase I

Once the initial safety of the drug candidate has been assessed, a series of extensive clinical trials in humans will begin. Before clinical trials can start, however, an Investigational New Drug application (IND in the U.S.) or a Clinical Trials Application (CTA in Europe) has to be submitted to the regulatory authority. These applications summarize the toxicological data and assess any potential risks to the human volunteers. Studies with human volunteers are conducted under the auspices of the Helsinki agreement, which requires that consenting volunteers must be fully informed of the risks of participation and they can withdraw from a study at any time.[4]

Phase I clinical trials are the first studies performed in humans. Studies usually consist of small numbers of healthy male volunteers (typically no more than 100 in total). Females are usually excluded, unless they are postmenopausal, as the reproductive toxicology of the drug is unlikely to have been fully assessed at this time. Single or multiple doses may be given. These initial studies monitor clinical effects, determine the therapeutic and maximum tolerated dose (MTD), and may study the effects of food on drug administration. Blood samples can be taken and analyzed to study how the drug concentration in the body changes over time (pharmacokinetics). The physiological or symptomatic effects of the drug over time are also examined (pharmacodynamics).

1.1.4 Phase II

Phase II clinical trials are conducted in small numbers of patients (total of around 100 to 300) suffering from the target disease. These studies are principally aimed at an initial assessment of the efficacy of the drug. Polymorphic effects (Section 1.5.3) might be examined as well as reactions with food and other drugs. As with phase I, blood samples can be taken to study the pharmacokinetics of the drug.

1.1.5 Phase III

Phase III clinical trials are usually performed in a number of countries (multicenter) with larger numbers of patients (low thousands to many thousands, depending on the drug class). Depending on local regulatory requirements, these trials would typically compare the test drug with a marketed drug or placebo comparator (as control) in a study where neither the patient nor the physician knows which dose is the drug and which is the control (this type of trial is known as a double-blind study). Further pharmacokinetic and pharmacodynamic measurements may also be made.

1.1.6 Drug Approval

The approval of a new drug by the regulatory agencies relies on a benefit–risk assessment based upon its therapeutic use and the target patient population, a process that is inevitably biased toward safety. The way the drug is developed is also influenced by its intended therapeutic use. For example, drugs used to treat cancer by their nature are cytotoxic and often have genotoxic potential. It would be unethical to administer such compounds to healthy volunteers (phase I), who would not receive any therapeutic benefit and, indeed, may be harmed by such compounds. Development programs may also differ, for example, for sex-specific therapies and aged populations. Moreover, many regulatory authorities have fast-track systems to bring lifesaving drugs to market sooner, thereby removing the need for certain studies.

1.1.7 Phase IV

Phase IV involves monitoring for adverse effects after a drug has been licensed for use (i.e., postmarketing surveillance). During the clinical trials, patients exposed to the drug may number a few thousand. Once the drug has been approved, however, hundreds of thousands or millions of patients may be exposed. Statistically, effects may arise after the drug is in use that were not detected during the clinical trials. Adverse reports during phase IV can result in the instigation of further studies being instigated or, on occasion, the withdrawal of the drug from the market. In 2004, it was reported that the Food and Drug Administration (FDA) requested postmarketing studies on 73% of recent new drugs in the U.S.[5]

1.1.8 The Future of Clinical Trials

The process of sequential clinical trials is being challenged, and it is likely that in years to come some radical changes will occur. Ideas such as the granting of provisional drug approval are currently being debated, whereby a drug will undergo less intensive clinical trials and more intensive postmarketing surveillance. Such ideas are controversial, but many believe that such a course of action is necessary to reduce the costs and time needed to bring a new drug to market. Moreover, there is a drive to radically shorten the approval time for drugs such as anti-infectives and vaccines, that may be required to battle bioterrorism.

In recent times, a new type of first-in-man study has emerged, the so-called human phase 0 studies. In these studies very small amounts of drug (a microdose) are administered to healthy human volunteers.[6] The amounts are below the level that have any pharmacological effect and are intended solely to study pharmacokinetics and metabolism. The advantage of such studies is that because the dose levels are so low, only limited preclinical toxicology is required to determine safety.

1.2 DRUG METABOLISM

The metabolic fate of the candidate drug is studied first *in vitro*, then in animal species (preclinical), and finally in humans (clinical). Studies to determine a drug's metabolism are conducted separately from the clinical studies outlined in Section 1.1.1 to Section 1.1.5. The timing of drug metabolism studies is covered in Section 1.7.1.

In order to understand the metabolic fate of a drug candidate, the physiological passage of what might be very low amounts has to be followed through an abundance of biochemical reactions. The chemical nature of the drug may also be altered as it passes through the body (i.e., metabolism or biotransformation), making detection even more challenging. These problems are overcome by labeling the drug candidate with a radioactive isotope (i.e., a radiotracer), and then following its metabolic route by means of radiodetection. Before we consider how radioactive isotopes are used as a tool in drug registration, however, we must first look at the origins of radiotracer studies. To do this, we will go back to the middle of the last century.

1.3 ORIGINS OF RADIOTRACER STUDIES

In the early 1930s, great advances were made in the understanding of anaerobic fermentation of sugar to lactic acid, ethanol, and carbon dioxide, but little was known about the metabolism of sugar in the living cell. It took another two to three decades to piece together the biochemical reactions that combine to make the distinct metabolic pathways vital to life. The citric acid cycle was the first major pathway to be elucidated, for which Hans Krebs received the Nobel Prize in 1953. Elucidation of the photosynthetic pathway by Melvin Calvin followed, along with his Nobel Prize in 1961. Untangling distinct metabolic pathways occurring within a living cell from myriad other reactions, all occurring simultaneously, was a formidable task. Calvin in his Nobel lecture described the problem thus:[7]

> One of the principal difficulties in such an investigation as this [the study of photosynthesis], in which the machinery which converts the CO_2 to carbohydrate and the substrate upon which it operates are made of the same atoms, namely carbon and its near relatives, is that ordinary analytical methods will not allow us to distinguish easily between the machinery and its substrate.

In 1940, Martin Kamen and Samuel Ruben[8] discovered a new isotope of carbon (^{14}C). All elements consist of more than one isotope, depending upon the number of neutrons in their atomic nucleus (Chapter 2). ^{14}C is an unstable isotope of carbon, decaying over time to ^{14}N and emitting radioactivity in the process. By 1945, sufficient amounts of ^{14}C were available to enable Calvin to carry out his investigations. In what are now a series of classical experiments, Calvin administered pulses of $^{14}CO_2$ to illuminated algal suspensions, which after a short period of time were then dropped into alcohol, thereby instantly stopping all biochemical reactions. (The apparatus he used for this experiment was called the Lollipop because of its shape.) Samples of the algal–alcohol extracts were analyzed using two-dimensional paper chromatography. The paper chromatograms were exposed to photographic film, and when the film was developed, a series of spots were revealed, each corresponding to a region on the chromatogram where radioactive compounds had eluted (Figure 1.2). As the time between the $^{14}CO_2$ pulse and the killing of the algae increased, so did the number of radioactive compounds seen in the chromatograms. Radioactive ^{14}C acted like a beacon incorporating itself into each compound in the pathway, distinguishing them from the plethora of other carbon-based substances present in the algal extracts. Calvin then undertook the formidable task of chemically identifying each radiolabeled compound, and by knowing the order of their formation from their appearance in the chromatograms, he was able to place each link into the chain of reactions, until the complete photosynthetic pathway was revealed.

Without radiotracers, the elucidation of many biochemical pathways would have been extremely difficult, if not impossible. (It is, however, interesting to note that Krebs did not use radiotracers in the elucidation of the citric acid cycle, although the pathway was subsequently confirmed using ^{14}C.) Although attention in the 1950s was focused on biochemical pathways essential for life, the first radiolabeled studies were also performed with xenobiotics.[9] By the 1960s, the first departments were set

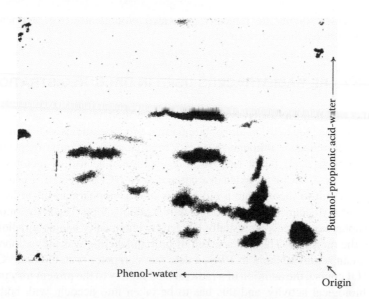

Phenol-water ←——————

Origin

Figure 1.2 Two-dimensional paper chromatogram of an extract of algae, 30 sec after delivering a pulse of $^{14}CO_2$. (This chromatogram appears in the Nobel lecture of Melvin Calvin, 1961. Copyright © The Nobel Foundation.)

up in pharmaceutical companies to investigate the metabolism of drugs in laboratory animals, and by the 1970s, such laboratories had become well established.[10] In a comparatively short span of time, we have gone from the paper chromatograms of Calvin to the highly sophisticated metabolism departments we see in the pharmaceutical industry today.

1.4 NEW CHEMICAL ENTITIES AND BIOPHARMACEUTICALS

Reasons for using radiotracers today are not much different from those of Calvin in the 1950s. Radiotracers are used to follow the metabolic fate of a drug through a test system where otherwise it would be difficult or impossible to distinguish the drug from its surroundings. A radiotracer can be used at any stage where it offers such an advantage. Of course, pharmaceuticals have more complicated chemical structures than $^{14}CO_2$, and so the synthetic effort to produce the radiolabeled compound is far more demanding. Today drugs in development can be divided into two broad categories: new chemical entities (NCEs) and biopharmaceuticals, although the distinction is somewhat blurred. NCEs have relatively low molecular weights and are typically of synthetic origin. These can also include some relatively low molecular weight natural products and natural products that have undergone a degree of chemical modification. Biopharmaceuticals are either peptides, polypeptides, or proteins. Peptides are usually synthesized by the condensation of a defined series of amino acids; polypeptides may be synthesized but are more commonly from natural sources. Proteins are typically generated biologically (e.g., fermentation) from genetically engineered organisms.

1.5 WHY ARE RADIOTRACERS USED IN DRUG REGISTRATION?

For the vast majority of NCEs, information on their metabolic fate is required for drug approval. Due to the nature of biopharmaceuticals, studies on their metabolic fate tend to be reduced, although there is a regulatory expectation (depending on the class of biological) for at least some evaluation. The use of radiotracers for biopharmaceuticals is not as extensive compared to NCEs because it can be synthetically difficult to incorporate a radiotracer into a biopharmaceutical by substituting a naturally occurring stable isotope with a radioisotope. The higher molecular weight biopharmaceuticals are usually labeled by chemically adding a radiolabeled moiety to the molecule. The first account of protein labeling was the radiobromination of human serum albumin in 1943, a date that competes with the first ^{14}C tracer studies.[11] Of course, the addition of a radiolabeled moiety to the protein may interfere with its biological activity, and this has to be taken into account with both study design and interpretation.

Most of the examples given here therefore refer to NCEs, but biologicals are covered when relevant. It has nevertheless been reported that as part of the U.S. safety assessment process, more than 80% of drugs used radiotracers in their testing program.[12]

For convenience, regulatory drug testing programs that utilize radiotracers can be divided into two groups: standard studies and explorative studies (Figure 1.3A and B, respectively). As a general rule, the standard studies are routinely conducted for the majority of NCEs, although the extent and design may vary, depending upon the drug class and specific circumstances. Explorative studies are not necessarily routinely required, but are performed to address specific questions. The importance of explorative studies, however, should not be underestimated; there are occasions when the development of a drug could not continue without them.

Radiotracers are used in animal and human studies. Perhaps not surprisingly, there are strict restrictions regarding the amounts of radioactivity that can be administered to humans, and this is discussed in Section 1.7.3.

1.5.1   *In Vitro* and *In Vivo* Studies

The standard package of studies, as shown in Figure 1.3A, consists of *in vitro* and *in vivo* experiments. Generally, *in vitro* studies are performed at an early stage in the drug development process and provide preliminary information for decision making and to assist in the design of *in vivo* studies. Because *in vitro* studies are conducted early in the development process, the radiolabeled drug may not have been synthesized by this stage. It is therefore not uncommon to perform *in vitro* studies without a radiolabeled compound. On the other hand, the conduct and interpretation of some of the *in vitro* studies is enhanced by the use of a radiolabeled compound, if available.

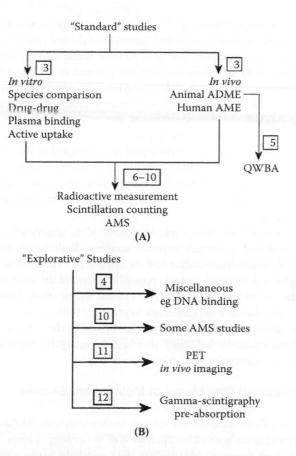

Figure 1.3 Schematic representation of the types of studies performed in drug registration, where radiotracers may be used. (A) Standard studies, performed for most NCEs. (B) Explorative studies, performed as required. The numbers in the boxes show the chapter numbers in this book where the topic is covered.

In vivo studies are conducted on laboratory animals and with human volunteers. Although there have been attempts to perform *in vivo* metabolism studies without a radiolabeled compound, given the complexity of living systems, this is particularly difficult and the use of the radiolabeled drug for these studies should be considered vital. All the experiments in the standard package follow the same basic experimental principles in that the radiolabeled drug is administered to laboratory animals or to humans, and samples are taken over time and analyzed for radioactivity and by radiochromatographic methods to determine the metabolic pathway.

1.5.2 Terminology

At this stage, certain terminology should be clarified. Where the metabolic fate of a drug is being studied, be it *in vivo* or *in vitro*, such studies are usually referred to as metabolism studies. The *in vivo* studies in animals provide information on the absorption, distribution, metabolism and excretion of the test compound, which gives these types of investigations the acronym ADME studies. In an ADME study, the amount of radioactivity administered and the amount recovered can be precisely measured, thus giving the assurance that everything is experimentally accounted for. Such studies are therefore sometimes known as balance studies or mass balance studies. When ADME (or balance) studies are performed in humans, these are sometimes referred to as AME (absorption, metabolism, and excretion) studies, as for obvious reasons, tissues are not dissected and collected at the end of the experiment. Other jargon can also be found, including terms such as ADMET and MET-PK. ADMET is a hybrid of ADME and metabolism; MET-PK comes from metabolism and pharmacokinetics. Such terms, however, all essentially refer to the ADME or AME type studies.

Metabolism studies are also sometimes referred to generically as radiolabeled studies, and this reveals a certain misunderstanding. Radiolabels are used as tools in the conduct of metabolism studies and should not be classified as a set of studies in their own right. Indeed, in theory it is possible to acquire the necessary metabolism data without the use of a radiolabel. Moreover, the use of stable isotope labels such as ^{13}C or ^{19}F might also be used (although beyond the scope of this book).[13] In short, there is no mandatory requirement to use radiolabels in the conduct of metabolism studies. The term *radiolabeled study* should only really be applied to a study in which radiolabel has actually been used.

1.5.3   The Principal Objectives of Metabolism Studies

Data obtained from metabolism studies are multifarious. Metabolism data can have an impact on the design and interpretation of toxicology studies, clinical studies, and the drug's dose regimen. Metabolism data can help explain toxic effects and answer questions on efficacy or the lack of it. The principal objectives of the metabolism studies are as follows:

1. Metabolism data help validate the animal species used for toxicological tests. If the drug is absorbed, metabolized and excreted in the animal species used for toxicological tests in a way similar to that in the human, then the animal species can be considered an appropriate model and toxicity results can then be extrapolated to humans with confidence. On the other hand, if human-specific metabolites are found, then these may have to undergo separate and costly toxicity testing.

2. The absorption (for drugs administered extravascularly) and metabolic stability of a drug are key to its efficacy and toxicology. A drug that acts systemically but is not absorbed when taken orally may not attain a sufficient concentration in blood to be efficacious. Conversely, a drug that is intended to act locally (e.g., a topical application) but is then extensively absorbed may lead to unacceptable toxicological effects. If an active drug is rapidly metabolized to inactive metabolites, there is little opportunity for the drug to exert its therapeutic effect. If the drug is metabolically stable and resides in the body for lengthy periods, this may lead to possible side effects and may influence the therapeutic dosing regimen.

3. Knowledge of the enzymes involved in the metabolism of a drug aids the understanding and prediction of possible drug–drug interactions or the effects of certain foods. In addition, the activity of some enzymes varies widely within certain populations (polymorphism), thereby leading to wide interpatient responses.

4. The total body burden is represented by the time a drug and its metabolites reside within the body. For example, a parent drug may be eliminated quickly, but metabolites may remain for prolonged periods. The metabolites might remain in systemic circulation, or they may accumulate in specific tissues or organs. It is possible that such metabolites are pharmacologically active, or could be responsible for undesirable toxicological effects. The metabolic pathway of a candidate drug is scrutinized for the presence of active groups known to be associated with toxicological effects; these are known as structural alerts. The distribution of the drug is important in understanding efficacy. For example, by using animal models (e.g., QWBA, Chapter 5) or human volunteers (e.g., PET, Chapter 11), the ability of a drug to cross the blood–brain barrier can be assessed.

5. Data acquired from the metabolism studies can influence the design of preclinical and clinical studies. For example, it may be necessary to determine the pharmacokinetics of metabolites as well as the parent drug in the clinical trials. This, of course, is only possible if the metabolites have been identified. Furthermore, it is often forgotten that a general knowledge of drug metabolism helps in the design of new drugs (i.e., discovery stage; see Section 1.1.1).

1.6 DETECTION OF RADIOACTIVITY

In order to follow and quantify the radiotracer through a test system, reliable detection methods are required. Undoubtedly, radiodetection technology has made huge advances in recent times. The methods of detection have not only made the job of the metabolism chemist much easier, but they have also opened new experimental opportunities hardly dreamt of in the time of Calvin. The measurement of radioactivity using liquid and solid scintillation counting is a routine laboratory method (see Chapters 6 and 8). Nowadays radiochromatography is a recognized expertise in its own right. Many of the constraints imposed by the use of ionizing radiation in humans have been alleviated with the use of accelerator mass spectrometry (AMS; Chapter 10). The use of imaging techniques such as quantitative whole-body autoradiography (QWBA) is now commonplace (Chapter 5). Explorative studies such as positron emission tomography (PET) and γ-scintigraphy (Chapters 11 and 12, respectively) are growing in their application. PET is an imaging technique that locates the radiotracer *in vivo*. Classically, PET has been used to verify that central nervous system drugs are able to cross the blood–brain barrier and measure the degree of receptor occupancy. The technique of γ-scintigraphy is applied to locating a drug prior to absorption and has therefore been used, for example, for inhaled formulations to ensure that the drug reaches the appropriate parts of the respiratory system. AMS is used as an ultrasensitive detection method for the conduct of standard studies, as shown in Figure 1.3A. AMS is also an enabling technology that can be applied to novel applications in drug discovery (Figure 1.3B).

1.7 THE REGULATORY POSITION ON METABOLISM STUDIES

The regulatory guidelines surrounding metabolism studies are divided into two categories. The first covers the data requirements for the regulatory submission. The second covers the administration of radioactivity to humans. Although sometimes the two categories are covered by the same regulatory authority, they are quite distinct and should not be confused.

1.7.1   Regulations for Data Requirements

Regulatory guidelines in the pharmaceutical sector today do not specify exactly how and when the metabolism studies on a candidate drug are performed; only general principles are set down. The ADME studies on animals are typically performed while phase I clinical trials are in progress, or at least prior to the start of phase II. The timing of a human AME study can vary widely but the study is often performed while the phase II clinical trials are run. It is common practice to perform the human AME study using healthy volunteers (i.e., a phase I type study). The regulatory guidelines, however, are very flexible, and pharmaceutical companies will adopt different strategies on developing their own drugs. As stated in Section 1.1.6, for a cytotoxic anticancer drug, phase I clinical trials would be omitted. Likewise, for this class of drug, an AME study in healthy human volunteers would also be omitted. There are, however, situations where an AME study might be conducted in consenting patients. Over the past few years, the pivotal nature of the metabolism studies has gained wider recognition and there has been a general trend for the pharmaceutical companies to perform the *in vivo* studies earlier than previously thought necessary.

1.7.2   Drug Registration: Some of the Major Authorities

The major regulatory authorities concerned with the registration and use of pharmaceuticals are listed below. Information and, for some authorities, copies of the guidelines can be obtained from the organizations' websites. There are two points to bear in mind, however: (1) the websites of these organizations are vast and can be very difficult to navigate, and (2) websites are ephemeral, and addresses can become out of date very quickly. Indeed, the regulations are revised and updated on a regular basis.

In the U.S. the authority is the Food and Drug Administration (FDA). Pharmaceuticals are evaluated by the Center for Drug Evaluation (CDER), and biologicals are evaluated by the Center for Biologics Evaluation (CBER). The FDA website (www.fda.gov) is of general interest and contains links to CDER (www.fda.gov/cder/) and CBER (www.fda.gov/cber/). It contains information on drugs registered in the U.S. as well as information on phase IV postmarketing study comments. Regulatory guidelines for NCEs can be found at www.fda.gov/cder/regulatory/.

In Europe the authority is the European Medicines Evaluation Agency (EMEA). The website is at http://www.emea.eu.int/home.htm, with a link to the human medicines site at http://www.emea.eu.int/htms/human/epar/a-zepar.htm, where information on drugs registered in the European Union can be found.

In Japan the authority is the Ministry of Health, Labor and Welfare (JMHLW). The website (in English) is www.mhlw.go.jp/english/. Pharmaceuticals in Japan are assessed by the Pharmaceuticals and Medical Device Agency (PMDA). The website (in English) can be found at http://www.pmda.go.jp/index-e.html. A very useful source of information is the Japanese Pharmaceutical Manufacturers Association (JPMA), with a website (in English) at http://www.jpma.or.jp/english/index.html.

In 1990, the International Conference on Harmonization of Technical Requirements for Registration of Pharmaceuticals for Human Use (ICH) was set up with the aim of bringing together the regulatory authorities of Europe, Japan and the United States and experts from the pharmaceutical industry in the three regions to discuss scientific and technical aspects of product registration. A number of the guidelines are therefore the same, irrespective if they are published by the FDA, EMEA, or PMDA. The ICH website can be found at http://www.ich.org/.

Regulatory guidelines are constantly updated and draft versions are frequently published for public review. It is therefore recommended that the reader obtain copies of current and draft guidelines from the relevant websites, to remain up to date. Moreover, although some of the toxicology guidelines are reasonably specific, guidelines that cover metabolism and pharmacokinetics are much more general. Indeed, there is very little about the use of radiotracers in the guidelines; they are more concerned with what questions require answering, rather than the methods used to answer them. (Here again, this reflects the science-driven process.)

1.7.3 Regulations Covering the Administration of Radioactive Compounds to Human Volunteers

Humans are exposed to radioactivity either occupationally or from natural background, and there are risks to health associated with such exposure. Consequently, governments set regulations limiting the amount of radioactivity to which their citizens should be exposed. The administration of radiotracers to human volunteers is permitted in many countries throughout the world, providing the levels of radioactivity administered do not exceed the stipulated limits. Some of the principal regulatory authorities are covered below. The limits that the agencies set and the calculations for radioactive dose are covered in Appendix 1, Chapter 5.

1.7.4 Administration of Radioactivity: Some of the Major Authorities

In the U.S., the FDA is the regulatory agency that controls the administration of radiotracers to humans in medical research (21 Code of Federal Regulations (CFR) 361: Title 21 — Food and Drugs, Chapter I, Food and Drug Administration, Department of Health and Human Services, Part 361, Prescription Drugs for Human Use Generally Recognized as Safe and Effective and Not Misbranded: Drugs Used in Research). The FDA delegates carefully defined responsibilities to local radioactive drug research committees (website: http://www.fda.gov/cder/regulatory/RDRC/review.htm).

In Europe, radioactive exposure to humans is regulated by the EURATOM directives (website: http://www.euratom.org/). Directive 96/29/EURATOM (Council Directive 96/29/EURATOM of May 13, 1996, covering basic safety standards for the protection of the health of workers and the general public against the dangers arising from ionizing radiation) is general and covers exposure, from medical x-ray through to air crews and the general public. Directive 97/43/EURATOM (Council Directive 97/43/EURATOM of June 30, 1997, on health protection of individuals against the dangers of ionizing radiation in relation to medical exposure and repealing Directive 84/466/EURATOM) stipulates the general rules for volunteers in research and introduces the acronym ALARA (as low as reasonably acceptable). It should be noted that at the time of writing, there are moves to update these directives. No specific dose limits for radiolabeled studies with humans are imposed by these directives; this is left to the individual member countries. In the U.K., for example, the Administration of Radioactive Substances Advisory Committee (ARSAC) is the relevant body (website: http://www.advisorybodies.doh.gov.uk/arsac/). ARSAC largely follows the guidelines of by the international bodies: the World Health Organization (http://www.who.int/en/)[14] and the Commission on Radiological Protection (http://www.icrp.org/).[15-16]

ACKNOWLEDGMENTS

I am grateful to Paul Baldrick, Paul Dow, and Laurence Bishop for their input and reviews of this chapter.

REFERENCES

1. DiMasi, J.A., Hansen, R.W., and Grabowski, H.G., The price of innovation: new estimates of drug development costs, *J. Health Econ.*, 22, 151–185, 2003.
2. Kola, I. and Landis, J., Can the pharmaceutical industry reduce attrition rates? *Nat. Rev. Drug Discov.*, 3, 711–715, 2004.
3. Schmid, E.F. and Smith, D.A., Is declining innovation in the pharmaceutical industry a myth?, *Drug Discov. Today*, 10, 1031–1039, 2005.
4. World Medical Association Declaration of Helsinki Ethical Principles for Medical Research Involving Human Subjects, adopted by the 18th WMA General Assembly, Helsinki, Finland, June 1964, and amended by the 29th WMA General Assembly, Tokyo, Japan, October 1975; the 35th WMA General Assembly, Venice, Italy, October 1983; the 41st WMA General Assembly, Hong Kong, September 1989; the 48th WMA General Assembly, Somerset West, Republic of South Africa, October 1996; and the 52nd WMA General Assembly, Edinburgh, Scotland, October 2000.
5. FDA request postmarketing studies in 73% of recent new drug approvals, *Tufts Center Study Drug Dev. Impact Rep.*, 6, 1–4, 2004.
6. Lappin, G. and Garner, R.C., Big physics, small doses: the use of AMS and PET in human microdosing of development drugs, *Nat. Rev. Drug Discov.*, 2, 233–240, 2003.
7. The website of the Nobel e-museum, http://www.nobel.se/index.html.

8. The website for the Enrico Fermi Award; Martin Kamen's citation is at http://www.pnl.gov/fermi/citations/kamen-cit.html.

9. Morris H.P., Weisburger, J.H., and Weisburger E.K., The distribution of radioactivity following the feeding of carbon 14-labeled 2-acetylaminofluorene to rats, *Cancer Res.*, 10, 620–624, 1950.

10. Alavijeh, M.S. and Palmer, A.M., The pivotal role of drug metabolism and pharmacokinetics in the discovery and development of new medicines, *IDrugs*, 7, 755–763, 2004.

11. Fine, J. and Seligman, A.M., Traumatic shock. IV. A study of the problem of the "lost plasma" in hemorrhagic shock by the use of radioactive plasma protein, *J. Clin. Invest.*, 22, 285–303, 1943.

12. Roberts, D. and Lockley, R., Radiosynthesis: a vital role supporting drug development, *Drug Discovery World*, Fall 2004, pp. 59–62.

13. Scarfe, G.B., Wright, B., Clayton, E., Taylor, S., Wilson, I.D., Lindon, J.C., and Nicholson, J.K., ^{19}F-NMR and directly coupled HPLC-NMR-MS investigations into the metabolism of 2-bromo-4-trifluoromethylaniline in rat: a urinary excretion balance study without the use of radiolabelling, *Xenobiotica*, 28, 373–388, 1998.

14. World Health Organization (WHO), U*se of Ionising Radiation and Radionuclides on Human Beings for Medical Purposes*, Technical Report Series, No. 611, Geneva, 1977.

15. International Commission on Radiological Protection (ICRP), *Radiological Protection in Biomedical Research*, ICRP Publication 62, Stockholm, Sweden, 1991.

16. International Commission on Radiological Protection (ICRP), *Recommendations of the International Commission on Radiological Protection*, Publication 60, Stockholm, Sweden, 1991.

CHAPTER 2

Radioactivity and Radiotracers

Graham Lappin

CONTENTS

2.1 ATOMS AND ISOTOPES

The nucleus of an atom contains neutrons (n) and protons (p$^+$) occupying a space of approximately 10^{-13} to 10^{-12} cm in diameter. Orbiting the nucleus, there are electrons (e$^-$), which occupy quantized orbitals or shells within the atom. Protons are positively charged, electrons are negatively charged and neutrons have no charge. The number of electrons equals the number of protons, thus the overall charge on the atom is neutral. The configuration of the electrons in the atom determines its propensity to react with other atoms to form molecules, which is the basis of the electronic theory of valance. Different elements are defined by the numbers of protons in the nucleus. Of the naturally occurring elements, the number of protons in the atomic nucleus varies between one (hydrogen) and 92 (uranium) (although this statement is qualified in 2.7).

Whilst the number of protons in the atomic nucleus is fixed for any given element, the number of neutrons can vary. The number of protons (Z) plus the number of neutrons (N) in the nucleus defines the atomic mass (A). Thus A=Z+N. Atoms of the same element with different numbers of neutrons are known as isotopes. Thus isotopes of the same element will have the same value for Z but a different atomic mass (A). (Frederick Soddy introduced the term isotope in 1914 and received a Nobel Prize in 1921).[1] Take hydrogen for example. The atom of the most abundant isotope of hydrogen (99.99%) has one proton (Z=1) and one electron but no neutrons (N=0) and hence it has an atomic mass of one (A=1). Deuterium (0.015% natural abundance) on the other hand has one proton (Z =1) and one neutron (N=1) and hence has an atomic mass of two (A=2). Isotopes are denoted by prefixing the atomic mass in superscript and the atomic number in subscript, thus $^A_Z X$. Hydrogen, for example is represented by the symbol $^1_1 H$. Deuterium is represented by $^2_1 H$. A third configuration of hydrogen exists where the nucleus contains two neutrons ($^3_1 H$ - tritium). (For completeness, isotopes of hydrogen above tritium are known but they have very short half-lives (2.7) and therefore are not relevant here).

Biochemists often depict isotopes without the subscripted atomic number. For example, $^3 H$ rather than $^3_1 H$. Physicists would no doubt say this is lazy notation but it is common practice amongst biochemists and so the atomic number is only included in this book where it is relevant.

2.2 ISOTOPE STABILITY

The nucleus is held together by the binding energy of the nucleus. Providing the binding energy exceeds the repulsive force between the positively charged protons, an equilibrium exists and the nucleus is stable. The presence of neutrons however, can upset the equilibrium and the atomic nucleus may become unstable. Although somewhat simplified, as a general rule the nucleus will become unstable when the number of protons and neutrons are uneven (Z ≠ N) resulting in incomplete spin-pairing. For example, deuterium ($^2 H$) has an equal number of protons and neutrons and is stable. Tritium ($^3 H$) however, contains two neutrons and one proton, and over time tritium decays to a more energetically-stable configuration and in the process releases radioactivity (Figure 2.1). Isotopes that undergo nuclear decay and emit radioactivity are known as radioisotopes. An atomic species whose nucleus is radioactive is known as a radionuclide.

2.3 TYPES OF RADIOACTIVE DECAY

There are different types of radioactive emission, depending upon the decay mechanism. The various types of radioactive decay are explained in 2.3.1 to 2.3.6. The descriptions focus on those aspects relevant to drug development and if the reader requires a wider understanding of radioactivity, then references are provided in Further Reading, at the end of this chapter.

2.3.1 Alpha (α) Decay

Alpha particles are equivalent to $_2^4He$ nuclei (two protons and two neutrons). It is usually the radioisotopes of heavy elements which emit α-particles. Drugs incorporating α-emitters may be used therapeutically (i.e., radiopharmaceuticals) but they are not generally used as radiotracers and as such are outside the scope of this book. An example of an α-emitter would be americium (^{241}Am) which decays to neptunium (^{237}Np), with the release of an α-particle ($_2^4He$) and 5.55 MeV of energy. (As an aside, the most common use of ^{241}Am is in smoke alarms).

2.3.2 Beta (β⁻) Decay

Isotopes that undergo β⁻ decay have an excess of neutrons, resulting in the transformation of a neutron to a proton, with the release of an electron and an antineutrino. β-decay is defined by equation 2.1 where n is a neutron, p⁺ is a proton, β⁻ is a beta particle (equivalent to an electron, or sometimes called a negatron) and $\overline{V}$ is an antineutrino.

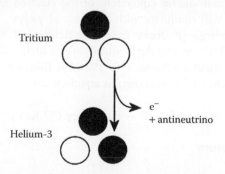

Tritium

e⁻
+ antineutrino

Helium-3

Figure 2.1 The tritium nucleus consists of one proton (●) and two neutrons (○). One neutron decays, forming a proton and releasing an electron and an antineutrino. Tritium therefore decays to form the stable isotope, helium-3 (³He). Note that ³He is rare on Earth. The most common isotope of helium is ⁴HE.

$$n \rightarrow p^+ + \beta\text{-} + \bar{V} + \text{energy } (E_{max}) \qquad (2.1)$$

The energy shown in equation 2.1 is measured in units of electron volts (1 eV = 1.6×10^{-19} J). In practice, β^- particles are easy to detect but neutrinos and antineutrinos (which are members of the lepton family of particles) interact with other matter only through gravitational and other weak forces, making them very difficult to detect experimentally.

The Nobel Laureate, Wolfgang Pauli said of the neutrino, in 1930, "I have done a terrible thing, I have postulated a particle that cannot be detected." He was almost correct; neutrinos were not shown to exist experimentally until 1953. The presence of the antineutrino was implicated before its discovery because β-particles are emitted with a range of energies during atomic decay. Since the process of atomic decay should release a precise and unvaried amount of energy per atom, the energy had to be shared between the β-particle and "something else." The "something else" turned out to be an antineutrino. Hence, the energy released during β-decay is defined as E_{max}, which is the β-particle's highest energy state. This phenomenon is relevant to scintillation counting and will be picked up again in Chapter 6. Of particular relevance to drug development are the β-emitters ^{3}H, ^{14}C and ^{35}S.

The decay of ^{14}C is shown in equation 2.2

$$^{14}C \rightarrow {}^{14}N + \beta\text{-} + \bar{V} + \text{energy } (156\text{KeV}) \qquad (2.2)$$

2.3.3 Beta (β^+) Decay

β^+ decay is essentially the reverse of β^- emission and is defined by equation 2.3 where β^+ is a positron and v is a neutrino.

$$p^+ \rightarrow n + \beta^+ + v + \text{energy } (E_{max}) \qquad (2.3)$$

A positron is the anti-matter equivalent of the electron and if a positron and electron collide, they will annihilate with a release of γ-rays.

Isotopes that undergo β^+ decay have a deficiency of neutrons. As with β^- emission, equation 2.3 tells us that the positrons are emitted with a range of energies. β^+-emitters are of particular relevance to Positron Emission Tomography (PET) (Chapter 11). The decay of ^{11}C is shown in equation 2.4.

$$^{11}C \rightarrow {}^{11}B + \beta^+ + v + \text{energy } (97 \text{ KeV}) \qquad (2.4)$$

2.3.4 Electron Capture

Isotopes with an excess of protons, can capture an electron from the inner shell of the atom, thereby attaining a stable configuration by converting a proton to a neutron. Electron capture is also sometimes known as K capture (as the K shell is closest to the nucleus and is mostly responsible for the supply of electrons). Electron capture is defined by equation 2.5

$$p + e^- \rightarrow n + v + energy \qquad (2.5)$$

Following electron capture, the nucleus is sometimes left in an excited state and emits further energy in the form of γ-radiation (2.3.5). The radioactive isotope of potassium (^{40}K) decays by both β^--emission ($^{40}K \rightarrow {}^{40}Ca$) and by electron capture ($^{40}K \rightarrow {}^{40}Ar$) in the ratio of approximately 9:1 in favor of β^--decay. Following electron capture, the unstable potassium nucleus releases γ-radiation with an energy of 1.46 MeV.

2.3.5 Gamma (γ) Decay

Gamma rays are electromagnetic radiation similar to radio waves or visible light. (The wavelengths of X-rays are between 10 and 0.01 nm. The wavelength of γ-radiation is less than 0.01 nm). Following nuclear decay by β, α or electron capture, the daughter nucleus can retain some of the disintegration energy. This energy is then emitted in the form of γ-radiation as the atom returns to the ground state. An example is the decay of ^{60}Co to ^{60}Ni by β^--decay, leaving the daughter ^{60}Ni nucleus in an excited state. The ^{60}Ni returns to the ground state almost instantaneously, emitting γ-photons at two characteristic energies (1.17 and 1.33 MeV).

In some cases, there is a delay in the release of the energy, in a process known as isomeric transition. In this case, the nucleus is left in a metastable state before excess energy is emitted. For this reason, the atomic number is followed by the letter m, for radionuclides that decay by this mechanism. An example is the decay of ^{99}Mo to ^{99}Tc as shown in equation 2.6

$$^{99}_{42}Mo \rightarrow {}^{99m}_{43}Tc + \beta^- \rightarrow {}^{99}_{43}Tc + \gamma \qquad (2.6)$$

2.3.6 Internal Conversion and Auger Electrons

In some cases, the excitation energy of a nucleus can be absorbed by an electron (usually from within the inner, K, shell). The excited electron is then ejected from the atom in a process known as internal conversion. Whilst β-emissions consist of a range of energies electrons emitted through internal conversion are mono-energetic. The space left by the ejection of an inner electron is filled by an electron from one of the outer shells and X-rays with a characteristic energy are emitted. In their turn, these X-rays may be absorbed by electrons in the outer shell, which are also ejected from the atom. These low-energy electrons are called Auger electrons (after Pierre Auger, a French Physicist, in the mid-1920s). Example of isotopes that emits Auger electrons are ^{80m}Br and ^{125}I.

2.4 SAFETY

There is a wealth of information in the literature on handling radioactivity safely and therefore these aspects will not be restated here. Suggestions for further reading are given at the end of this chapter. Some shielding may be required for certain radioactive sources. ^{14}C does not require shielding but higher energy β-emitters such as ^{32}P (1.71 MeV) and γ-emitters such as ^{131}I do. With higher energy β-emitters an effect known as "braking radiation," or to give it its proper name Bremsstrahlung radiation occurs, which results in the emission of X-rays. When shielding for β-emitters is necessary, the shielding materials are of low density thus reducing the energy of the Bremsstrahlung radiation. Acrylic sheet at a thickness of 1 cm will stop all β-particles that are of interest in this publication and relevant screens are easily purchased for this use. Gamma-emitters however may require either thick acrylic or lead shielding, depending upon the level of activity.

Monitoring for contamination, in the case of most β and γ emitters, is conducted by the use of hand held radiation monitors which are either Geiger Muller tubes or NaI detectors. In the case of tritium it is necessary to monitor by swabbing the affected area and then analyzing by liquid scintillation counting (Chapter 6) as tritium does not have sufficient energy to be detected by the hand held monitoring devices.

2.5 UNITS OF RADIOACTIVITY

The basic unit of radioactivity is the number of decay events per unit of time (irrespective of the mode of decay). This is expressed as disintegrations per second (dps) or disintegrations per minute (dpm).

Other units of radioactivity are derived from the dps or dpm value. Two are in common usage, the Curie (Ci) and the Becquerel (Bq). Strictly speaking, the Bq is the SI unit, although both Bq and Ci are very commonly used together. (From experience, industrial laboratories are split about equally in the use of Bq or Ci). Examples in this book will use Bq with Ci in parenthesis if appropriate.

$$1Bq = 1 \text{ dps and therefore } 1MBq = 6 \times 10^7 \text{ dpm}$$

$$1Ci = 2.22 \times 10^{12} \text{ dpm, thus } 37MBq = 1mCi$$

2.6 UNITS OF DOSE

The radioactive dose is the amount of radiation energy absorbed by matter. A dose of 1 Gray (Gy) equals one Joule (J) of energy absorbed by one Kg of a substance (1 Gy = 1 J/Kg). The Gray is known as the unit of absorbed dose.

Radiation interacts with matter, ultimately leading to the formation of excited and ionized atoms. In brief, radiation energy upon collision with an atom is transferred to the electrons. This dissipation of energy leads to an electron "jumping" out of the atom, forming an ion pair (a negatively charged electron and a positively charged atom); a process known as ionization. For example, the collision of β^+ with water forms H_2O^+ + e^-. (In some cases, the electron can return to the atom in a process known as atomic excitation). These ionized chemical species will readily react with their surroundings and are a major cause of autoradiolysis (2.13). If reactive species are formed inside the living cell they will react with macromolecules such as protein or DNA and thereby cause cellular damage. This damage may result in cell death, or may trigger uncontrolled cell division and lead to the formation of tumors.

Different modes of radioactive decay (2.3.1 to 2.3.6) have different propensities to cause biological damage. This arises because the energy density distribution differs from one form of radioactivity to another. To use an analogy; β-radiation can be likened to a shot gun with the total energy of the discharge spread over a wide angle. In contrast, α-radiation is more like a high velocity rifle bullet, with all its energy concentrated in a small region. The geometric spread of energy is accounted for by the use of a Quality Factor (QF). The QF for α-radiation is 20 and for β and γ-radiation it is 1. The absorbed dose (Gy) multiplied by the Quality Factor (QF) gives the dose equivalent, in units of Sieverts (Sv).

The use of the SI units, the Gray and the Sievert are relatively recent and the literature often quotes the "old" units of the rad and the rem. The relationship between the various units is shown in Table 2.1. Calculation of radioactive dose is conducted experimentally and is dealt with in Chapter 5, Appendix 1.

2.7 HALF-LIFE

Radioactive decay is random. To illustrate this, we will conduct a short thought experiment. Imagine one atom of ^{14}C. The atomic nucleus contains 6 protons and 8 neutrons and is unstable. It "wants" to decay to the more energetically stable element ^{14}N (with 7 protons and 7 neutrons). We are now watching this single atom, waiting for the decay process to occur but when will it decay? Now? In the next few minutes? A thousand years from now? Ten thousand years from now? The fact is that it is impossible to predict the time it will take for an individual atom to decay. Now let us image we have one mole of ^{14}C before us. Avogadro's number says that one mole of an element will contain 6.0221×10^{23} atoms. With such a huge population, statistically, some of the atoms will decay immediately and some will not decay for a very long time. With large populations, statistical calculations can be applied to predict what will happen to that population over time. Radioactive decay is perfectly random and so the statistics of random populations can be readily applied (which, as Chapter 7 explains, makes the mathematics reasonably straightforward).

Historically, the idea that atomic decay is random was a difficult concept to grasp. Indeed, no lesser person than Albert Einstein was unhappy about this type of randomness in nature. This led to his famous quote "I am convinced that He [God] does not play dice" (although he was referring to Heisenberg's uncertainty principle, rather than radioactive decay specifically). The rate of decay therefore, is expressed in terms of a population, not single atoms. Looking at our one mole of ^{14}C (all

Table 2.1   Relation between units of dose

Measurement	Old unit	Symbol	Modern unit	Symbol	Conversion
Dose	rad	rad	gray	Gy	1 rad = .01 Gy
					100 rad = 1 Gy
Dose equivalent	rem	rem	sievert	Sv	1 rem = .01 Sv
					100 rem = 1 Sv

6.0221×10^{23} atoms), we start our stopwatch and wait until half of the atoms have decayed to ^{14}N. By the time the number of remaining ^{14}C atoms reaches 3.0110×10^{23}, 5730 years would have elapsed. Another 5730 years later and 1.5056×10^{23} atoms of ^{14}C will remain and so on: 5730 years is therefore the radioactive half-life $(t_{1/2})$ of ^{14}C.

The concept of half-life is applied to areas other than atomic decay, which can cause confusion (see pharmacokinetics Chapter 3, Appendix 3). For clarity therefore this book qualifies the type of half-life being referred to (in the present context, radioactive half-life will be used).

The fundamental mathematical equation describing $t_{1/2}$ is shown in equation 2.7. (The derivation of this equation is not important here and for more information the reader is referred to the Further Reading list at the end of this chapter).

$$N = N_0\, e^{-\lambda t} \tag{2.7}$$

N_0 = the number of nuclei at time zero, N = the number of nuclei after time t has elapsed, λ = radioactive decay constant, e = is the exponential number (=2.7172).

The radioactive decay constant is related to radioactive half-life as follows: $\lambda = e/t_{1/2}$ and the amount of radioactivity (A), expressed in any given units = λN. Substituting the expressions and rearranging gives equation 2.8.

$$A = A_0\, e^{-0.693t/t_{1/2}} \tag{2.8}$$

A_0 is the amount or radioactivity at time zero and A is the amount of radioactivity remaining after time t.

For practical purposes, equation 2.8 is very useful. For example, assume you are conducting an experiment with ^{35}S, which has a half-life of 87.4 days. Let us assume that at time zero, there are 2.5 MBq of ^{35}S and the experiment takes 25 days to complete. How much radioactivity remains after this time?

$$A_0 = 2.5 \text{ MBq}$$

$$t = 25 \text{ days}$$

$$t_{1/2} = 87.4 \text{ days (note, keep the units of time consistent)}$$

Thus:

$$A = 2.5 \times 2.7172^{-0.693 \times 25/87.4}$$

$$A = 2.05 \text{ MBq}$$

In the case of isomeric transition (2.3.5), the two stages of decay have their own radioactive half-lives. Equation 2.6 can therefore be rewritten as equation 2.9.

$$\,^{99}_{42}\text{Mo} \rightarrow \,^{99\text{m}}_{43}\text{Tc} + \beta^- \left(t_{\frac{1}{2}} 66\text{h}\right) \rightarrow \,^{99}_{43}\text{Tc} + \gamma \left(t_{\frac{1}{2}} 6\text{h}\right) \qquad (2.9)$$

It is interesting to note, that the four elements $_{43}$Tc, $_{61}$Pm, $_{85}$At and $_{87}$Fr each have a number of isotopes but none of them are stable. Of the isotopes of these elements, $^{98}_{43}$Tc has the longest radioactive half-life of 4.2 million years. Consequently, any amount of these elements formed with the Earth, 4.5 billion years ago, has now decayed away. The statement that there are 92 "naturally occurring" elements (section 2.1) is therefore not entirely correct, as the above four of the 92 cannot be found in nature.

2.8 SPECIFIC ACTIVITY

The specific activity of a radiolabeled compound is expressed in units of radioactivity per mole or weight of compound. For example, a compound with a molecular weight of 182, radiolabeled with ^{14}C, might have a specific activity of 100 MBq/mmole. Expressed as a weight, the specific activity is 100 MBq/182 mg or 0.549 MBq/mg.

Superficially therefore, the concept of specific activity is straightforward, but it is complicated somewhat by the fact that the value is based on an average. This is explained as follows. For some compounds the position of the radioisotope can be precisely defined. This is illustrated in Figure 2.2A by the compound benzophenone, labeled in carbon-1. When synthesized, in theory, it is possible to substitute all the atoms at carbon-1 for ^{14}C (i.e., all the molecules of benzophenone have ^{14}C at carbon-1). The specific activity of benzophenone shown in Figure 2.2A will be 2.3 GBq/mmole. (This can be calculated mathematically as is explained in section 2.9, but for the moment, just take this as read). Since the molecular weight of benzophenone is 182, then this is equivalent to 12.6 MBq/mg. If equal weights of [^{14}C]-benzophenone and non-labeled benzophenone were mixed, then the specific activity would be 6.3 MBq/mg and half the molecules would have a ^{14}C at carbon-1. The overall specific activity of the mixture is therefore an average of all the molecules contained within it.

The example becomes more complicated as illustrated in Figure 2.2B. Here the benzophenone is labeled in the benzene rings. (Note that benzophenone is a symmetrical molecule and therefore it is not possible to distinguish between the rings). If all twelve carbon atoms in the benzene rings were ^{14}C then the specific activity would be 151.2 MBq/mg (i.e., 12.6 MBq/mg x 12). If, on the other hand, the specific activity of benzene ring labeled benzophenone was 12.6 MBq/mg, then on average each molecule would contain one ^{14}C. If it were possible to pluck single molecules out of the pot of labeled benzophenone and examine them, then some might have 12 ^{14}C atoms within the benzene rings, some may have none and others would have every combination in between. Since only a proportion of the carbon atoms within the rings consisted of ^{14}C then the precise position of the radiolabeling becomes less well defined and is therefore depicted by a "*", as shown in Figure 2.2B.

Alternatively, the benzophenone could be referred to as "[U-^{14}C]-benzene ring labeled benzophenone" (the U standing for universal). Also note the use of square brackets, which is the convention when defining an isotopically enriched compound.

2.8.1 Natural Abundance

With a radioactive half-life of 5730 years, any ^{14}C around when the Earth was formed 4.5 billion years ago has long since decayed away. Nitrogen in the upper atmosphere however, is bombarded with cosmic radiation leading to the formation of approximately 2.5 ^{14}C atoms per cm^3 of air per second. There is therefore, a natural background of ^{14}C; every 1.18×10^{12} atoms of carbon contains one atom of ^{14}C. (Note that I have seen values higher than this in the literature ranging from 0.001 to 0.1%. These values are far too high for ^{14}C). As a consequence carbon has a natural specific activity of 13.56 dpm/g. (The average human contains about 222,000 dpm of radioactivity due to natural background ^{14}C). Similarly tritium is formed in the upper atmosphere and its natural abundance is approximately one ^{3}H atom per 10^{18} H atoms. The background levels quoted above also contain contributions from the atom bomb tests of the 1950s.

2.9 MAXIMUM THEORETICAL SPECIFIC ACTIVITY

The maximum specific activity for a radioisotope is related to its radioactive half-life and can be calculated mathematically. The specific activity for pure ^{14}C ($t_{1/2}$ = 5730 years), for example, is 2.3 GBq/mmole and that for ^{3}H ($t_{1/2}$ = 12.26 years) is 1.08 TBq/mmole (see below).

For a radiolabeled organic compound one, or in some cases several, of the atoms will consist of the radioisotope and the remainder will be non-radioactive (ignoring any insignificantly small amounts of background, 2.8.1). For simplicity, consider the case where one atom per molecule is substituted for a radioisotope; thus 1 mmole of the organic compound will contain 1 mmole of the isotope. For ^{14}C, 1 mmole of the organic compound, containing one ^{14}C per molecule, will therefore have a specific activity the same as 1 mmole of pure ^{14}C, namely 2.3 GBq. Under these circumstances the isotopic abundance is referred to a 2.3 GBq/mg atom, or 2.3 GBq/milliatom (abbreviated to matom). Of course, organic molecules, could contain two or more atoms of the radioisotope per molecule. If the organic compound contained two ^{14}C per molecule then the specific activity would be 4.6 GBq/mg atom. The maximum theoretical specific activity for any radioisotope can be calculated from equation 2.10.

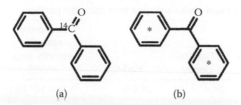

(a)   (b)

Figure 2.2   Benzophenone (A) labeled with ^{14}C in carbon-1 and (B) uniformly labled with ^{14}C in the benzene rings. Since the precise position of the ^{14}C label cannot be defined, it is represented by "*".

$$\left(dpm / mole\right) = \frac{\ln 2}{t_{\frac{1}{2}}} \times 6.0221 \times 10^{23} \times n \qquad (2.10)$$

ln2 is the natural logarithm of 2 (0.693). n = average number of isotopes per molecule. The units for the specific activity in equation 2.10 are dpm/mole. The units for half-life ($t_{\frac{1}{2}}$) are therefore also minutes. 6.0221×10^{23} is Avogadro's number number, i.e., the number of molecules in 1 mole of the radiolabeled substance. Note that equation 2.10 calculates the specific activity at time zero, it takes no account of radioactive decay over time.

Let us take an example. The maximum specific activity for any ^{14}C labeled compound (based on one ^{14}C per molecule, n = 1 in equation 2.10) is 2.3 GBq/mmole (i.e., 2.3 GBq/matom). This is calculated as follows:

The half-life ($t_{\frac{1}{2}}$) of ^{14}C is 5730 years (3.03×10^9 minutes) therefore,

$$\left(dpm / mole\right) = \frac{0.693}{3.03 \times 10^9} \times 6.0221 \times 10^{23} = 1.377 \times 10^{14} \ dpm/mole$$

Converting dpm to Bq (see section 2.5, 1 MBq = 6×10^7 dpm) 1.377×10^{14} dpm/mole = 2.3×10^6 MBq/mole. Conventionally, the specific activity would be quoted as 2.3 GBq/mmole.

Table 2.2 gives some properties of selected radioisotopes, including the half-life and maximum theoretical specific activity.

2.10 UNIVERSAL QUANTIFICATION

One of the great advantages of radiotracers is that radiodetection offers a universal method of quantification. The majority of non-radiotracer based analytical methods require a reference standard and often a standard curve in order to translate a detector response into an actual quantity of compound. Take Liquid-Chromatography Mass-Spectroscopy (LC-MS) for example. In LC-MS, following separation by HPLC, analytes are ionized in an ion source and the ions are separated by virtue of their mass over charge ratio (3.5.12). The ions are detected with the detector response

Table 2.2　Commonly used radioisotopes and their properties

Isotope	Decay product	Type of decay	Half-life	Maximum specific activity (mg atom)	Typical application
^{76}Br	^{76}Se	β^+ EC	16.2 h	7.16×10^3 TBq	PET
^{11}C	^{11}B	β^+ 99% EC 0.2%	20.4 min	3.41×10^5 TBq	PET
^{14}C	^{14}N	β^-	5730 y	2.3 GBq	Common general tracer
^{41}Ca	^{41}K	EC (X-ray)	103,000 y	128 MBq	Calcium flux (AMS)
^{45}Ca	^{45}Sc	β^-	165.1 d	29.3 TBq	Calcium flux
^{36}Cl	^{36}Ar ^{36}S	β^- 98.1% EC (X-ray) 1.9%	300,000 y	44.1 MBq	Chlorine tracer
^{171}Er	^{171}Tm	β^- (γ)	7.52 h	1.55×10^4 TBq	γ-scintigraphy
^{18}F	^{18}O	β^+ 97% EC 3%	109.8 min	6.32×10^4 TBq	PET
^{52}Fe	^{52}Mn	β^+ 56% EC (γ) 44%	8.3 h	1.4×10^4	Potentially PET
^{59}Fe	^{59}Co	β^- (γ)	44.5 d	107 TBq	Iron flux
^{3}H	^{3}He	β^-	12.35 y	1.08 TBq	Common general tracer
^{123}I	^{123}Te	EC (γ)	13.02 h	8.92×10^3 TBq	γ-scintigraphy
^{124}I	^{124}Te	EC 75% β^+ 25%	4.15 d	1.21×10^3 TBq	Potential PET
^{125}I	^{125}Te	EC (γ)	60.25 d	81 TBq	Iodination
^{129}I	^{129}Xe	β^- (γ)	1.57×10^7 y	8.27 MBq	Iodine tracer (AMS)
^{131}I	^{131}Xe	β^- (γ)	8.04 d	601 TBq	Iodination iodine flux
^{111}In	^{111}Cd	EC (γ)	2.83 d	1.73×10^3 TBq	γ-scintigraphy
^{40}K	^{40}Ca	β^- 89% EC (γ) 11%	1.26×10^9 y	1.02 TBq	Potassium flux
^{13}N	^{13}C	β^+	9.9 min	6.96×10^5 TBq	PET
^{22}Na	^{22}Ne	β^+ (90%) EC (10%)	2.6 y	5.09 TBq	Na-flux PET
^{15}O	^{15}N	β^+ >99% EC 0.1%	2.0 min	3.48×10^8 TBq	PET
^{32}P	^{32}S	β^-	14.28 d	338 TBq	General phosphorus tracer (DNA binding)
^{33}P	^{33}S	β^-	25.3 d	189 TBq	As ^{32}P
^{35}S	^{35}Cl	β^-	87.4 d	55.3 TBq	General sulfur tracer
^{153}Sm	^{153}Eu	β^- (γ)	46.8 h	2.48×10^3 TBq	γ-scintigraphy
^{99m}Tc	^{99}Tc	IT (γ)	6 h	1.93×10^4 TBq	γ-scintigraphy

being proportional to the number of ions striking it. The degree to which any compound ionizes in the ion source depends upon the structure of the analyte and so the detector signal for a given amount of one analyte may not be equal to the same amount of another analyte. In other words, quantification of the analyte is compound-dependent. Consequently, in order to quantify an analyte (1) the identity of the analyte must be known and an authentic standard must be available. (2) It is usual practice to generate a standard curve where the concentration of analyte is plotted against the detector response. The detector response observed for an unknown amount of analyte is then determined from the standard curve to provide a concentration.

But what if the chemical identity of the analyte is unknown or if standards are not available? In such circumstances analytical quantification can be very challeng ing. If however, the analyte (of known or unknown chemical identity) is radiolabeled, then measurement of radioactivity is independent of the chemical structure. Moreover, the rate of decay for any given radioisotope is constant irrespective of its environment (e.g., concentration, pressure, temperature, pH etc). Radioactivity therefore, offers a universal quantification method with standard curves and authentic chemical standards being unnecessary.

The concept of universal quantification is an important one and is a major advantage of radiolabels. In drug metabolism studies for example, the chemical identity of metabolites is not always known but it is still possible to quantify them, based on radiodetection techniques. There are certain pitfalls and these are discussed in 2.11.

2.11 CALCULATION OF LIMITS OF DETECTION (LOD)

Because the use of radiotracers offers a universal quantification method, the limits of detection (LOD) can be calculated on a generic basis, irrespective of the chemical structure of the analyte. For biological samples, the LOD is expressed as an amount of drug per weight of sample. To calculate a LOD for any analyte present in any sample, only the following information is required:

1. The limit of detection for the measuring instrument
2. The amount of sample analyzed by the instrument
3. The specific activity of the radiolabeled compound being quantified

The limit of detection for the measuring device is an innate limit dependent upon the detection technology. For example, routine liquid scintillation counting (Chapter 6) can detect down to about 10 dpm for ^{14}C but realistically in a metabolism laboratory the LOD is more likely to be around 50 or 100 dpm. Techniques such as Accelerator Mass spectrometry (AMS) (Chapter 10) can detect down to a few hundredths or, under the right conditions, a few thousands of one dpm.

The amount of sample analyzed will depend upon the method used and may depend upon the type of sample under analysis. For example, some samples may have limited amounts available and therefore this will limit the sample size available for analysis. For the sake of an example, let us assume that we are working with a liquid scintillation counter with a LOD of 50 dpm and a sample size of 0.5 g.

Specific activity was discussed in 2.8 above. Let us assume, for the sake of argument that we are working with $[^{14}C]$-benzophenone (Figure 2.2) with a specific activity of 2.3 GBq/mmole or 12.6 MBq/mg (which is equivalent to 7.56×10^8 dpm/mg).

Thus, from the specific activity, if 7.56×10^8 dpm is equivalent to 1 mg, the LOD will be the weight of benzophenone equivalent to the LOD for the detection device (50 dpm): $(50/7.56 \times 10^8) \times 1$ mg = 66 pg. The sample size was 0.5 g, thus 66 pg can be detected in 0.5 g, which is equivalent to 132 pg/g.

This seems straightforward but there is a slight complication that needs to be addressed. What if $[^{14}C]$-benzophenone had been administered to some biological system and formed a metabolite of unknown chemical identity. More than this, what if the biological sample contained benzophenone and several metabolites (labeled with ^{14}C) but of unknown chemical identities and of unknown proportions? This introduces the concept of weight equivalent. To explain this, we will stay with our example of $[^{14}C]$-benzophenone with a specific activity of 12.6 MBq/mg (7.56×10^8 dpm/mg), but let us assume that 1 g of sample was analyzed and found to contain 1,000 dpm. The 1,000 dpm would represent a mixture of compounds, not a single component and would contain $(1,000/7.56 \times 10^8) \times 1$ mg = 1.33 ng equivalents of benzophenone per g sample: or to express it in the accepted shorthand 1.33 ng equiv/g. Thus the concentration of the mixture in the sample is expressed relative to the starting compound, benzophenone in this case.

There are certain occasions however, where weight equivalents can be misleading. The assumption is that the specific activity does not change from parent to metabolites. Generally speaking this is true, except, that is, if the number of radioisotope substitutions per molecule changes. This can happen in one of two ways. (1) If a dimer is formed during metabolism. (2) If a compound is labeled with the same radioisotope in two separate positions within the molecule and the molecule is metabolically cleaved. This is illustrated in Figure 2.3. Figure 2.3A represents a compound containing one radioisotope (represented by ★). Assume for the sake of the illustration that the starting compound in A has a specific activity of 1 MBq/mmole. When metabolized, the compound forms a dimer and therefore mole for mole, the dimer contains twice as many radioisotopes than did the parent compound. Hence its specific activity is now 2 MBq/mmole. If the weight equivalents are calculated based on the specific activity of the parent, then the true concentration will be half of that actually measured.

Figure 2.3B shows the opposite situation. Here the parent compound consists of two moieties each containing a radioisotope, joined by a metabolically labile bond (represented by ----). Here assume the specific activity is 2 MBq/mmole. If the bond is cleaved during metabolism and one moiety is eliminated whilst the other remains, then mole for mole, the remaining moiety contains half the number of radioisotopes than did the parent compound. Hence its specific activity is now 1 MBq/mmole. If the weight equivalents are calculated based on the specific activity of the parent in this case, then the true concentration will be twice that actually measured. This latter example illustrates why in dual labeling experiments, it is unwise to label two halves of the same molecule with the same isotope (2.10).

A historical example of where a metabolic change in the number of isotopic substitutions led to misleading results can be seen in terpenoid biosynthesis. This example is not drug related, as it concerns the anabolism of natural products in

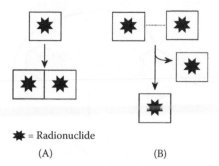

✹ = Radionuclide

(A)   (B)

Figure 2.3   An illustration of how the specific activity can change during metabolism (A) the formation of a dimer. (B) If the drug is labeled in two parts of the molecule with the same isotope and the compound is metabolically cleaved.

plants but nevertheless, it does illustrate how it is easy to misinterpret what otherwise might appear to be obvious. The monoterpene geraniol pyrophosphate (GPP) is formed from the condensation of isopentyl pyrophosphate (IPP) and dimethylallyl pyrophosphate (DMAPP). DMAPP itself is formed from the reversible isomerization of IPP (Figure 2.4). (GPP is the precursor of geraniol, which gives geraniums their characteristic smell).

It might be supposed therefore that [^{14}C]-IPP would lead to the formation of GPP with two equal ^{14}C substitutions in positions C-1 and C-6. This however, does not happen. GPP is formed with the ^{14}C predominantly in the C-1 position; that part of the molecule derived from IPP (see Figure 2.4). The reason for this is uncertain but is likely to be due to the upset of endogenous pools of IPP and DMAPP, thrown out of equilibrium by the experimental addition of precursor.[2]

2.12 SYNTHESIS OF RADIOLABELED COMPOUNDS

The introduction of a radioisotope into a molecule can be achieved in one of two ways. First, the compound under study can be synthesized so that a certain number of its atoms are substituted for those of a corresponding radioactive isotope (i.e., same element, different isotope). For example, one or more ^{12}C are substituted for ^{14}C. Historically this is known simply as isotopic labeling. There is a range of radioisotopes available, depending upon the structure of the compound under study. Isotopes of most relevance to drug development are ^{14}C, ^{3}H, ^{35}S, and ^{32}P, since these represent those elements most commonly found in organic xenobiotics. Oxygen and nitrogen are also commonly found in organic compounds but these elements only have radioisotopes with short half-lives; ^{15}O has a radioactive half-life of 2 minutes and ^{13}N 10 minutes. Nevertheless these isotopes have uses in positron emission tomography (PET) studies (Chapter 11) as they are β^{+} emitters.

The other method of introducing a radiotracer into a compound is by addition to the molecule. In this case, unlike substitution, the compound is structurally altered. A common example is where therapeutic proteins are under study (1.4). Proteins

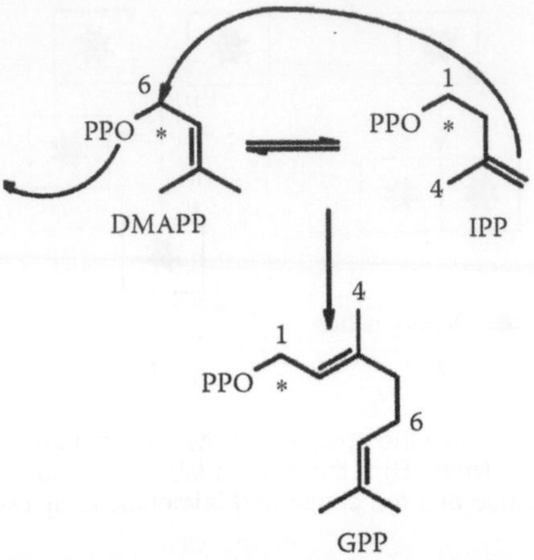

Figure 2.4   The condensation of isopentyl pyrophosphate (IPP) with dimethylallyl pyrophospate (DMAPP) to form geranyl pyrophosphate (GPP). Labeling IPP at carbon-1 and DMAPP at carbon-6 would be expected to result in GPP labeled equally at C-1 and C-6. This does not occur however, C-1 retains the majority of the label.

are obtained from biological sources and since they are not chemically synthesized, substituting a stable isotope with a radioisotope other than ^{3}H is very difficult. The alternative is therefore to iodinate the protein with ^{125}I, or sometimes with ^{131}I, although a range of isotopes have been used from Bromine to Samarium.[3] It may be necessary under such circumstances to demonstrate that the iodinated protein is an adequate surrogate for the intended therapeutic product. This is typically undertaken with a protein-receptor binding assay. Historically this method is known as non-isotopic labeling. The terms isotopic and non-isotopic labeling have however, become less common in recent years. Indeed the terminology has become confused as non-isotopic labeling is sometimes used for fluorescent labels, or other methods where isotopes are not relevant.

Detailed radiosynthetic chemistry is outside the scope of this book but a general appreciation of how radiolabeled drugs are synthesized is useful and provides an understanding of both the skill of the synthetic chemist as well as the technical limitations. For the synthesis of non-radiolabeled compounds, there is a wide choice of starting materials, many derived from petrochemical or other natural sources. Such starting materials are molecular in nature and as such are already a step towards the complexity of the desired product. The starting material for radiosynthesis however, is the isotope itself. From the isotope, some simple building blocks are made, followed by increasing degrees of complexity to the completed product. The synthetic routes for the non-radiolabeled and radiolabeled compounds can therefore be very different. As a point of interest, because many starting materials for chemical synthesis are derived from petrochemical sources, which are of immense age, they are virtually devoid of any ^{14}C and hence do not contain the background levels described in 2.8.1. Only if the drug is obtained from at least a partial natural source (eg fermentation-derived antibiotics) will it contain small natural levels of radioisotope.

2.12.1 ^{14}C

^{14}C is manufactured by neutron bombardment of ^{14}N, usually in the form of beryllium nitride or aluminum nitride, resulting in ^{14}CO$_2$, typically stored as Ba^{14}CO$_3$. From here, a number of building blocks can be made, the most useful being carboxylic acids (particularly acetic acid), cyanide, methyl iodide and acetaldehyde. Carboxylic acids are frequently brominated or chlorinated. From these basic building blocks, more complex radiolabeled molecules are synthesized. As an illustration, we will take two examples. Pyruvic acid, which is itself a precursor of more complex structures, can be made from a reaction of acetyl bromide with cyanide over a copper catalyst (Figure 2.5). There are three possible combinations of ^{14}C-labeled reactants, each resulting in pyruvic acid labeled in a different carbon atom. If [U-^{14}C]-pyruvic acid were required, then the three forms shown in Figure 2.5 would be mixed to provide a statistically uniform product, but no one molecule of pyruvic acid would be labeled in all three carbon atoms (see 2.8 regarding the relevance of this to specific activity).

The second example, shown in Figure 2.6 is more complex and illustrates a cyclization reaction as a step in the synthesis of cephalosporin antibiotic.[4] Note that the radiolabeled intermediate is simply potassium thiocyanate (KS^{14}CN).

More recently, there has been a demand for optically-pure ^{14}C-compounds, as opposed to racemic mixtures. So called asymmetric synthesis has been a challenge for the synthetic chemist. Enantioselective synthesis is possible, proving optically pure intermediates are available. Such intermediates are in short supply and so synthesis of the racemic form, followed by chiral separation is still commonly used.

Non labelled reactant		Labelled reactant		Intermediate		Product
CH$_3$COBr	+	Cu$_2$(^{14}CN)$_2$	→	CH$_3$CO^{14}CN	→	CH$_3$CO^{14}COOH
Cu$_2$(CN)$_2$	+	CH$_3$^{14}COBr	→	CH$_3$^{14}COCN	→	CH$_3$^{14}COCOOH
Cu$_2$(CN)$_2$	+	^{14}CH$_3$COBr	→	^{14}CH$_3$COCN	→	^{14}CH$_3$COCOOH

Figure 2.5 Synthesis of [^{14}C]-pyruvic acid, with the ^{14}C-label in three different positions.

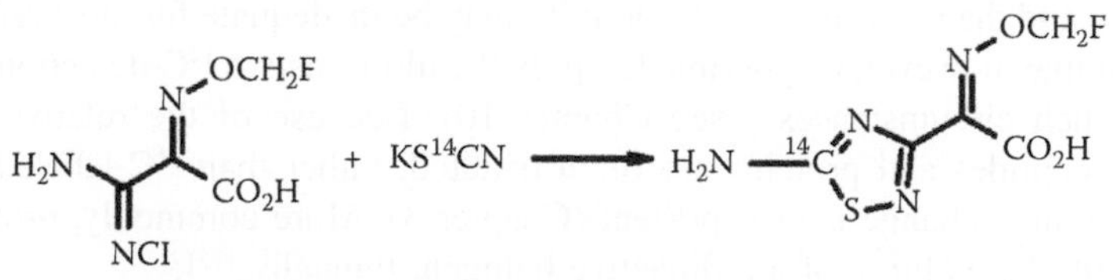

Figure 2.6 An example of a cyclization reaction, incorporating ^{14}C into a ring structure using a simple KS^{14}CN reagent.

2.12.2 ³H

Overall, tritiation of a compound is more straightforward than ^{14}C labeling and often incorporation of ^3H can be achieved in a single, or at least a limited number of reaction steps. On the other hand, ^3H is more easily lost from the molecule (see tritium exchange, 3.2.1). Tritium gas is generated during the neutron bombardment of ^6Li. Tritium gas or ^3H_2O can be used to directly tritiate compounds, often in the presence of a catalyst or even using microwaves. This results in a wide distribution of tritium in the molecule and is known as exchange labeling or non-specific labeling. Synthetic tritiation or specific tritium labeling on the other hand, is where tritium label is inserted at a specific structural position within the molecule. Synthetic tritiation is achieved by incorporating specific tritiated moieties into the synthesis. For example [^3H]-methyl magnesium iodide to produce tritiated tertiary alcohols from esters; [^3H]-Na[^3H]-BH$_4$ to produce tritiated primary alcohols from the ester. A number of advances have been made in synthetic tritiation over recent years. ^3H-Alkaline metal borohydrides, for example, are widely used as semi-selective tritiating agents. Tritiated diphenylsilane has been used in the reduction of ketones and aldehydes.[5]

Therapeutic proteins can be tritiated as it is very difficult to label by ^{14}C substitution. Tritium gas has been used for this as well as reagents such as pyridoxal phosphate-sodium boro- [^3H]-hydride.[6]

2.12.3 Radiosynthesis of Peptides and Proteins

Peptides and small polypeptides can be manufactured using automated solid and solution phase synthesizers. Consequently the introduction of a [^{14}C]-amino acid into the sequence is, in theory relatively straightforward. Peptides are synthesized from the C-terminus and therefore if the ^{14}C amino acid is at or close to the N-terminus, the majority of the peptide can be synthesized under non-radioactive conditions; leaving just the final stages where the radiolabel is added. This makes the synthesis simpler and therefore, cheaper. The converse is also true; if the C-terminus is labeled, then the synthesis becomes more expensive.

Monoclonal antibodies are manufactured by the fermentation of genetically engineered organisms and therefore in theory the fermentation medium can be enriched with a [^{14}C]-precursor. In practice however, the efficiency of incorporation is very low and the resulting specific activity may be inadequate for most radiotracer studies. (It may however, be possible to apply the ultrasensitve ^{14}C-detection method AMS in such circumstances - see Chapter 10). Because of the relative ease of synthesis, peptides and proteins are often tritiated, rather than ^{14}C-labeled but the risk of tritium exchange is ever present (Chapter 3). More commonly, proteins are labeled with the addition of a radioactive halogen, typically ^{125}I.

The iodination of proteins is conducted using a variety of methods, which are divided into two categories. Those that add iodine directly to the protein are known as direct methods (for obvious reasons). The other is known as a conjugation method, whereby the halogen is attached to a chemical species that then reacts with the protein. Direct methods can produce high specific activities and yields but they sometimes lead to the denaturing or inactivation of the protein and so generally the more specific conjugation methods are favored. An example of a direct method is the sodium N-monochloro derivative of p-toluene sulfonamide, forming the $^{125}I^+(H_2O)$ radical in the presence of the isotope, leading to the iodination of tyrosine residues. (This is known as the chloramine-T method). Conjugation methods are more specific and therefore reagents can be selected to avoid amino acid residues around the active site. Yields and specific activities however, tend to be lower compared to direct methods. There is a wide range of conjugating reagents available. The most commonly used are active esters, which react with free amines (Figure 2.7) and maleimides, which react with thiols at pH ≤7 and with amines at a pH around 9-10 (Figure 2.8). One of the most frequently used conjugating reagents is the Bolton-Hunter reagent[7] which targets free amines and is shown in Figure 2.9.

2.13 RADIOPURITY AND AUTORADIOLYSIS

After synthesis, the radiochemical purity of the labeled compound must be determined. Radiochemical purity is measured by a radiochromatographic technique such as radio-HPLC (Chapter 8). The radiolabeled compound should be as pure as possible, typically 98% or better.

In practice, it is difficult to state precisely what percentage radiopurity is acceptable. For example, Figure 2.10A shows a typical radio-HPLC chromatogram of a radiochemical with a high radiopurity (98%). Figure 2.10B shows a radiochromato-

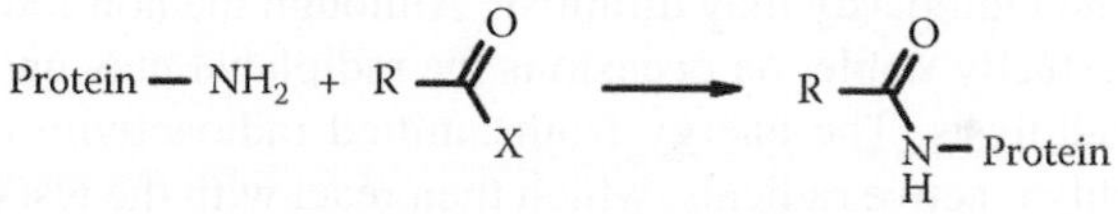

Figure 2.7 Conjugation of activated ester with amine groups on proteins. R is some organic moiety containing the radioisotope, typically ^{125}I.

pH 7 or lower

pH 9–10

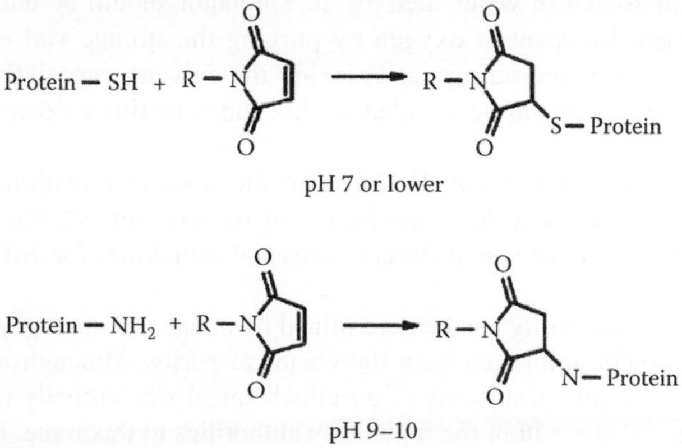

Figure 2.8 Conjugation of maleimide reagent with either thiol or amine groups on proteins. R is some organic moiety containing the radioisotope, typically ^{125}I.

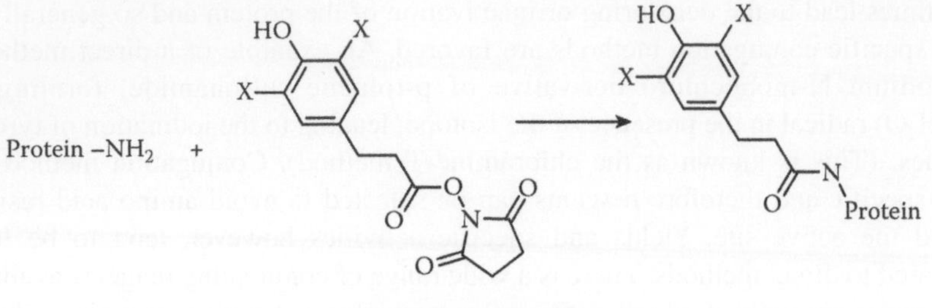

Bolton-Hunter reagent

Figure 2.9 The Bolton-Hunter reagent. X represents the radioisotope, typically ^{125}I.

gram with a small but distinct impurity, but the radiochemical purity of the compound of interest is still 98%.

Would the radiopurity as shown in Figure 2.10B be acceptable? The answer depends upon the experimental questions being asked. Consider, for example, a situation where the radiolabel was administered to laboratory animals and the results showed that 2% of the administered dose was retained for a considerable period of time in one specific organ. In terms of tissue retention, 2% is a very large proportion of the dose. If the compound as shown in Figure 2.10B had been administered, the question would immediately arise: what if all of the impurity had been retained and none of the actual compound of interest? On this basis, even though the radiochemical purity was 98%, it would nevertheless seem sensible to repurify the compound shown in Figure 2.10B to remove the minor peak.

On storage, the radiopurity may diminish. Although the non-radiolabeled compound may be perfectly stable, on occasions the radiolabel may undergo a process known as autoradiolysis. The energy from emitted radioactivity can lead to the formation of highly reactive radicals, which then react with the test chemical (2.6). Autoradiolysis tends to be more prevalent with high-energy radionuclides and high specific activities but overall it is very difficult to predict. Storing the radiolabel in dilute solution, ideally in aromatic solvent, can reduce autoradiolysis. If the compound is dissolved in water then 10-20% ethanol should be added as a free radical scavenger. Removal of oxygen by purging the storage vial with nitrogen can also help reduce autoradiolysis. Freezing the solvent, especially water with tritiated compounds, should be avoided as this can sometimes exacerbate autoradiolysis.

The stability of the radiolabeled drug in the dose formulation (Chapter 3) should be established for at least the period of the experiment. This is achieved by measuring the radiopurity at different times and sometimes for different storage conditions.

Although the radiopurity can be determined by a radiochromatographic method, this does not provide information on the chemical purity. Although in years gone by, the issue of the chemical purity of a radiochemical was virtually ignored, there is a growing awareness within the regulatory authorities to this issue. In Europe for example, there are now requirements for radiolabeled compounds destined for administration to humans, to be synthesized under Good Manufacturing Practices.

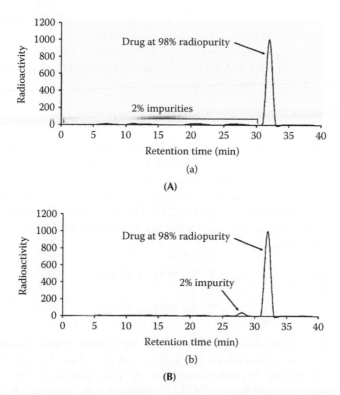

Figure 2.10 Both radiochromatograms (A and B) show a radiopurity of 98%. In example A, the 2% impurities are indistinct, whilst in (B) the 2% is a single component.

2.14 KINETIC ISOTOPE EFFECTS

When conducting radiotracer work, it is assumed that the chemical behavior of the radiolabeled compound is the same as that of its unlabeled equivalent. This however, is not necessarily true as the vibration frequency of chemical bonds is dependent upon the mass of the bonded isotopes; a phenomenon known as the kinetic isotope effect (KIE).

Compare hydrogen (^1H) and tritium (^3H) for example. Tritium is three times as heavy as hydrogen, consequently, the $C–^3H$ bond has a lower zero-point energy than the $C–^1H$ bond and a higher activation energy is required for bond-cleavage. Hence, the rate of a reaction involving $C–^3H$ is slower than the same reaction with $C–^1H$. The kinetic isotope effect only influences the rate of a reaction; the products are unchanged irrespective of the isotopic make-up. The KIE can be seen during chemical reactions and physical interactions. For example, deuterated compounds may sometimes have slightly different retention times when separated using high performance liquid chromatography (HPLC) compared to the undeuterated counterpart. The kinetic isotope effect becomes less significant the larger the atomic mass, as the relative difference in atomic weight between the light and heavy isotopes decreases. For example, the difference in atomic weight between ^1H and ^3H is 300% whereas the difference between ^{12}C and ^{14}C is only 14%.

A chemical reaction can be represented by equation 2.11, where X and Y are reactants, Z is the product and TS is the transition state. The overall rate of the reaction is defined by the rate constant k.

$$X + Y \leftrightarrow [TS] \rightarrow Z \; (k) \qquad\qquad (2.11)$$

Let us assume that the reactants X and Y are organic compounds and contain only a light isotope (L) (equation 2.12). Now let us assume that the light isotope in reactant X is replaced with a heavy isotope (H) (equation 2.13). Due to the kinetic isotope effect, the rate of the reaction represented by equation 2.13 will be somewhat slower than that represented in equation 2.12. The magnitude of the kinetic isotope effect is simply defined as the ratio of the rate constants based upon the light (k^L) and heavy (k^H) isotopes.

$$X_L + Y_L \leftrightarrow [TS] \rightarrow Z \; (k^L) \qquad\qquad (2.12)$$

$$X_H + Y_L \leftrightarrow [TS] \rightarrow Z \; (k^H) \qquad\qquad (2.13)$$

The kinetic isotope effect $= k^L/k^H$. Mostly for reasons of experimental convenience, the majority of studies on the kinetic isotope effect of carbon have been conducted with ^{12}C and ^{13}C, rather than with ^{14}C. For example, the kinetic isotope effect has been calculated for $^{12}C/^{13}C$-CO_2 fixation by the enzyme ribose 1,5-bis-phosphate carboxylase (in the citric acid cycle) and found to be in the region of 1.0178. In other words, $^{12}CO_2$ was fixed by the enzyme approximately 1.0178 times faster than $^{13}CO_2$.[8]

Whereas the kinetic isotope effect with $^{12}C/^{14}C$ is relatively small, effects with $^1H/^3H$ can be significant. For example, the kinetic isotope effect for the peroxidation of $^1H/^3H$-ethanol by liver catalase was reported to be as high as 2.52; that is the reaction with ^1H-ethanol was over two and half times faster than with ^3H-ethanol.[9]

KIE values are determined for specific reactions and the situation *in vivo* is far more complex, involving a variety of reactions and enzymes. A metabolic pathway can be affected by a series of KIEs, for each individual enzyme; in which case this is known as the metabolic isotope effect (MIE). For example, differences in the metabolism of different isotopes of nitrogen are known to occur in plants.[10]

Whilst care must be taken with deuterium and tritium, where the KIE and MIE can be significant, in contrast typical values for $^{12}C/^{13}C$ are in the region 1.04, for $^{12}C/^{14}C$ around 1.07 and for $^{32}S/^{35}S$ 1.01. It is therefore reasonable to state that the presence of these isotopes or others of similar atomic weight or higher, will have no discernable effect on the reaction rates of the test compound *in vivo*, especially in light of the fact that biological systems themselves will exhibit a degree of variation which is likely to be greater than any kinetic isotope effect.

FURTHER READING

L'Annunziata, M. F. (2003) Handbook of Radioactivity Analysis 2nd Edition. Academic Press

Billington, D., Jayson, G. G. and Maltby, P. J. (1992) Radioisotopes. Introduction to Biotechniques. Bios Scientific Publishers.

Theodórsson, P. (1996) Measurement of Weak Radioactivity. World Scientific Publishing

ACKNOWLEDGMENTS

My son Paul for working through the equations and calculations.

REFERENCES

1. The Nobel Lecture by Frederick Soddy can be found on the website of the Nobel Foundation on http://nobelprize.org/chemistry/laureates/1921/soddy-lecture.pdf.
2. Allen, K. G., Banthorpe, D.V, Charlwood, B.V., Ekundayo, O. and Mann, J., Metabolic pools associated with monoterpene biosynthesis in higher plants, *Phytochemistry* 15, 101-107, 1976.
3. Boniface, G. R., Izard, M. E., Walker, K. Z., McKay, D. R., Sorby, P. J., Turner, J. H., and Morris, J. G., Labeling of monoclonal antibodies with samarium-153 for combined radioimmunoscintigraphy and radioimmunotherapy, *J Nucl Med* 30 (5), 683-91, 1989.
4. McCarthy, K. E., Recent advances in the design and synthesis of carbon-14 labelled pharmaceuticals from small molecule precursors, *Curr Pharm Des* 6 (10), 1057-83, 2000.
5. Saljoughian, M. and Williams, P. G., Recent developments in tritium incorporation for radiotracer studies, *Curr Pharm Des* 6 (10), 1029-56, 2000.
6. Howard, R. J., Barnwell, J. W., and Kao, V., Tritiation of protein antigens of Plasmodium knowlesi schizont-infected erythrocytes using pyridoxal phosphate-sodium boro [^{3}H]hydride, *Mol Biochem Parasitol* 6 (6), 369-87, 1982.
7. Bolton, A. E. and Hunter, W. M., The labelling of proteins to high specific radioactivities by conjugation to a ^{125}I-containing acylating agent, *Biochem* J 133 (3), 529-39, 1973.
8. Roeske, C. A. and O'Leary, M. H., Carbon isotope effect on carboxylation of ribulose bisphosphate catalyzed by ribulosebisphosphate carboxylase from Rhodospirillum rubrum, *Biochemistry* 24 (7), 1603-7, 1985.
9. Damgaard, S. E., Tritium effect in peroxidation of ehtanol by liver catalase, *Biochem J* 167 (1), 77-86, 1977.
10. Evans, R. D., Physiological mechanisms influencing plant nitrogen isotope composition, *Trends Plant Sci* 6 (3), 121-6, 2001.

CHAPTER 3

The Study of Drug Metabolism
Using Radiotracers

Graham Lappin

CONTENTS

3.1 INTRODUCTION

In bringing a new pharmaceutical to market, a series of toxicology studies are performed, each of them designed to examine the effects a drug has on a biological system. (Ultimately, the effect on humans is the important question, although for this, to some extent, extrapolations from animal models may be used.) While toxicology studies examine the effects of the drug on biological systems, metabolism studies examine the effect biological systems have on the drug. The term *biological system* is used here, as experiments can be conducted with isolated cells or cellular extracts (i.e., *in vitro* systems), animals, humans, or plants and microorganisms.

The general principles behind the performance of a drug metabolism study are the same as those described in Chapter 1, where Calvin used $^{14}CO_2$ to elucidate the photosynthetic pathway. The drug, labeled with a suitable radiotracer, is administered to a biological test system, and samples are taken over time and analyzed for radioactivity and by radiochromatography, thus revealing both qualitative and quantitative effects of the test system on the drug.

The subject of this chapter is how radiotracers are applied to the conduct of drug metabolism studies (*in vitro* and *in vivo*). The chapter is not overly concerned with the mechanisms of drug metabolism, although these are covered in appendices. Methods for the detection and quantification of radioactivity are covered in Chapter 6 and Chapter 8 (scintillation counting) and Chapter 10 (accelerator mass spectrometry).

Metabolism studies are routinely performed with small molecules (new chemical entities (NCEs); see Section 1.4). With therapeutic proteins, there is less of a demand for metabolism studies, although data are sometimes required, depending upon the specific protein being developed. There is a need for pharmacokinetic data with proteins, and radiolabels are occasionally necessary, if, for example, the protein occurs naturally in the body and cannot be distinguished from constitutive proteins using other methods, such as enzyme-linked immunosorbent assay (ELISA) (Section 4.3). This chapter therefore concentrates on NCEs, unless otherwise stated.

This chapter assumes a certain knowledge of pharmacokinetics and the types of biotransformations commonly seen in drug metabolism. If the reader is unfamiliar with these areas, then Appendices 1 and 3 provide some general background. In addition, Appendix 2 provides some examples of drug metabolism studies from the literature.

3.2 CHOICE OF RADIOLABEL

Of key importance is the position of the radioisotope within the molecular structure of the drug. Generally, the radioisotope is incorporated into a metabolically stable position within the molecule, so that it remains with that part of the molecule under study. To fully appreciate the meaning of this requires the reader to have some familiarity with the types of metabolic processes that commonly occur with xeno-biotics. A general review of metabolism and examples from the literature are covered in Appendices 1 and 2, respectively.

The most commonly used radioisotopes in drug metabolism studies are ^3H, ^{14}C, ^{35}S, ^{32}P, ^{33}P, and ^{125}I. By far the most commonly used radioisotope is ^{14}C. (This list excludes the isotopes used for positron emission tomography (PET) and γ-scintigraphy — Chapter 11 and Chapter 12, respectively.)

3.2.1 Tritium (^3H)

Tritium is a commonly used radiotracer in drug metabolism. It is relatively straightforward to label a molecule with ^3H, although it is equally as easy to lose the label in a process known as tritium exchange, whereby the tritium label exchanges with ^1H in physiological water. This can lead to the ubiquitous labeling of water within the test system.

The extent of tritium exchange can be estimated by comparing the amounts of radioactivity present in a sample before and after freeze drying. The freeze-drying process removes water (tritiated or otherwise), and therefore, if no radioactivity is lost, then no tritium exchanged occurred. This does, of course, assume that the parent compound and its metabolites are not volatile.

Tritium can exhibit a significant kinetic isotope effect (Section 2.14), and there-fore results concerned with rates of reactions should be treated with caution. Some-times ^3H is simply a cheaper option, particularly in the early stages of compound development. Tritium is also used where it is difficult to incorporate other radiotrac-ers in the molecule of interest, for example, ^{14}C into naturally occurring compounds such as steroids. In addition, proteins are commonly labeled with tritium.

Tritium has a radioactive half-life of 12.4 years, which is sufficiently long, so that no corrections are required for specific activity over the duration of an experi-ment, although corrections may be necessary if the radiolabeled test compound or biological samples are stored for prolonged periods.

Very high specific activities, and hence low limits of detection, can be achieved with tritium (Section 2.8). High specific activities are possible because of both the relatively short half-life (Section 2.9) and the ability to incorporate multiple ^3H atoms within the molecule.

If metabolites are separated using radiochromatography, then ^3H can be useful purely to chromatographically locate a metabolite. Freeze drying can be incorporated as part of the sample preparation process prior to chromatography, thus serving the triple purpose of estimating the amount of tritium exchange, removing extraneous ^3H_2O, and concentrating the sample.

3.2.2 ^{14}C

For *in vivo* drug metabolism studies, the first choice of radiolabel is ^{14}C. Above all other radioisotopes, ^{14}C can be incorporated into the general skeleton of an organic chemical, such as aromatic rings, as these are rarely subject to metabolism in mammalian systems (the same is not true for certain bacteria).

On the other hand, incorporating ^{14}C into a metabolically labile position can lead to the labeling of general metabolic pathways and the widespread labeling of naturally occurring compounds, such as sugars, amino acids (and then proteins), lipids, etc. Also remember that at the outset, the metabolism of the drug is not known, and therefore the choice of where to label the compound depends largely upon expert opinion (Appendix 2).

The radioactive half-life of ^{14}C is 5730 years, and therefore there is no significant degradation of specific activity over the period of an experiment. The radioactive half-life, however, limits the specific activity to about 2.3 GBq/mg atom (Section 2.9), which in some cases can lead to experimental constraints due to the limit of detection (Section 2.11).

3.2.3 ^{35}S

Sulfur labeling is used only occasionally, if, for example, a sulfur-containing moiety is of specific interest. Sulfur-containing aromatic rings such as thiophenes are better labeled with ^{14}C. The radioactive half-life of ^{35}S is 87 days, so corrections to the specific activity are likely to be necessary over the duration of an experiment (Table 2.2). ^{35}S is occasionally useful as a label for glutathione or sulfate (Appendix 1). in which case, instead of incorporating the label directly into the drug, ^{35}S is used to label a potential conjugate.

3.2.4 ^{32}P and ^{33}P

Out of the two phosphorus radionuclides, traditionally ^{32}P has been favored. In fact, ^{33}P probably has more to offer and should be given serious consideration. It has a longer half-life (and where half-lives of a few tens of days are concerned, the extra few days can make all the difference). ^{33}P has a lower energy and so is a safer option, and its maximum specific activity is still perfectly acceptable for most applications. The reason why ^{33}P has been overlooked is probably because ^{32}P has been widely used in postlabeling DNA binding studies (Section 4.2.7). The biggest drawback of ^{32}P or ^{33}P is their short half-lives (14 and 25 days, respectively). For this reason, phosphorus is only used in experiments where the phosphorus-containing moiety is of specific interest. There are also safety issues with the use of phosphorus isotopes, and shielding is necessary (Section 2.4).

3.2.5 ^{125}I

Therapeutic proteins are large complex molecules, and it is difficult, if not impossible, to incorporate radiolabels into their structures in the same way as with small molecules (NCEs). Instead, labels are added on to the structure of the protein, the theory being that given the large size of the protein, the attachment of a few additional chemical species will not make any difference to its activity and metabolic behavior. This is, however, an assumption, and at least some form of bioactivity assay should be performed following labeling.

After ^{3}H, the most commonly used isotope for labeling proteins is ^{125}I (Section 1.4). Proteins can be directly iodinated, resulting in a protein–iodine product. Alternatively, the protein can be reacted with a conjugating reagent containing the iodine label, resulting in a protein–conjugate–iodine product (Section 2.12.3).

The principal disadvantage of ^{125}I is its half-life of only 59.6 days, and therefore there is limited time to conduct any experiments following synthesis. ^{125}I is also a γ-emitter, and therefore a degree of shielding is necessary as a safety precaution. In addition, proteins iodinated with ^{125}I can often undergo significant autoradiolysis (Section 2.14).

In addition to ^{125}I, ^{131}I may also be used, although ^{131}I emits more penetrating γ-radiation and is therefore more hazardous to use. The radioactive half-life of ^{131}I is only 8 days, and therefore ^{131}I is rarely chosen over ^{125}I. There are difficulties with the administration of all iodine radioisotopes to humans because of safety issues relating to the γ-emission and the fact that any free iodine will concentrate in the thyroid.

3.2.6   Dual Labeling

A test compound can be simultaneously labeled with more than one radioisotope to study separate parts of the molecule as part of a single experiment. The most common form of dual labeling is ^{14}C and ^{3}H. In reality, the two radiolabeled compounds are synthesized separately and mixed prior to administration, thus providing a statistically uniform mixture. If it was possible to pluck any single molecule from this mixture, it would contain either ^{14}C or ^{3}H, but never both. This way the specific activities for both radiolabels can be independently controlled. ^{14}C and ^{3}H can be measured separately in the same sample by liquid scintillation counting, as they can be distinguished by their different energy windows (Section 6.4). Not all isotopes can be distinguished in this way; for example, the energy windows for ^{14}C and ^{35}S overlap and cannot be readily deconvoluted.

True dual-labeling studies use two different isotopes to independently label separate parts of the molecule. Labeling different parts of a molecule with the same radioisotope is not classed as dual labeling; in any case, this can lead to artifacts and should only be undertaken with great care (see Section 2.11 for an explanation). If different parts of the same molecule require labeling with the same radioisotope, then the experiment should be conducted as separate dosings, each dose using a different radiolabeled form. Such studies are termed double labeling, rather than dual labeling.

3.3 TEST SYSTEMS

There are three types of test systems where radiotracers might be used in the drug registration process.

1. *In vitro* studies
2. *In vivo* studies with laboratory animals
3. *In vivo* studies with human volunteers

At the beginning of developing a new drug, very little is known about the compound or its behavior in biological systems. Over time, knowledge and data are built up in series of steps, each step adding or refining the knowledge. *In vitro* systems offer a relatively straightforward, inexpensive, and rapid method of gathering early data. They provide useful rather than precise information, but nevertheless, at the early stages approximate data are all that is needed to throw light into an otherwise dark void.[1] As the development program continues, some of the earlier decisions may in retrospect be deemed inappropriate, and investigations may have to be repeated as a consequence. In general, therefore, *in vitro* experiments are at some stage superceded by the *in vivo* studies.

3.4 *IN VITRO* STUDIES

The use of radiolabel for *in vitro* investigations is not universal but can offer certain advantages, which are discussed below. The *in vitro* studies are largely relevant to small molecules (NCEs) rather than therapeutic proteins.

3.4.1 Species Comparison Studies

If a drug is metabolized in the animal species used for toxicological tests, in a way similar to that in the human, then the animal species can be considered an appropriate model and toxicity results can be extrapolated to humans with confidence. *In vitro* studies are used as an initial screen to select the toxicological species and sometimes to select metabolites for analysis in clinical trials. Using *in vitro* techniques, a number of species can be screened (e.g., mouse, rat, rabbit, dog, minipig, monkey, and man) in parallel by using relatively simple experimental protocols. What can be done *in vitro* in a few days would take many weeks or months *in vivo*. There are risks in predicting drug metabolism from *in vitro* models, as they are not always predictive of the metabolism *in vivo*.

Because *in vitro* systems are simpler and generally produce "cleaner" samples than *in vivo* systems, it is technically possible to conduct metabolic screening across species using nonlabeling techniques, such as liquid chromatography–mass spectrometry (LC-MS; Section 3.5.12) or nuclear magnetic resonance spectroscopy (NMR; Section 3.5.13). LC-MS and NMR data can be interrogated for the presence of spectra that might be drug related, or estimates can be made on what sort of biotransformations are likely, and then specific searches are made for these putative metabolites. *Ad hoc* searching for metabolites without the use of a tracer, however, can be very error-prone, as it is sometimes difficult to make accurate predictions as to how a drug might be metabolized (see the examples in Appendix 2). Judicious use of radiolabel can ensure that all the metabolites are fully accounted for.

Different pharmaceutical companies will take different views on the use of radiolabeled compound for *in vitro* experiments. I know of some companies that would never use radiolabel in *in vitro* studies, some would use ^{3}H, and others would synthesize a ^{14}C label very early and use it in as many *in vitro* experiments as appropriate. I know of one company that routinely uses [^{3}H]-drug even earlier in the discovery stage. (All the above experience is based the top 20 pharmaceutical companies in the world.)

3.4.2   *In Vitro* Dose Administration

For administration to *in vitro* systems, the radiolabeled test compound is typically added as a solution in a suitable solvent. An organic solvent can be used, but the volume should be as low as possible ($\leq$1% v/v) to minimize its effect on the *in vitro* test system. The choice of solvent therefore largely depends upon the solubility of the compound. Typical concentrations of drug in an *in vitro* incubation are around 0.5 to 1 μm; however, if the *in vivo* concentrations are known, then this may be adjusted to achieve a more physiologically relevant concentration.

3.4.3   *In Vitro* Preparations for Metabolite Profiling

There are four principal *in vitro* systems used for species comparison studies: S9 fraction, microsomes, hepatocytes and organ slices. Overall, the most commonly used are microsomes and hepatocytes. A description of each of the four systems is given below. Methods of preparation have been described previously and can be found in Evans (2004).[2]

The *in vitro* system is incubated in the presence of the test drug and samples are taken periodically for metabolic profiling. Metabolite profiling (irrespective if it is associated with *in vitro* or *in vivo* studies) is the process whereby samples, taken from a biological system administered a radiolabeled drug, are analyzed by radio-chromatography and the extent of metabolism is assessed (Section 3.5.9). The number of metabolites and their relative magnitude over time are studied, although the precise structural identity may not be known at the stage of the *in vitro* investigations. The experiment conducted by Calvin as described in Chapter 1 was a metabolite profile, albeit using the relative primitive chromatographic method of paper chromatography.

3.4.4   Submitochondial Fraction (S9)

A crude preparation of liver homogenate, centrifuged at 9000 *g* to remove particulate matter, is known as the S9 fraction. The S9 fraction contains cytosolic enzymes as well as fragments of membrane with membrane-bound enzymes such as CYP P450s (these enzymes are explained in Appendix 1). The preparation can be stored frozen (cryopreserved) over reasonable periods.

3.4.5 Microsomes

Microsomes are fragments of endoplasmic reticulum in the form of vesicles, but lacking the sophistication of the intact cell. They contain membrane-bound enzymes such as CYP P450, and with the addition of appropriate cofactors, they have some conjugation activity (e.g., glucuronidation; see Appendix 1). As with S9, microsomes can be cryopreserved. They may also be purchased commercially, derived from a range of species, including human. Human microsomes are pooled from a number of donor livers to ensure genetic homogeneity.

3.4.6 Hepatocytes

Hepatocytes are isolated parenchymal cells of the liver. They contain a wider range of active enzymes than do S9 or microsomes, including CYP P450s and conjugating enzymes along with cofactors. There are two schools of thought on cryopreserved hepatocytes. One school says that hepatocytes should be prepared fresh, as they are liable to lose their CYP P450 activity over time. The other school favors cryopreserved hepatocytes, since they can be pooled across donors and can be used on multiple occasions. Several suppliers now sell well-characterized cryo-preserved hepatocytes from a wide range of species.

3.4.7 Organ Slices

Organ slices contain intact and, to some extent, morphologically organized whole cells from the organ from which the slice was obtained. Liver slices contain CYP P450s and conjugating enzymes. Slices can also be prepared from other organs, such as kidney or lung, if required.

3.4.8 Determining the Metabolic Profile and Responsible Enzymes

The initial investigations are typically performed in liver microsomes. The test compound is administered, incubated for a given period, extracted with suitable solvents, and analyzed by radiochromatography.

At its simplest level, the radiochromatographic profiles are directly compared between species to determine whether any species-specific metabolites are formed, particularly in humans. In addition to a simple profile, the enzymology and kinetics can be studied. In particular, it is important to understand which CYP P450 enzymes are involved in the metabolism of the drug, as this provides a better understanding of potential drug–drug interactions (Section 3.4.13) and polymorphisms (Section 3.4.15). In these experiments the turnover of the test drug *in vitro* should be limited to <20%, which is achieved by varying the incubation time and protein concentration. Once the major metabolites are established, incubation conditions are optimized to ensure linear kinetics, in terms of incubation time and enzyme concentration. The kinetic parameters (k_m and V_{max}) governing the formation of each metabolite of interest may then be determined. Incubations are typically performed at eight or more drug concentrations, over a logarithmic scale. The data are plotted in a linear transform to determine K_m

and V_{max}, such as 1/rate against 1/substrate concentration (Lineweaver–Burk plot) or rate against rate/substrate concentration (Eadie–Hofstee plot).

There are three generally accepted approaches to phenotyping CYP P450-mediated metabolism. None of the approaches are definitive in isolation; rather, two or more methods are used in combination to form a consensus on which P450s are involved:

1. Incubations are performed in pooled human liver microsomes at one or more appropriate concentrations, and the rate of production of the metabolite of interest is determined in the presence and absence of enzyme inhibition. The specific CYP P450 isozymes are individually inhibited by known chemical inhibitors (at potent yet selective concentrations). For example, CYP 2D6 is inhibited with quinidine. Alternatively, inhibitory antibodies can be used.
2. Heterologously expressed cloned human CYP P450 enzymes are commercially available. The test article is incubated with each individual CYP P450, and production of metabolites of interest is monitored. It should be noted that this is an isolated system, and false positive results are common.
3. The test article is incubated with a library of extensively characterized individual human liver microsomes from at least 10 donors. The rate of metabolite production is then plotted against each CYP P450 activity, and correlation analysis is performed. For example, for a drug only metabolized by CYP 3A4, a plot of the rate of metabolite production vs. the CYP 3A4 activity level in each of the microsomes used will be linear. Conversely, if the same graph is drawn against CYP 2D6, for example, then there will be no obvious correlation.

3.4.9   Metabolite Factories

Microsomes, hepatocytes, and sometimes organ slices can be used as "metabolite factories." This application is often overlooked but can nevertheless be very useful. An *in vitro* system is fed with the radiolabeled drug, and following incubation, metabolites are isolated using semipreparative chromatography. The resulting isolated radiolabeled metabolites are rarely highly pure, and they are only produced in small quantities, but at a much lower cost than synthetic chemical methods. They can be very useful, for example, as chromatographic markers when profiling metabolites from *in vivo* studies.

3.4.10   Permeability Using Caco-2, MDCK, or PAMPA

The degree to which a drug intended for oral administration is absorbed through the gastrointestinal tract can be assessed using *in vitro* models. There are three such models in common use: Caco-2, MDCK, and PAMPA.[3,4]

The Caco-2 cell line is derived from a human colonic adenocarcinoma and is grown as a monolayer on a permeable support, to model the intestinal epithelium.

Drugs can be absorbed through the gastrointestinal tract by passive diffusion or by active transport mechanisms. Caffeine and mannitol are examples of compounds that are transported by passive diffusion. The Caco-2 cell line expresses a range of active transport carriers, including absorptive transporters such as the bile acid and peptide transporters, and efflux transporters, such as MRP1 to MRP6, MDR1 (P-gp), MDR3, and BCRP.

The MDR-1 (more commonly known as P-glycoprotein or P-gp)-mediated efflux pump limits transepithelial absorption of many drugs (e.g., vinblastine and cyclosporine) by actively pumping the compound out of the cell. Compounds such as verapamil can be used to inhibit P-gp, and such compounds can be used as inhibitors *in vitro* to study whether P-gp is involved in the active transport of the candidate drug. (Attempts have also been made to use such inhibitors *in vivo* to increase the concentrations of anticancer drugs in tumors.)[5] In addition, fexofenadine has been widely used as a probe for intestinal and hepatic P-gp activity.[6]

The MDCK cell line, which is derived from canine kidney, does not express P-gp to the same extent as Caco-2. The advantage of MDCK is that it requires a shorter time to achieve mature monolayers.

Parallel artificial monolayer permeability assays (PAMPA) is a non-cell-based isolated active transport system. This system is usually used in drug discovery, and hence radiolabel is rarely available.

The use of radiolabel is by no means essential for *in vitro* permeability determination, but negates the need to develop a sensitive analytical method for quantification of test article (exploiting the universal detection and quantification properties of radiolabels; Section 2.10).

3.4.11 Plasma Protein Binding and Blood Cell Partitioning

Drugs that bind strongly to plasma protein or the cellular fraction of blood are not necessarily then systemically bioavailable. Such binding can therefore have effects on efficacy and, if the binding persists, can have toxicological consequences.

The extent of blood binding and blood cell partitioning can be tested *in vitro*. The compound can be simply mixed with blood or plasma and, in the case of blood, the cellular fraction separated by centrifugation. In the case of plasma, the protein can be separated through a molecular weight filter (ultrafiltration). In many cases, however, the degree of nonspecific binding to ultrafiltration apparatus is significant, making the technique unreliable. Equilibrium dialysis, on the other hand, allows the study of binding under conditions of equilibrium. Plasma is fortified with a known amount of drug and added to the donor half of a dialysis cell. A semipermeable membrane separates the donor side from the receptor side containing isotonic buffer. Drug not bound to plasma protein will equilibrate across the membrane, while the portion bound to the protein remains trapped on the donor side. The extent of protein binding is determined by comparing drug concentrations in both cell halves after equilibrium is achieved. Such experiments can be conducted using nonradiolabeled compound (measuring parent compound or a suitable surrogate), but the use of radiolabel not only makes the experiments more straightforward, but also allows an accurate recovery to be calculated. Blood cell partitioning is also studied *in vivo* (Section 3.6.4).

3.4.12 Dermal Absorption Models

The extent and rate that a drug penetrates the skin can be studied *in vitro*. Skin, obtained from laboratory animals or human sources, is placed over a cell and drug is applied to the surface. On the other side of the skin is a buffer receptor fluid. Samples of the buffer are taken over time to monitor the rate of penetration through the skin. There are two types of dermal absorption model: one uses a static fluid receptor, and the other uses a flow-through cell, thereby simulating blood circulation (Figure 3.1A and B). The former system is simpler and easier to use. The latter system, it can be argued, provides a better model for the *in vivo* situation. Such systems are particularly useful at investigating the effects of different formulations on dermal absorption. As with other *in vitro* systems, in theory it is possible to conduct dermal absorption studies without radiolabeled compound, but this would be unusual in the industry, as an overall recovery is often an important factor in the experiment. Moreover, ^{3}H water is commonly used to check for the integrity of the skin prior to dose application (although electrical resistance methods are also available). In general, *in vitro* dermal absorption systems overestimate absorption through the skin when compared to the *in vivo* situation.[7]

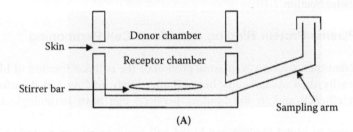

(A)

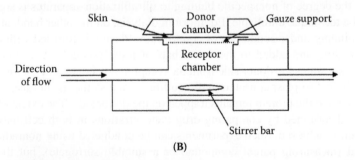

(B)

Figure 3.1   Systems for the study of dermal absorption *in vitro*. (A) Flow-through cell and (B) unoccluded static Franz cell. (Diagrams with permission from Covance Laboratories.)

3.4.13 Drug–Drug Interaction Studies Using *In Vitro* Systems

Drug–drug interactions are caused by the effect one drug has on certain enzymes or transporters within the body (Figure 3.2). The effect on the enzyme can be inhibition, but some drugs cause an increase in protein synthesis, thereby leading to enzyme induction. The enzymes of concern are mostly the CYP P450s (Appendix 1), although not exclusively so. Transporter systems can also be involved in drug–drug interactions (see below).

Drug–drug interactions can be divided into two types: (1) those where the drug under development has an effect on an enzyme that causes a change in the metabolism of an existing drug (2) and those where an existing drug has an effect on an enzyme that causes a change in the metabolism of the development drug. In the industry, the two cases are often depicted in terms of "the guilty party." In Figure 3.2, drug 1 is the guilty party in respect to drug 2, and drug 2 is the guilty party in respect to drug 1.

Where the development drug is the guilty party, *in vitro* systems are used to examine inhibition or induction of enzymes, such as the CYP P450s. In order to assess inhibition, the drug is administered to either microsomes or sometimes hepatocytes along with a probe substrate for a particular enzyme. For example, midazolam is a probe substrate for CYP 3A4 and bufuralol is a probe substrate for CYP 2D6.[8] The rate of disappearance (or more usually the rate of formation of a specific metabolite) for the probe substrate is monitored in both the presence and absence of the development drug. If the development drug inhibits the enzyme, then the rate of metabolism of the probe substrates falls.

To assess induction, cultured human hepatocytes are exposed to the drug (usually three concentrations) for typically 72 h. The relative rates of metabolism for probe

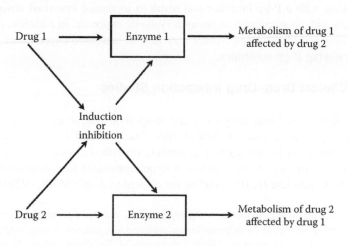

Figure 3.2 Schematic representation of drug–drug interactions.

substrates in cultures with and without the test drug are compared to determine the fold induction of CYP P450. The baseline CYP activity and the inducibility of human hepatocyte preparations are, however, highly variable. Therefore, at least three donors are usually investigated and prototypical inducers are investigated alongside the development drug as comparators.[9] For example, phenobarbital can be used to induce CYP 2B enzymes. An induction of >40% of that of the prototypical control is considered significant.

In some cases, the development drug is dosed, often repeatedly, to animals, and then microsomes or hepatocytes are generated from those animals. Comparisons of the rate of metabolism of the probe substrate from *in vitro* systems generated from dosed and control animals are then made. This technique is often better at detecting induction. CYP P450 enzymes, however, are not always the same in animals and humans (e.g., the human-specific CYP 2C subfamily), nor does an induction in animals necessarily predict an induction in humans.

Since, in the above experiments, the metabolism of a probe substrate is being examined, the substrate and products are known, so there is little need for radiotracers.

Where the coadministered drug is the guilty party, the situation is more complicated. Here it is necessary to know what enzymes are responsible for the metabolism of the candidate drug. If, for example, the candidate drug is metabolized extensively by one particular CYP P450, then any coadministered drug inhibiting or inducing this enzyme is likely to have an interaction. Furthermore, certain foods[10] and herbal remedies[11] can inhibit or induce drug-metabolizing enzymes. To study these effects, a thorough understanding of the metabolism of the drug is necessary, and here radiotracers play an important role. Knowledge of the enzymology is also key to understanding possible polymorphic effects (see Section 3.4.15).

A potential for drug–drug interactions exists, if the test article is either a substrate for or an inhibitor of the P-gp efflux pump (Section 3.4.10). Coadministration of a P-gp substrate with a P-gp inhibitor can result in increased intestinal absorption of the substrate with an associated increase in systemic exposure. In addition, inhibition of P-gp within the blood–brain barrier may lead to increased exposure of the brain to any circulating P-gp substrates.

3.4.14   Clinical Drug–Drug Interaction Studies

It should be noted that drug–drug and drug–food interaction studies are often performed as part of the phase I clinical trials. The need and design of such studies is heavily influenced by the early experiments described above. The International Conference on Harmonization of Technical Requirements for Registration of Pharmaceuticals for Human Use (ICH) guideline for clinical trials (CPMP/ICH/291/9) states:

> If a potential for drug-drug interaction is suggested by metabolic profile, by the results of non-clinical studies or by information on similar drugs, studies on drug interaction during clinical development are highly recommended. For drugs that are frequently co-administered it is usually important that drug-drug interaction studies are performed in non-clinical and, if appropriate, in human studies.

Clinical drug–drug interaction studies do not involve the use of radiotracers, but are mentioned here for the sake of completeness and illustrate how results of metabolism studies impact upon the wider aspects of drug development.

3.4.15 Polymorphism

The human population is genetically heterogeneous, and the activities of certain drug-metabolizing enzymes can vary widely from one individual to another. Such variations in the population are known as polymorphisms, and the study of the genetic heterogeneity in the human population is known as pharmacogenetics. Perhaps the best known example is the polymorphic enzyme CYP 2D6 and its substrate, the antihypertensive debrisoquine.[12] The systemic elimination of debrisoquine relies on the formation of the 4-hydroxy-metabolite, a reaction catalyzed by CYP 2D6. About 5 to 10% of the Caucasian population, however, have deficient CYP 2D6 activity and are classed as poor metabolizers. CYP 2D6 in poor metabolizers has a markedly reduced affinity for debrisoquine, and so the rate of formation of the 4-hydroxy-metabolite is reduced, thus slowing its systemic clearance. If normal repeat dosages are taken by poor metabolizers, systemic concentrations build up and toxic symptoms quickly develop. Legend has it that the debrisoquine effect was discovered when the head of the pharmacology unit in England that was testing debrisoquine collapsed with vascular hypotension on taking a trial dose of the new drug. He was later found to be a poor metabolizer. Thus, it is not only important to understand the metabolic pathway by which a drug is metabolized, but also something of the enzymology. Drugs that rely on polymorphic enzymes for their elimination harbor greater risks than those that do not.

Other polymorphic P450s are CYP 2C19 (3 to 5% of Caucasians and Afro-Caribbeans and 18 to 23% of Asians are poor metabolizers) and CYP 1A2 (12 to 13% of Caucasians and Afro-Caribbeans are poor metabolizers). Drugs metabolized by CYP 2C19 include omeprazole (Prilosec — used to treat frequent heartburn by decreasing the amount of acid produced in the stomach) and for CYP 1A2, caffeine and acetaminophen (paracetamol).

3.5 *IN VIVO* STUDIES: EXPERIMENTAL ASPECTS

3.5.1 An Overview

The use of radiotracers for *in vivo* experiments is more prevalent than for *in vitro* experiments. *In vivo* metabolism studies are conducted with laboratory animals and human volunteers. There are many similarities in the conduct of laboratory animal and human metabolism studies, and so they will be covered together here, with differences in approach dealt with appropriately.

With animal studies, the amounts of radioactivity that can be administered are limited only by the specific activity of the radiolabeled compound. When administering radiotracers to humans, however, there are strict regulatory limits on the amounts of radioactivity that can be given. Limits are defined in terms of the radioactive dose equivalent (Section 2.6), which is dependent upon the amount of radioactivity administered and the duration of exposure. Since the duration of exposure is dependent upon the time the drug resides within the body, experiments have to be conducted on a compound-by-compound basis to determine how much radioactivity can be safely administered. These experiments are known as dosimetry studies and are covered in Appendix 1 to Chapter 5.

In recent times, human metabolism studies have been designed around the use of accelerator mass spectrometry (AMS; Chapter 10), as opposed to liquid scintillation counting. AMS is an ultrasensitive technique for measuring isotopes (including ^{14}C) and allows very low doses of radioactivity to be administered, without the loss of analytical sensitivity. This technique opens the experimental design of human studies, allowing, for example, multiple doses of radiolabeled drug to be administered. Although the use of AMS in human studies is growing, it is not yet universal.

In Chapter 1, the terminology for various types of *in vivo* metabolism study was explained, and it is worth reiterating here. The *in vivo* studies in animals provide information on the absorption, distribution, metabolism and excretion of the test compound, which gives these types of investigations the acronym ADME studies. Since a precise amount of radioactivity can be administered in an ADME study, it is possible to recover this radioactivity at the end of an experiment, to be certain that everything is experimentally accounted for. Such studies are therefore sometimes known as balance studies or mass balance studies. A schematic representation of a typical ADME study, illustrating a mass balance, is shown in Figure 3.3.

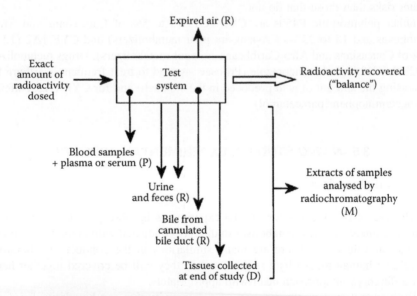

Figure 3.3   Schematic of a typical ADME study, showing the primary contribution of each sample type. P, pharmacokinetics; R, rates and routes of excretion; D, distribution; M, metabolism.

For both laboratory animal and human studies, after the administration of the radiolabeled compound, samples of blood, urine, and feces are collected. Bile is also a possible route of elimination, and with animals, it is therefore possible to collect bile by surgically cannulating the bile duct. Some compounds are eliminated *via* the breath, and therefore expired air can be passed through traps to collect volatiles. At the end of the experiment, laboratory animals may be killed and tissues dissected. It is possible, although in practice quite rare, to collect biopsies from human volunteers.

There are two routes of elimination that are rarely investigated, but they may on occasions be significant: sweat and saliva.[13]

An average human will produce around 1 liter of sweat per day. Distribution of sweat glands in mammals differs, depending upon the species. The dog has few sweat glands, and rats mainly regulate their temperature *via* the tail.

It is not uncommon to see radioactivity accumulate in the salivary glands in quantitative whole-body autoradiography studies (Chapter 5), but overall there have been very few studies examining elimination in saliva or sweat. For these reasons, these routes of elimination are not considered further in this text, but this does not mean that they do not represent possible routes of elimination.

Samples, once collected, are then analyzed for radioactivity, followed by extraction and analysis by radiochromatography (i.e., metabolic profile). The metabolites present in the radiochromatographic peaks can undergo further analysis, such as mass spectrometry (Section 3.5.12) or nuclear magnetic resonance spectroscopy (Section 3.5.13) in order to elucidate their chemical structures. For many purposes, the elucidation of the metabolic pathway of a drug is the key objective of a metabolism study. The use of radiotracer for this purpose is central, ensuring that a complete picture is obtained.

While animal studies are conducted with the animal in a metabolism cage, human volunteer studies are conducted in a clinical facility, and occasionally human studies are performed with consenting patients in hospitals.

3.5.2 Dose Preparation

Although a variety of radioisotopes might be used to study drug metabolism, ^{14}C will be referred to here for simplicity. Only rarely is pure [^{14}C]-drug administered. More often, the [^{14}C]-drug is mixed with nonradiolabeled drug to achieve the required dose level. To take an example, a typical level of radioactivity administered to the laboratory rat is around 1 MBq per animal (4 MBq/kg). Let us assume that the gravimetric dose is 25 mg per animal and that the specific activity of the pure [^{14}C]-drug is 10 MBq/mg (see Section 2.8 for an explanation of specific activity). The required specific activity for dosing is 1 MBq/25 mg or 40 KBq/mg. Thus, nonradiolabeled drug has to be mixed with pure [^{14}C]-drug in the ratio of 250:1. (As an aside, the enthusiastic reader could use the information in Section 2.11 to calculate the limit of detection (ng equiv/g) for a specific activity of 40 KBq/mg dosed. Based on a limit of detection for a scintillation counter of 50 dpm and a 0.5-g sample size, the answer is 41.6 ng equiv/g.)

In the preparation of the dose, two key points must be considered:

1. For isotopic labeled compounds (Section 2.12) the radiolabeled and nonradiolabeled compound must be chemically identical. Some radiolabeled drugs may be supplied as different derivatives compared to the nonradiolabeled variety. For example, one may be a free base or acid, while the other is a methylated or ethylated derivative. Prior to dose administration, both the radiolabeled and nonradiolabeled forms must be converted to the same derivative. In other cases, the radiolabeled and nonlabeled drugs might be supplied as different salt forms, for example, free base and a potassium or sodium salt. If the radiolabel is the free base and the nonlabeled form is added in excess, then the mere act of mixing may form an equilibrium, but this should not be assumed.
2. The radiolabeled and nonradiolabeled compounds should be in the same physical form. If the drug is administered as a solution, then the radiolabeled and nonradiolabeled forms, being dissolved, will be in the same physical form. If, however, they are administered as a suspension or in capsules, then differences may occur in, for example, particle size, and these differences can have profound effects on absorption. It should be remembered that the routes of synthesis of the radiolabeled and nonradiolabeled drug are likely to be different, and this can result in slightly different physical properties, which are commonly attributed to different physical forms of the compound (Section 2.12). Therefore, if the drug is to be administered as a suspension, ideally the radiolabeled and nonradiolabel drugs should first be dissolved together in a suitable solvent, and then the mixture of labeled and nonradiolabeled compounds recrystalized (for example, by evaporation of the solvent).

The situation with proteins is different in that the radiolabeled protein is either directly halogenated or halogenated *via* a chemical conjugate.

3.5.3   Routes of Administration

There are numerous routes by which drugs can be administered to animals or humans. These include intravenous, intra-arterial, oral, sublingual, vaginal, rectal, intramuscular, subcutaneous, intraperitoneal, inhalation, ocular and topical. In metabolism studies the radiolabeled drug is typically administered *via* the intended route of administration. Experimentally, the drug may also be administered intravenously (at least in animal studies), as this route is not complicated by the dynamics of absorption. Ideally, the drug is administered by the intravenous route in humans, as well as the intended route for clinical administration. In this case, however, toxicology studies are required to determine a safe dose level of the intravenous route. Such studies are expensive, and so for reasons of practicality and economics, intravenous administration is often omitted in human studies unless of clinical relevance.

For many drugs, the most convenient dose route is oral. This text therefore concentrates on the oral and intravenous routes, but other routes are mentioned when appropriate. By definition, the intravenous and intra-arterial routes introduce the drug directly into the circulation. Routes that do not introduce the drug directly into the circulation (e.g., oral, intramuscular, subcutaneous, inhalation, etc.) are generically known as extravascular.

3.5.4 Dose Administration

For *in vivo* studies using oral administration, ideally the dose is administered as a solution. Where this is not possible, the dose is prepared as a suspension, sometimes in the presence of suspending agents such as carboxymethyl cellulose or Gum Arabic. Hydroxypropyl-β-cyclodextrin is popular for solubilizing water-insoluble drugs. The dose may also be added to a support, such as starch or cellulose, and included in capsules (particularly when dosing dogs). On occasions, the dose is formulated to simulate therapeutic administration, but the purpose of the radiolabeled studies is rarely to mimic therapeutic conditions; such information is better obtained from the clinical trials. In metabolism studies it is often desirable to dose under conditions of maximum absorption on the grounds that the metabolism of the drug can only be studied once it is absorbed. Oral doses (solutions or suspensions) are typically administered to animals by gavage, but for human studies, the solution is simply drunk. In human studies, therefore, the issue of palatability must be considered, and it may be necessary to add flavorings.

Intravenous doses are prepared in physiological saline, glucose, or certain specialized formulations specifically designed for intravenous administration. For intravenous administration to humans, the preparation must be sterile. Particularly in human studies, the drug must be completely dissolved in the intravenous vehicle, with no chance of precipitation in the blood during dosing. For this reason, intravenous doses are often administered as an infusion over time, rather than a bolus dose.

Other routes of administration, such as dermal or inhalation, are specialized, and the formulation of the dose will depend very much on the specific circumstances of the study. For dermal administration, the choice of formulation may have profound effects on absorption. For inhalation, the particle or droplet size is important.

Doses can be administered on the basis of a fixed dose (e.g., 1 mg), a dose per kilogram of body weight (e.g., 1 mg/Kg), or a dose per body surface area (e.g., 1 mg/m^2). This latter method of dosing is applicable to cytotoxic compounds (e.g., anticancer therapies), as cytotoxic drug disposition is only partially affected by body mass and dosing on the basis of body surface area reduces interpatient variability.[14]

There are limits to the volume of dose that can be administered, and a general guide is shown in Table 3.1.[15]

Unlike the larger clinical trials, it is not common practice to statistically justify the number of animals or volunteers used on metabolism studies. For rats, typically about 10 animals are used (5 male and 5 female). The number is reduced for the dog and increased for the mouse, partly for convenience and partly because of sample size. It is generally accepted that four is the minimum number of healthy human volunteers used in a metabolism study, and six to eight is more common. Usually only male volunteers are used, but this depends upon the intended use of the drug. With humans it is possible to phenotype subjects to either select or reject, for example, poor or extensive metabolizers (Section 3.4.15). (Modern technology is now allowing genotyping as well as phenotyping to be carried out.) If studies are conducted in patients, then usually larger numbers are enrolled (typically 10 to 12), as there will be greater variability in the results compared to healthy volunteers.[16]

Table 3.1   A General Guide to the Maximum Volumes that can be
Administered for the Main Routes of Administration

	Route of Administration			
Species	Oral (mL/Kg)	IV Bolus (mL/Kg)	IV Infusion (total mL)	IM (mL/Kg)
Mouse	10	5	25	0.05
Rat	10	5	20	0.1
Rabbit	10	2	10	0.25
Dog	5	2.5	5	0.25
Marmoset	10	2.5	10	0.25
Human	3	0.5 over 1 min	12.5 mL/Kg/h	0.05

Note: IV = intravenous; IM = intramuscular.

Single or repeat administrations of radiolabeled drug can be given, although single-dose studies are more common. Repeat-dose studies are performed either to examine possible accumulation of drug or metabolites in tissues or to examine the possibility of additional metabolites being formed as repeat dosing continues (as it would in the clinical setting). Repeat-dose studies are not necessarily required for all drugs, although some pharmaceutical companies will perform them routinely. The need for repeat-dose studies is triggered if, for example, the half-life of the drug in certain tissues exceeds that of plasma. Repeat dosing might be considered if during the regular pharmacokinetic studies (nonradiolabeled) the measured half-life after repeat dosing is significantly longer than that predicted from a single dose. In addition, histopathological findings in toxicology studies may also trigger repeat-dose studies to see if the toxicological effect is related to the tissue concentration of drug or drug–metabolite.

Repeat dosing can be conducted in one of two ways: (1) Repeat doses of radiolabeled drug are administered. (2) Repeat administrations of nonradiolabeled drug are administered over several days, followed by a single dose of radiolabeled drug.

Repeat doses of radiolabeled drug are applicable to animal studies where accumulation in tissues is being examined. Questions on tissue accumulation are typically answered using quantitative whole-body autoradiography (Chapter 5). A single radiolabeled dose following a series on nonradiolabeled doses is used to examine possible enzyme saturation or induction effects. This experimental design can be applied to animal or human studies.

3.5.5   Sample Collection

With both animal and human studies, samples of blood, urine and feces are collected over time. Blood is typically collected at 0.5, 1, 2, 4, 6, 8, 10, 12, 18, 24, 36, and 48 h and then 24 hourly until the end of the study. Blood samples can be analyzed as whole blood, but more often they are centrifuged to produce plasma, or clotted and centrifuged to produce serum. For small animals, the number of samples that can be taken is limited by the total blood volume. For this reason, blood samples are often collected from overlapping groups of animals. For example, two groups of five animals might be used: group 1 being bled from 0.5 to 6 h, group 2 from 8 to 24 h, group 1 from 36 to 72 h and then finally group 2 from 96 to 168 h. This type of overlapping sampling alleviates the stress of blood taking, but the concentration–time curves are not necessarily as smooth as those where only one group of animals is used for all samples.

Although different laboratories will operate under their own rules, as a general guide for animal work, withdrawal of blood within a 24-h period should not exceed 15% of the total blood volume. Over 28 days, the total volume withdrawn should not exceed 20% of the total blood volume.[17] The rat contains about 64 mL blood/Kg body weight; the rabbit, 56 mL/Kg; the dog, 85 mL/Kg; and the monkey, between 56 and 70 mL/Kg. The adult human contains about 70 mL blood/Kg body weight, and about 9% of this volume can be safely removed on a single occasion. Most clinics will allow the removal of a total of 500 mL of blood from a 70-Kg human, for studies lasting less than 4 weeks.

Urine is typically collected over periods of 0 to 6 h, 6 to 12 h and 12 to 24 h and then 24 hourly to the end of the study. Similarly, feces are collected 24 hourly. The weight or volume of excreta at each collection time is recorded. For animal studies, the collection vessels on the cages are normally surrounded by solid carbon dioxide so that excreta are collected frozen. With human studies, excreta are collected and pooled over the designated time periods, then stored frozen.

On occasions it is necessary to collect exhaled volatiles. If radioactivity is exhaled as $^{14}CO_2$, then this can be trapped either by a solution of sodium hydroxide or in a mixture of 2-ethoxyethanol:ethanolamine (3:1 v/v). Although some laboratories use potassium hydroxide, others avoid it, as potassium exhibits a relatively high radioactive background. In small animal studies, particularly with the laboratory rat, metabolism cages can be designed for the total collection of exhaled air. A schematic showing a CO_2 collection system is shown in Figure 3.4. The inlet to the cage is fitted with a device to absorb CO_2, so as not to saturate the traps with atmospheric CO_2. On the outlet of the cage there are two traps arranged in series. The first trap will efficiently retain $^{14}CO_2$, and therefore the second trap should be devoid of radioactivity. If the first trap becomes saturated with exhaled CO_2, then radioactivity

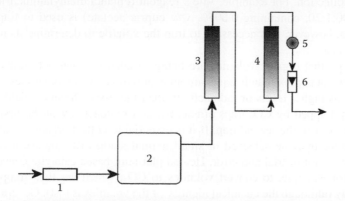

Figure 3.4   Schematic of an expired collection system: (1) carbon dioxide scrubber, to remove CO_2 from atmospheric air, (2) metabolism cage, (3) CO_2 trap 1, (4) CO_2 trap 2, (5) air pump and (6) flow gauge and alarm in case of failure.

will appear in the second trap. If radioactivity is found in the second trap in any appreciable quantity, then there is a chance that the whole trapping system became saturated and some $^{14}CO_2$ was lost to the atmosphere. The total volume of each trap is recorded, and from the analysis of aliquots of known volume, the total radioactivity present in the traps can be calculated.

In larger laboratory animal species, such as the dog, it is possible to collect samples of breath over short periods using a face mask, although this is a somewhat specialized technique.

In human studies, a slightly different approach is taken to CO_2 collection. Unless very specialized systems are available, it is not possible to collect and trap CO_2 from humans over prolonged periods.[18] Instead, the volunteer blows into an exact amount of sodium hydroxide solution containing an indicator such as phenolphthalein (or sometimes hyamine hydroxide with thymolphthalein as an indicator). The volunteer blows into the vial for only a short period, until the indicator changes color, showing that the sodium hydroxide is saturated. Every 2 mol of sodium hydroxide will trap 1 mol of carbon dioxide ($2NaOH + CO_2 \rightarrow Na_2CO_3 + H_2O$); thus, by knowing how many moles of sodium hydroxide there are in the solution, the number of moles of trapped carbon dioxide can be calculated.

An aliquot of the trap is analyzed, and the radioactive concentration is measured. To determine the amount of radioactivity exhaled over a given period, the breath rate and percentage carbon dioxide in the breath are measured, and the percentage of dose expired is then extrapolated from these values. Samples are taken at frequent intervals (e.g., one sample of breath once per hour to start with, then once every 6 to 12 h as the study proceeds). This technique does require that the clinic conducting the study has facilities to measure breath rate and the carbon dioxide concentration of the breath. It is important to keep the volunteer at rest during the collection periods, to ensure a constant breath rate.

Breath may contain radiolabeled species, other than $^{14}CO_2$, such as small organic molecules. These types of volatiles can be notoriously difficult to trap. If the chemical nature of the volatile is known, then traps can be specifically designed for their collection. For example, Vile's reagent (ethanol:diethylamine:triethanolamine, 1000:1:20, containing 0.005% w/v cupric acetate) is used to trap CS_2. In most cases, however, it is necessary to trap the volatile to determine its identity in the first place.

One sign that organic volatiles are being exhaled is when both traps in series contain low but approximately equal amounts of radioactivity (sometimes the second trap contains higher levels of radioactivity than the first). Organic volatiles are not necessarily trapped by CO_2 traps efficiently, and radioactivity in the first trap can be sparged over to the second trap. If it is essential to collect organic volatiles, then this can sometimes be achieved in small animal studies (the mouse and rat), but often entails a lot of trial and error. Heated platinum-based catalytic converters can be used, for example, to convert volatiles to CO_2, which are then trapped in the normal way (although the chemical identity of the volatiles is lost). Generic trapping systems, such as cold traps utilizing liquid nitrogen, are never 100% efficient. In some cases, activated charcoal will trap volatiles, which can then be flushed from the trap with organic solvents. Efficient collection of unknown organic volatiles from humans is particularly difficult.

Tissues can be dissected at the end of an animal study, and occasionally biopsies are taken in human studies. For animal studies, the distribution in tissues is usually investigated by quantitative whole-body autoradiography (Chapter 5), as this technique is more straightforward than dissecting individual tissues, and it "sees" the whole animal. On occasions, however, it may be necessary to dissect tissues, extract them, and produce radiochromatographic profiles.

3.5.6 Bile Duct Cannulation

Some compounds are eliminated from the body in bile. To study this, it is possibly to surgically prepare animals with a cannula inserted into the bile duct. Bile then flows out of the cannula for collection. With the right surgical methods, the animals are allowed to recover and bile can be collected for reasonable periods (2 days, perhaps up to 3 days). Bile duct-cannulated animals are depleted of bile, and this can cause some stress. Dehydration can be alleviated by feeding the animals a dilute solution of glucose and saline. A more sophisticated surgical method is available where artificial bile salts are infused into the duodenum of the animal *via* a second cannula. Although bile duct cannulation can be conducted in virtually any laboratory species, it is most commonly performed on the laboratory rat. A typical bile flow from a cannulated rat is 28 to 47 mL bile/Kg body weight/day. Unlike urine and feces, bile is collected over wet ice, as collection over solid carbon dioxide will cause the cannula to freeze and block.

It would be unusual to administer more than a single dose of radiolabeled drug to bile duct-cannulated animals, due to both the stress involved and the shorter duration of the experiment.

Bile duct cannulation has been performed in the human, but in patients fitted with a T-tube drain following an operation; therefore, data are sparse.

3.5.7 Lactation Studies

Lactating mothers taking medication may inadvertently expose their offspring to the drug or its metabolites in their milk. A typical amount of milk ingested by an infant is around 0.15 L/Kg/day. The newborn and infants up to about 18 months show lower clearance rates than adults and are therefore at particular risk.

Drug transfer from maternal plasma to milk is typically by passive diffusion. Transfer is likely to be more prominent if the drug is lipid soluble and has low plasma binding. In addition, since milk is slightly acidic, basic drugs often transfer into milk more readily.

The risk to the infant is assessed using animal models (typically the laboratory rat), where the animal is administered radiolabeled drug and milk samples are taken for analysis. Under such circumstances, it is particularly important to account for the drug and its metabolites. Even if the metabolism of the drug is known, the metabolites present in milk may be different than those detected in, for example, excreta, and therefore the use of radiolabeled drug becomes all the more important.

Transfer of drug or metabolites to the infant through the mother's milk can also be investigated using quantitative whole-body autoradiography (Chapter 5).

3.5.8 Sample Preparation and Analysis of Radioactivity

The distribution of radioactivity in feces may not be uniform, and therefore it is important to homogenize the whole sample and then take aliquots of the homogenate for analysis. Feces are typically homogenized in water, or occasionally with a thickening agent such as Gum Arabic using a mechanical blender.

Tissues and remaining carcass are also homogenized prior to analysis. Tissues are either homogenized in a mechanical blender or solubilized by dissolving in a mixture of methanol and 5 *M* sodium hydroxide or using a commercial solubilizing reagent (Chapter 9). If the carcass of small laboratory animals is solubilized, this is normally conducted under reflux. Solubilization techniques work well for total radioactivity analysis, but any radiochromatography is ruled out. If metabolite profiles of tissues are required, then solvent extraction is necessary (see below).

Urine and bile do not usually require any sample preparation, unless sample concentration is necessary.

Results of sample analysis are normally expressed as dpm/mL or g, which are then converted to drug concentration in weight equivalents (e.g., ng equiv/g) from the specific activity (Section 2.11). For excreta, the total amount of radioactivity excreted for each collection period is calculated by multiplying the radioactive concentration (dpm/mL or g) by the amount of urine or feces collected. The result is usually expressed as the percentage of administered dose excreted. For graphical representation, results are usually expressed as the cumulative percentage of administered dose excreted.

3.5.9 Metabolite Profiling

The metabolic profile is produced by suitable radiochromatographic methods. typically thin-layer chromatography (TLC) or high-performance liquid chromatography (HPLC). (TLC is a more sophisticated version of the paper chromatography used by Calvin in the first radiotracer studies ever performed; see Section 1.3.) The workings of these techniques are beyond the scope of this book; refer to Evans (2004).[2] The principles behind radio-TLC and radio-HPLC are no different than the conventional use of these analytical methods, except detectors are designed to locate and quantify radioactivity. Although TLC is considered an old technology, it still holds great value in radiotracer work. Because the sample is applied to a flat surface, when the chromatogram is developed and the radioactivity visualized, all of the sample applied can be accounted for. TLC is often used to gather preliminary information to assist in the development of HPLC separations. Radiodetection applicable to TLC is discussed further in Section 5.4.5, and a discussion of radiodetectors used in radio-HPLC can be found in Section 6.15 and Section 8.9.

For HPLC analysis, individual samples of excreta or plasma can be analyzed, but it is also common practice to pool samples from animals or human volunteers across collection times. For example, there might be one plasma sample for each time point (at 0.5, 1, 2 and 4 h, etc.) consisting of a pool made by taking an equal volume from each animal or volunteer in the study. Such pooling averages out interanimal variation and makes the data much easier to interpret.

For excreta and bile, pools are not made from equal volumes, but from a constant proportion of the sample excreted over the given collection period. For example, let us assume that four animals were used in an experiment, and in the period 0 to 6 h, they excreted 100, 150, 170, and 180 mL of urine, respectively. Then to make the 0- to 6-h pool, 1, 1.5, 1.7, and 1.8 mL of urine would be pooled from each animal, respectively (using a constant 1%).

Prior to radiochromatographic analysis, extraction of the sample may be necessary, to extract the radiolabeled drug and its metabolites from the biological matrix. (Some samples, such as urine and bile, do not usually require extraction). Extraction methods vary, depending upon the compound under study, but typically plasma is treated with an organic solvent such as acetonitrile to precipitate proteins, followed by centrifugation and analysis of the supernatant. Drug and metabolites are sometimes separated from plasma and occasionally urine or bile, using solid-phase extraction columns.

Feces are extracted with various organic solvents. For some compounds, the pH is adjusted prior to extraction, and for others, extractions may have to be undertaken at several pHs. With feces, an initial extraction with hexane can often be beneficial. The hexane is not intended to extract the drug or metabolites (although this has to be confirmed experimentally), but removes lipid from the sample, making further extractions more straightforward. Alternatively, feces can be extracted with polar solvents and then the extracts partitioned with hexane.

It is important that the solvents do not react with any of the metabolites being extracted. For example, extremes of pH can lead to the hydrolysis of certain conjugates, particularly glucuronides. Tissues can be extracted in solvents, but it may be necessary to use more aggressive methods, such as Soxhlet.

The extraction efficiency is defined as the percentage of radioactivity in the extract compared to the original sample. Typically, extraction efficiencies of 80 to 90% are considered adequate. Feces and tissues are often difficult to extract, and the more aggressive the extraction method, the more likely that the extraction procedure will chemically alter the drug or metabolites. In such cases, a compromise has to be reached and lower extraction efficiencies may have to be accepted. It should be borne in mind, however, that if a compound is metabolized to metabolites with a range of polarities, the extraction efficiency of each metabolite might be different. Under these circumstances, it is possible that an extraction efficiency of 80% means that 80% of the metabolites have been extracted and a metabolite representing 20% of the profile remains unextracted and therefore undetected.

3.5.10 Profiling and Bioanalysis

It is important to understand the difference between radiochromatographic analysis of samples from a metabolism study and the analysis of samples in bioanalytical studies. Bioanalysis, typically conducted using LC-MS, is routinely performed on clinical studies (phases I, II, and III; see Section 1.1) and sometimes on animal

samples from toxicology studies, and therefore does not involve the use of radiolabels. Samples are analyzed for target analytes, usually parent drug and a number of
specific metabolites. Bioanalysis results are used to generate pharmacokinetic data
from large numbers of human subjects participating in the clinical trials.

Bioanalysis requires a standard for the analyte and an appropriate internal standard. The internal standard is added as an exact and constant amount to each sample
prior to extraction. Internal standards are structurally related to the analyte; the ideal
internal standard is considered to be deuterated or sometimes a $[^{13}C]$-labeled analyte,
with a very similar chromatographic retention time, and is distinguished on LC-MS
by virtue of its increased molecular weight (Section 3.5.12). A calibration curve is
constructed from a range of concentrations of analyte, all containing the same amount
of internal standard. The concentration of the analyte is accurately known by weigh-
ing out amounts of highly pure compound. The analyte concentration is plotted on
the x-axis, and the ratio of the chromatographic peak area for the analyte and internal
standard is on the y-axis. The amount of analyte in a sample is then determined by
measuring the ratio of peak areas for the sample analyte and internal standard and
correlating this with the concentration using the calibration curve. If any loss of
analyte occurs in the preparation process, then this is corrected for by equal losses
of the internal standard.

The situation with metabolism studies is different from bioanalysis in that no
internal standards are used; the process is instead absolute, and quantification relies
on either 100% extraction efficiency or at least knowing what the extraction efficiency is. In bioanalysis, true extraction efficiencies are rarely known. For chromatographic analysis, there is sometimes a tendency to use the same method of sample
preparation for metabolism studies as that developed for bioanalytical analysis.
Although in principle there is no reason why this should not be done, it can transpire
that the extraction efficiency thereby achieved in the metabolism study is in practice
relatively low. Under these circumstances, it is best if the bioanalytical method is
abandoned and a more appropriate method is developed for an absolute extraction.

It is fairly common (although not invariably so) to analyze plasma samples from
human metabolism studies for parent and selected metabolites using a bioanalytical
method. It is more unusual, however, with animal studies, perhaps because of the
small volumes of sample obtained, at least in the case of rodents.

3.5.11 Identification of Metabolites

This topic warrants a book all to itself, and so only the barest of principles can
be outlined here. A fuller account of the methods and instrumentation can be found
in Evans (2004).[2] There are many analytical techniques available for the identification of metabolites, but mass spectrometry (MS) and nuclear magnetic spectroscopy
(NMR) are used most frequently; these are summarized below.

3.5.12 Liquid Chromatography–Mass Spectrometry

In LC-MS, analytes are separated using conventional HPLC methods and the
eluate from the HPLC is passed into the ion source of a mass spectrometer. Here

the analytes are ionized by one of a variety of ionization techniques. Depending upon the energy of the ionization, some molecular fragmentation of the analyte may occur. The ions, either positively or negatively charged, are extracted from the ion source by virtue of their charge. In addition to charge, the ions also have mass depending upon the molecular weight of the analyte or the fragment. These are separated in magnetic or quadrupole fields according to the mass of the ion (m) divided by the charge (z). In most cases, particularly with small molecules, z = 1 and the resulting mass spectrum (Figure 3.5) reveals the molecular weight of the analyte. Depending upon the type of ionization employed, positive ions are often formed by the addition of H^+, and therefore the ion representing the molecular weight (i.e., the molecular ion) is depicted as $[M + 1]^+$. The opposite is also true: negative ions are formed by the extraction of H^+, and hence the molecular ion is depicted as $[M - 1]^-$.

Some instruments have two mass spectrometers in series, with a gas collision cell in between. These are known as tandem mass spectrometers. Where the mass spectrometers are quadrupoles, they are known as triple-quadrupole mass spectrometers. Ions enter the collision cell from the first mass spectrometer (parent ions) and are fragmented, the fragments being detected with the second mass spectrometer (daughter ions). This is known as LC-MS/MS. By selecting parent and daughter ions, a more precise chemical structure can be constructed.

There is also an instrument known as an ion trap that can fragment an analyte step by step a number of times (MS/MS^n, where n is the number of steps). In the ion trap, fragmentation takes place in the ion source, not in sequential mass spectrometers. Ion traps have proved to be particularly useful in metabolite identification.

Mass spectra show the absolute molecular weights of the ions. For example, the average molecular weight of 2-hydroxy-2-pyrrole-quinoline, taking the abundance

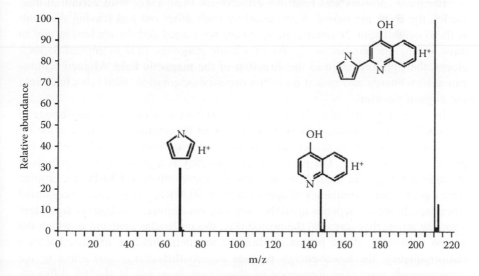

Figure 3.5 Mass spectrum of 2-hydroxy-2-pyrrole-quinoline, ^{14}C-labeled in the benzene ring. The molecular ion $[M + 1]^+$ is seen at m/z 211.

of each isotope of carbon, hydrogen, nitrogen, and oxygen into account, is 210.24. The mass spectrometer, however, detects each individual isotope abundance. For 2-hydroxy-2-pyrrole-quinoline (Figure 3.5) the isotope abundance of carbon predominates, and therefore the $[M + 1]^+$, m/z 211, ion is based on ^{12}C.

The ion at m/z 212 is based on ^{13}C, and the ion at m/z 213 is based on ^{14}C. The natural abundance of ^{14}C is very small, at about $1.5 \times 10^{-10}\%$, and so the ^{14}C-related ion is also very small. In the example of 2-hydroxy-2-pyrrole-quinoline, however, the compound is enriched with ^{14}C in the benzene ring, and hence the ion seen at m/z 213 is significant. In Figure 3.5 two fragment ions are illustrated. The molecular ion and the quinoline fragment both show the enhanced ^{14}C ion, but the pyrolle ion at m/z 68 contains no ^{14}C enrichment, and therefore the abundance of the ^{14}C ion is much lower.

The level of enrichment of the radioisotope can be determined precisely using accurate isotope ratio mass spectrometers.

Mass spectrometry is a sensitive technique. Interpretable spectra can be obtained from just a few nanograms (10^{-9}) of analyte, and the limits of detection for quantification can do down to picogram (10^{-12}) levels.

A common reaction seen in drug metabolism is hydroxylation of aromatic rings (Appendix 1). There are usually several options for the position of substitution on the ring, but all products will have the same molecular weight. Therefore, mass spectrometry is sometimes only capable of determining that a substitution has occurred, without being able to reveal the precise position of substitution on the molecule; for that, nuclear magnetic resonance spectroscopy is required.

3.5.13 Nuclear Magnetic Resonance Spectroscopy

Electrons, protons and neutrons all spin on their axes. With certain atomic nuclei, the spins are paired, thus canceling each other out and leaving the atom with no overall spin. In others, the spins are not paired and the nucleus is said to have a quantum number of $1/2$. When a static magnetic field is applied to such atoms, their protons align in the direction of the magnetic field. Aligned protons can absorb energy and pass it on to the opposite orientation, then relax back into the aligned position.

In addition to the spin, the proton also exhibits a "wobble" — analogous to the wobble on a spinning top as it turns around its central axis. The wobble on the proton is known as precessional motion, and its frequency is known as the precessional frequency. The precessional frequency is affected by the strength of the external magnetic field. At a magnetic field strength of 1.4 Tesla (T), protons have a precessional frequency of approximately 60 MHz. The precise precessional frequency, however, depends upon the magnetic environment, and this is dependent upon the atoms that surround the proton (i.e., the molecular structure in which the proton is nested). If the proton, within the magnetic field, is irradiated with a radiofrequency, the lower-energy protons absorb this energy and move to the higher-energy state. The frequency of absorption, however, is slightly different, depending upon the position of the proton within the molecule. A plot of the

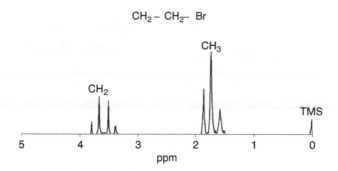

Figure 3.6 The ^{1}H-NMR spectrum of ethyl bromide.

absorption of the radiofrequency vs. the strength of the signal constitutes the NMR spectrum (Figure 3.6).

Standards are used in NMR to define certain positions on the spectrum (e.g., tetramethyl silane, TMS). The degree to which the signals shift from the standard is known as chemical shift and is measured in δ units (parts per million, ppm). It is therefore possible to build up a complete picture of the structure of the molecule by examining the interactions and shifts exhibited by the protons.

Radiofrequency is measured in hertz, and the more powerful the NMR, the higher the radiofrequency. In the 1960s, a state-of-the-art NMR was around 60 MHz; now they have exceeded 1 GHz. Naturally, the higher the radiofrequency, the stronger the magnetic field has to be. Modern NMR instruments therefore use superconducting magnets, cooled with liquid helium to reach field strengths in excess of 20 T.

The most useful isotopes in NMR are ^{1}H, ^{13}C, ^{19}F, and ^{31}P. All these isotopes are stable, and ^{1}H in particular is very abundant. For this reason, ^{1}H-NMR is used most frequently. The downside of ^{1}H-NMR is that the analyte has to be dissolved in a solvent devoid of, or at least heavily depleted of, ^{1}H. Carbon tetrachloride can be used, but if the analyte is not soluble in this solvent, then deuterated solvents have to be used. An example of an NMR spectrum of ethyl bromide is shown in Figure 3.6. Note how the resonance signals divide into a triplet for the CH_3 and a quadruplet for CH_2 due to spin orientations. This is key to NMR interpretation but is outside the scope of this book.

NMR is not as sensitive as mass spectroscopy, and as a rule of thumb, 1 to 100 µg of reasonably pure analyte is required for analysis (based on modern NMR instruments). This usually involves quite complex sample preparation. The most modern instruments can work with as little as 100 ng.

If the drug contains fluorine, then ^{19}F-NMR is a powerful analytical technique. ^{19}F is the most abundant isotope of fluorine, and so ^{19}F-NMR is very sensitive. ^{19}F acts as a stable tracer, and drug metabolism studies have been conducted using ^{19}F-NMR without the use of a radioisotope.[19] ^{13}C-NMR can be conducted using the natural abundance of ^{13}C (1.1%), but it is limited by its low sensitivity. Sometimes drugs are synthesized with a ^{13}C label, which enhances the usefulness of ^{13}C-NMR spectroscopy (and is used as a marker in mass spectrometry). Another technique

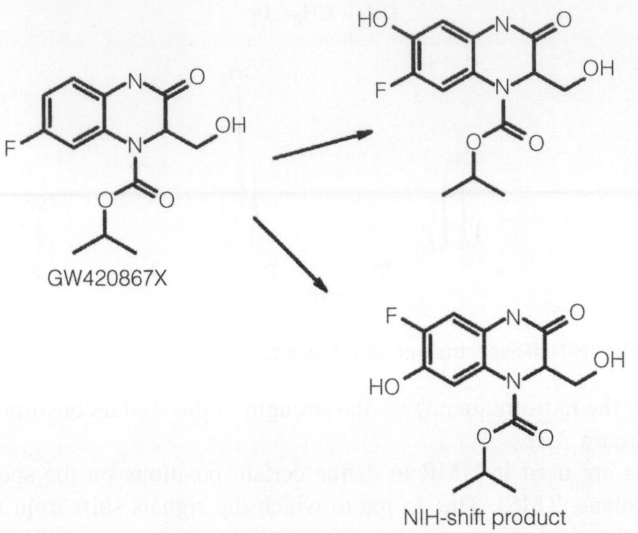

Figure 3.7   Example of NIH shift, elucidated with ^{19}F and ^{1}H-NMR.

that is sometime used is two-dimensional NMR, where the relationship between two isotopes is mapped.

In recent times, NMR has been interfaced to HPLC (LC-NMR), which has simplified the isolation procedures and has increased sensitivity. LC-NMR, however, is expensive and requires powerful instrumentation and the use of deuterated HPLC solvents (for ^{1}H-LC-NMR). NMR can also be conducted with tritium; ^{3}H-NMR is used to locate the position of ^{3}H labels during their synthesis.

The elucidation of NIH shift* products in the metabolism of GW420867X (a reverse transcriptase inhibitor intended as an anti-HIV drug) serves as an example where LC-^{1}H-NMR and ^{19}F-NMR were used to elucidate the structures of the metabolites.[20] (The NIH shift is explained in Appendix 1, Table 3.4). In the present example, the NIH shift involved the migration of a fluorine atom on an aromatic ring, as shown in Figure 3.7. The two products could be separated on HPLC, but they had virtually identical mass spectra. The chemical shifts in the ^{18}F-NMR and ^{1}H-NMR spectra allowed unambiguous identification.

The most recent advancement in metabolite identification technology is the coupling of HPLC, MS, and NMR, and this is reviewed by Lindon *et al.* (2003).[21]

3.6 *IN VIVO* STUDIES: DATA INTERPRETATION

3.6.1   General Considerations

Interpretation of data will always depend upon the specific circumstances of the drug under development. Some general aspects are discussed below, and some

---

* NIH stands for the National Institute of Health, where the shift was discovered.

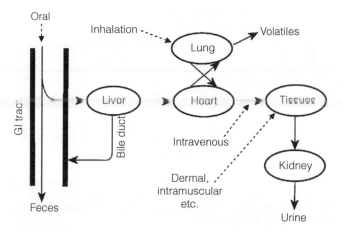

Figure 3.8 Key routes of administration (indicated by dotted arrows) and key routes of elimination.

examples from the literature are then examined in Appendix 2. Key routes of administration and routes of elimination are illustrated in Figure 3.8.

3.6.2 Recovery

The recovery of radioactivity from animal studies can be 90% or better. Recovery with human studies can be just as high providing excretion is complete by the time of the last sample collection. Recoveries can, of course, only be calculated when the exact dose administered is known. This is straightforward for intravenous and oral doses. For dermal administrations, the remaining dose must be washed off the skin and any dressings to achieve a recovery. For inhalation studies where the dose is administered in an atmosphere over time, the administered dose is more difficult to measure, as some will be absorbed and some will be immediately exhaled.

All excreta are collected, as is bile. Exhaled CO_2 can be collected for animal studies, and the total amount exhaled can be extrapolated in human studies (Section 3.5.5). Blood, however, is sampled, and so the percentage of dose present in the relatively small volume of blood sample is not normally added to the recovery. In animal studies the same applies to certain tissues. For example, all of the radioactivity in liver can be measured, as liver is a distinct organ. Muscle and fat, however, are just sampled, and so the total amount in the animal for these tissues is unknown. In practice, in animal studies the amount of blood, fat, and muscle removed for analysis is insignificant and makes no real difference to the recovery compared to the amounts remaining in the carcass, which is analyzed and included.

There are occasions, with laboratory animals, where there is a need to estimate the total amount of radioactivity located in blood, fat, and muscle. This can be done by extrapolation from the concentration found in the small sample taken. It is possible to make estimates, based on published figures, for the amount of fat, muscle, and blood in the body. A laboratory rat is approximately 6.4% blood, 45.5% muscle,

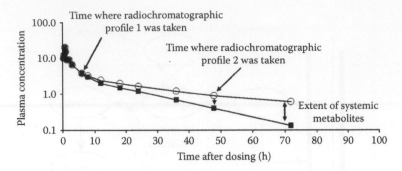

Figure 3.9   Comparison of total radioactive concentration (○) in plasma vs. the concentration of parent drug (■) following a single dose of radiolabeled drug. Samples taken for radiochromatographic profiling at the times indicated (6 and 48 h) gave the results shown in Figure 3.10.

and 7.08% fat (and the skin represents about 18%). These values were obtained from an old publication,[22] and different laboratories may use their own figures.

3.6.3 Systemic Samples

Total radioactivity measurements in blood, plasma, or serum provide information on the systemic concentrations of the drug and its metabolites over time. (For simplicity, this text will refer to plasma.) In this section a general understanding of pharmacokinetics is assumed. For the reader unfamiliar with the terminology, brief descriptions of relevant pharmacokinetic parameters are described in Appendix 3.

Pharmacokinetic parameters such as plasma half-life ($t_{1/2}$)*, clearance (Cl), and volume of distribution (V) should all be expressed in terms of a single compound, usually the parent drug. Detection of radioactivity in a sample only provides information on the presence of the radiotracer first introduced into the experiment; it does not provide any information on the presence of the drug itself. When pharmacokinetic calculations are applied to total radioactivity measurements, remember that no distinction is made between drug and metabolites, and therefore interpretation of the data is limited.

To calculate pharmacokinetic parameters correctly, the concentration of parent (and individual metabolites, if appropriate) has to be measured in each individual plasma sample. For reasons explained in Section 3.5.9, however, this is not always appropriate in metabolism studies, as it is often pools that are radiochromatographically analyzed. In human studies, and perhaps for some larger animals (e.g., dog), sufficient plasma may be available for the analysis of parent and selected metabolites by LC-MS, or another suitable nonradioactive bioanalytical method. A combination of data for the concentration of total radioactivity and for the parent drug can be useful. Take Figure 3.9: here the concentration of parent drug (measured by, for example, LC-MS and expressed as ng/mL) is compared with the total radioactive concentration (expressed as ng equiv/mL — the term *equivalence* is explained in Section 2.11).

* Plasma half-life is used so as not to confuse this pharmacokinetic parameter with radioactive half-life.

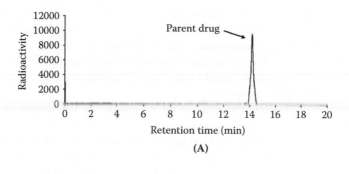

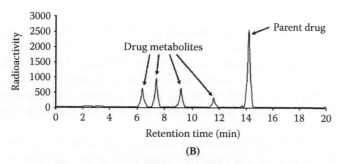

Figure 3.10 (A) Radiochromatographic profile of plasma sampled at 6 h. (B) Radiochromato-graphic profile of plasma sampled at 48 h. See Figure 3.9.

In Figure 3.9, up to the 8-h time point, the parent drug concentration and equivalent drug concentration based on total radioactivity are approximately the same. Up until 8 h, therefore, analysis of the plasma by radiochromatography would only reveal parent drug (Figure 3.10A). After 8 h, the concentration of parent and equivalent concentration for total radioactivity diverge. The line for total radioactivity therefore represents some parent drug, but also some unknown metabolite(s) (Figure 3.10B). As the drug is metabolized over time, so the two lines continue to diverge. Interpretation of metabolite profiling is picked up again in Section 3.6.8.

Data acquired from plasma are of particular concern to the regulatory authorities, as they represent systemic exposure. The formation of metabolites that exhibit no therapeutic activity are, in effect, undesirable baggage and ideally should be eliminated from the body as quickly as possible. This is not always the case, as situations are not uncommon where the parent drug demonstrates high plasma clearance, while one or several metabolites exhibit lower clearance.

Plasma concentrations, however, may not necessarily reflect the situation in the rest of the body. Consider a case where the parent drug is metabolized to form a metabolite, and at a given point in time, there are equal amounts of parent and metabolite in the body. Assume that the parent has a volume of distribution of 100 L and the metabolite has a volume of distribution of 1200 L (see Appendix 3 for an explanation of volume of distribution). Under these circumstances, although the total amounts of parent and metabolite in the body are the same, the concentration of the metabolite in plasma would be 12 times lower than that of the parent. The metabolite might therefore appear insignificant or, indeed, may not be detected in plasma at all. For such a difference in the volume of distribution to occur, the metabolite must be sequestered in a body compartment, such as a tissue or organ.

These effects may be detected in the tissue distribution studies (e.g., quantitative whole-body autoradiography, Chapter 5) and may necessitate the extraction of tissues for radiochromatographic analysis.

The volume of distribution is a useful parameter in the design of *in vivo* radiotracer studies. The volume of distribution for the parent drug may well be known from clinical trials or animal studies by the time the metabolism studies are performed. Let us say, for argument's sake, that the volume of distribution for a particular drug was 100 L. If 3.7 MBq (2.22×10^8 dpm) was administered intravenously, then the plasma concentration at time zero (assumed to be the first sampling point after intravenous administration) will be 3.7 MBq in 100 L or 2220 dpm/mL. This radioactive concentration is easily detectable by liquid scintillation counting (Chapter 6). Imagine a situation, however, where 370 KBq of a drug with a volume of distribution of 1500 L was administered. Here the plasma concentration will be 14.8 dpm/mL, and this is likely to be too low to measure with liquid scintillation counting; another technique, such as accelerator mass spectrometry (Chapter 10), may be necessary.

The volume of distribution does, of course, relate to the parent drug, whereas concentration based on radioactivity represents drug and any metabolites. Although it is likely that in the very earliest of sample times (perhaps 10 min after dosing) the majority of the radioactivity will still be the parent drug, it is recognized that this is only an approximation. It is nevertheless a useful estimate for study design.

3.6.4 Blood Cell Partitioning

Blood cell partitioning was mentioned under the *in vitro* section (Section 3.4.11). *In vitro* studies however, are conducted by adding parent compound (or occasionally metabolites if they are available) directly to blood. The drug, however, may be metabolized *in vivo*, forming a metabolite that binds strongly to either blood cells or plasma protein. Unless the metabolite was tested *in vitro*, the *in vitro* model might underestimate the extent of binding.

The extent of blood binding, and sometimes plasma protein binding, is therefore examined in the *in vivo* studies. There can be marked species differences in the degree of blood binding. Rodent hemoglobin, for example, is known to contain a reactive cysteine-125 residue, and consequently, blood binding in these species can be significantly higher than in the human.[23]

The extent of blood binding is assessed by measuring the total radioactive concentration in whole blood and comparing this with the concentration in a plasma sample taken at the same collection time. In calculating the extent of binding to the cellular portion of blood, account has to be made of the change of volume when blood is centrifuged to produce plasma. The extent of the cellular component after centrifugation is known as the hematocrit, and a typical hematocrit for humans is

0.45 (i.e., 45% of the blood consists of cells and 55% plasma). Calculation of the percentage of blood binding is shown in Equation 3.1:

$$1 - \left(\frac{plasma}{blood} \right) \times (1 - h) \times 100 \tag{3.1}$$

The amount of radioactivity in plasma is dived by the amount in blood; h is the hematocrit. Thus, if a blood sample contained 1000 dpm and when centrifuged ($h = 0.45$) the plasma contained 800 dpm, then the degree of blood binding would be 11%.

Samples of plasma can be subjected to ultrafiltration or equilibrium dialysis (Section 3.4.11) and the degree of protein binding assessed by measuring the amounts of free and bound radioactivity.

3.6.5 Absorption, Distribution, and Excretion

Following oral dosing of a drug, a portion may be adsorbed through the gastrointestinal (GI) tract (Figure 3.11). Once absorbed, the drug enters the capillaries surrounding the GI tract and goes into the hepatic portal vein. This vein carries the blood to the liver, which is generally considered the principal organ of metabolism within the body. There are two routes out of the liver for the drug, either into systemic circulation or into bile. The route taken largely depends upon the molecular weight of the compound and the presence of polar ionic groups. The molecular weight values are generally known as the biliary molecular weight threshholds. At these values approximately 10% of the compound would be expected to be excreted in the bile; as the molecular weight increases above the threshhold, so more compound is eliminated in bile. For rat, the threshhold is 325

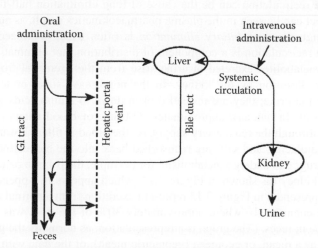

Figure 3.11 Schematic showing routes of excretion in urine, feces and bile.

± 50, and for the rabbit, it is 475 ± 50. Compounds with molecular weights above 500 are likely to be excreted in bile for most species.[24,25] The threshhold for humans is usually quoted as 500, but the evidence for this value is less compelling than that for the rat and rabbit. Proteins, although well over the 500 molecular weight threshhold, tend not to be found in the bile.

Although the drug itself may have a low molecular weight, conjugation in the liver with, for example, glutathione (Appendix 1) increases the molecular weight significantly, and therefore increases its chance of being eliminated in the bile.

As shown in Figure 3.11, if the drug or its metabolites are excreted in bile, then they proceed down the bile duct and into the duodenum. Note that the drug was absorbed from the GI tract, only to end up back in the same place. At this point, the drug or its metabolites may be excreted in feces. The feces may also contain a proportion of the unabsorbed drug, passing straight through the GI tract. What is evident from this, however, is that excretion in feces does not necessarily represent unabsorbed drug (indeed, fecal excretion *via* bile can readily occur from an intravenous dose).

Once excreted back into the GI tract, conjugated metabolites such as glucuronides might be hydrolyzed back to the aglycone. Hydrolysis is likely to be a result of the action of the gut microflora. The deconjugated compound (the aglycone) may then be reabsorbed through the GI tract back to the liver. (In the case of glutathione conjugates, further metabolism can occur in the bile duct itself; see Figure 3.23, which appears in Appendix 1.) Once back in the liver, the drug can be reconjugated and the whole process starts over again. This process is known as enterohepatic recirculation.

A classical example of enterohepatic recirculation is the indicator phenolphthalein. Phenolphthalein undergoes glucuronidation in the liver and is excreted in bile into the duodenum. Here the glucuronide moiety is cleaved and the free phenolphthalein is reabsorbed, to go back to the liver to start the process all over again.[26] Enterohepatic recirculation can be the cause of long elimination half-lives. Sometimes the effect can be seen in the plasma pharmacokinetics graph, as an oscillating curve. Although the term *biliary elimination* is often used, pharmacokinetically, enterohepatic recirculation is a component of distribution, not elimination.

Drug or metabolites excreted in urine arise from their removal from systemic circulation by filtration by the kidney. In the nondisease state, proteins are not eliminated in the urine; they are instead broken down to amino acids, probably in the kidney itself. In humans, approximately 600 mL of blood enters each kidney each minute, through the renal artery supply. As the blood is filtered, water, glucose, vitamins, amino acids, and salts are reabsorbed back into the bloodstream. As they are filtered, drugs can undergo metabolism; for example, the β-lyase pathway is very active in the kidney (as shown in Figure 3.23, which appears in Appendix 1).

The data presented in Figure 3.12 represent excretion from a normal animal (i.e., not bile duct cannulated), where approximately 30% of the dose was excreted in urine and 65% in feces. (The graph is a representation, as normally the graph would be presented as a mean, or geomean (geometric mean), of the data with error bars.)

In order for 30% of the dose to be excreted in urine, at least this proportion of the dose must have been absorbed. Was the 65% excreted in feces unabsorbed,

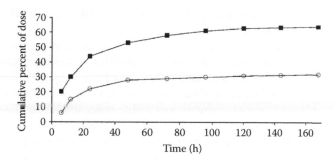

Figure 3.12 Cumulative percent of dose excreted in urine (○) and feces (■) from a normal (non-bile duct-cannulated) animal, following a single oral dose of radiolabeled drug.

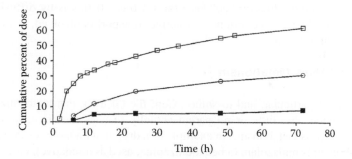

Figure 3.13 Cumulative percent of dose excreted in urine (○), bile (□), and feces (■) from a bile duct-cannulated animal, following a single oral dose of radiolabeled drug.

passing directly down the GI tract, or was it absorbed and then excreted in feces *via* bile? Figure 3.13 shows the data from the bile duct-cannulated animal. It is only possible to maintain bile duct-cannulated animals for limited periods (in the example in Figure 3.13, 72 h); therefore, excretion was not complete by the end of the experiment. Nevertheless, approximately 28% of the dose was excreted in urine, only about 5% in feces and 65% in bile. Based on these results, the drug was well absorbed and the radioactivity found in feces was almost certainly a result of biliary excretion. (As an aside, the separation of excreta in animal cages is never perfect, and when just a few percent of the dose are excreted in feces, this may be due to contamination with urine.)

To study enterohepatic recirculation, bile collected from one animal dosed with radiolabeled drug can be administered to another (recipient) animal, usually intraduodenally, or into the stomach, *via* a tube passing down the esophagus. Samples are taken from the recipient animal and analyzed in the normal way. Sometimes the recipient animal is also bile duct cannulated. A more sophisticated surgical technique involves the linking of two animals through bile duct cannulae. The bile duct of one animal (the donor) is cannulated, the animal is dosed, and bile is collected. Small aliquots of bile, along with excreta samples, are taken for analysis, and the remainder of the bile is pooled. The pooled bile is then infused *via* an infusion pump into the bile duct of a second animal (recipient). Samples are collected from the recipient, which may also be cannulated.

These types of experiments are somewhat rare because of the surgical skills required and not all laboratories have such capabilities. When conducting experiments where bile from a donor animal is administered to a recipient animal, it must be remembered that the bile being dosed is a pool from the donor. The experiment lacks the possible dynamics of changing metabolite concentration in bile over time.

With all bile duct cannulation experiments, it should be appreciated that the animals have undergone surgery, and this is bound to have some effect on absorption and metabolism. The lack of bile salts in the duodenum of a bile duct-cannulated animal may cause a reduction in drug absorption. Drug-metabolizing enzymes may be affected by the anesthetic used during surgery.

Radioactivity once absorbed can travel back into the GI tract by an alternative route to bile. Radioactivity in the blood feeding the tissues of the GI tract can travel from the blood directly back into the GI tract. If this is by diffusion, then the amounts are likely to be minimal. If active transport is involved, however, this route can be significant.

3.6.6 First-Pass Metabolism

The liver in particular, and to some extent the GI tract, can metabolize a drug to such an extent that little or no parent actually reaches the circulation. This is known as first-pass metabolism. An example of a drug that undergoes extensive first-pass metabolism is midazolam (a benzodiazepine, used as a sedative). Orally administered midazolam is metabolized by CYP 3A4 in the GI tract and in the liver to an inactive hydroxylated metabolite. Thus, by the time the drug-related material reaches the systemic circulation, a significant proportion is metabolized, thereby reducing the systemic concentration of the active parent drug.

The first-pass effect can be complicated by the action of, for example, stomach acid, which might break down the drug prior to absorption. Under such circumstances, a good proportion of what is absorbed may be breakdown products, not parent drug. There are situations where a derivative of an active drug is administered, which is then metabolized to the active drug. These are known as prodrugs, and they are often used in cases where the active drug is poorly absorbed. An example is codeine, which is the O-methyl derivative of morphine. Morphine is poorly absorbed from the GI tract. Codeine, however, is well absorbed through the GI tract, and once absorbed, a proportion is O-demethylated to form the active drug, morphine, by first-pass metabolism. Morphine is eliminated *via* bile, principally as morphine-3-glucuronide, and some enterohepatic recirculation is evident.[27]

First-pass metabolism and biliary excretion can occur together. For example, a drug may undergo first-pass metabolism by conjugation to be eliminated in the bile. On the other hand, first-pass metabolism can occur in the absence of biliary excretion, and so the two entities should not be confused.

An intravenous dose enters the systemic circulation directly, and therefore does not exhibit any first-pass effects that may result from oral administration. For this reason, midazolam can be administered intravenously, so that the maximum amount of the active drug is available systemically. Nevertheless, as the drug circulates, it continually passes through the liver and other tissues and is therefore exposed to drug-metabolizing enzymes. An intravenous dose, like an oral dose, can therefore be eliminated in the bile and then excreted in the feces or undergo enterohepatic recirculation.

First-pass metabolism can be studied by examining plasma concentration data for total radioactivity and parent drug for both the oral and intravenous routes of administration. Such experiments ideally require two radiolabeled doses to be given (one intravenous, one oral), and so the ideal design for this type of experiment is a crossover study. Animals or human volunteers are given the drug by one dose route, and following a suitable period of time to allow elimination of all radioactivity, the same animals or volunteers are given the drug by the other dose route. The advantage of the crossover design is that any interanimal or intersubject variation is minimized. It is possible to administer two radiolabeled doses to animals, but because of restrictions concerning radioactive exposure, humans have traditionally been limited to one radioactive dose. This situation is now changing, however, with the introduction of accelerator mass spectrometry (Chapter 10).

In animal studies, sufficient plasma has to be collected in order to carry out the bioanalysis for parent compound, and therefore this may not be possible with smaller animal species.

The concentration time curve for total radioactivity is composed of the parent and metabolites; it is the quantitative sum of the concentrations of all components containing the radiolabel present in the plasma. Figure 3.14A shows the plasma concentration vs. time for total radioactivity and for the parent drug, after oral administration. Following absorption, the drug underwent first-pass metabolism, and so from the earliest sampling time, the concentration of the parent drug was significantly lower than the concentration of total radioactivity. The concentration of the parent drug in plasma was approximately one tenth, at C_{max}, of that of total radioactivity.

When the drug was administered intravenously (Figure 3.14B), it did not undergo first-pass metabolism, and therefore at the earliest collection times, the concentrations of the parent drug and total radioactivity were approximately the same. After a short time (approximately 1 h in the example), the intravenous dose underwent metabolism, and so the parent concentration began to fall compared to total radioactivity. (This, of course, was not first-pass metabolism, but a result of the drug encountering drug metabolism enzymes as it circulated systemically.)

In human studies, it may not be possible to administer an intravenous dose, and so the extent of first-pass metabolism may have to be assessed based on data from an oral dose only. A situation could be envisaged where the concentrations of parent and total radioactivity in the early time points for both the oral and intravenous doses were dissimilar. Under these circumstances, first-pass metabolism may not be occurring, but the drug is simply undergoing rapid systemic metabolism. Such a situation would not be detected without the administration of the intravenous dose, but it is likely to be a fairly unusual case.

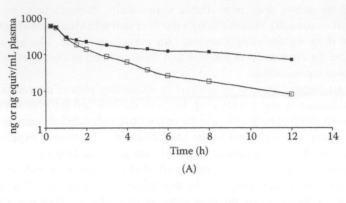

(A)

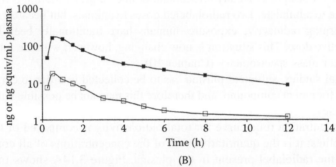

(B)

Figure 3.14 Effect of first-pass metabolism by plotting the concentration of radioactivity (■) and the concentration of parent drug (□) for (A) a single oral dose and (B) a single intravenous dose of radiolabeled drug.

3.6.7 Bioavailability

By comparing the area under the plasma concentration time curves (AUCs) for the parent drug between the oral and intravenous administrations, the absolute bioavailability is obtained (Appendix 3). If a drug is poorly absorbed, the AUC of the oral administration will be significantly lower than the AUC for the intravenous administration (relative to the dose given), thus demonstrating low bioavailability. The drug may, however, be well absorbed and then undergo first-pass metabolism. This will also result in the AUC measured for the parent for the oral administration being lower than that for the intravenous administration (relative to the dose given), again demonstrating low bioavailability. Low bioavailability of the parent drug therefore can be caused by poor absorption or by first-pass metabolism.

Figure 3.15 plots the same data shown in Figure 3.14, with the plasma concentrations of the parent resulting from the oral and intravenous administrations compared. If, for the sake of the example, we assume the oral and intravenous doses were the same, then comparison of the respective AUCs shows the bioavailability to be approximately 10% (F = 0.1, Appendix 3). From the data presented in Figure 3.15, however, it is not possible to tell if the low bioavailability was caused by poor

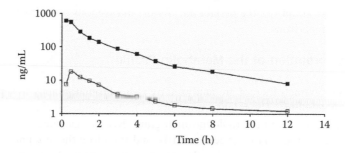

Figure 3.15 Plasma concentration of parent drug resulting from a single intravenous dose (■) and a single oral dose (□). By comparing the AUC for the two curves (relative to dose), the absolute bioavailability can be calculated (Appendix 3). Assume in this example that the oral and intravenous doses were the same, then the bioavailability is low (about 10%).

absorption or by first-pass metabolism. Comparison of parent drug concentration with that of total radioactivity (Figure 3.14) shows that in this example it was due to first-pass metabolism.

For certain types of drug, low bioavailability is desirable. For example, where topical or ocular treatments are designed to have a local effect, any drug absorbed into systemic circulation has the potential to cause toxicity. What is required under these circumstances is a measure of total exposure to drug and all its metabolites (i.e., everything in circulation that arose from the drug application). If the bioavailability of such drugs were assessed by measuring only parent compound in plasma, this could underestimate the degree of bioavailability if the drug is rapidly metabolized once in systemic circulation. This type of bioavailability study can therefore be conducted by determining the AUCs based on the total radioactivity concentrations following administration by the extravascular and intravenous routes, as the total radioactivity will represent all radiolabeled components of the drug (parent and metabolites).

Comparison of the AUCs based on total radioactivity is valid providing that there is no metabolism or degradation of the drug prior to it reaching the site of measurement. Take a topical drug as an example (i.e., dosed onto the skin). If a proportion of the drug was absorbed through the skin and entered the bloodstream entirely as the parent drug, then the AUCs based on total radioactivity can be compared for the dermal and intravenous doses to correctly determine the total absolute bioavailability. This is because what entered the bloodstream for the dermal and intravenous dose routes was the same (namely, parent drug). The same applies if the drug was metabolized in the skin but the metabolites remained in the skin, with only the parent being absorbed. If, however, the drug was metabolized in the skin and the metabolites (perhaps a mixture of metabolites and parent drug) were absorbed, then the AUCs for the dermal dose and intravenous dose would be based on different chemical entities and the AUCs cannot be compared to determine absolute bioavailability. Experiments should therefore be conducted to verify that it is the parent drug that is absorbed from the extravascular route. If metabolites are absorbed, then it may be necessary to administer the metabolites by the intravenous route in order to make the correct comparisons.

3.6.8   Interpretation of the Metabolic Profile

Excreta or extracts thereof are analyzed by radiochromatography to separate the individual metabolites. The relative amounts of metabolites can then be calculated from their proportions in the radiochromatogram. Recall that radioactivity offers a universal detection technique (Section 2.10), and therefore the amount of radioactivity present is directly related to the amount of compound, irrespective of its chemical structure.

Figure 3.16A and B represents radiochromatograms of samples taken at different times in a study (note the appearance of a time-dependent metabolite). The area for each peak was expressed as a percentage of the total for the radiochromatogram. Inevitably, some radioactivity is unaccounted for, and this, along with the percentages for each metabolite, is shown in Table 3.2.

It is important to determine the recovery of radioactivity from the chromatographic column. Because radioactive tracers are used, this can be readily achieved by simply knowing the amount injected and the amount recovered from the HPLC column. A consistently low column recovery means that a certain proportion of the radioactivity is uneluted, and therefore not accounted for. For this reason, many researchers will start the separation process using TLC rather than HPLC, as all the radioactivity on the TLC plate can be visualized.

It is also possible to express the quantity of each metabolite in terms of the percentage of dose. If, for example, 20% of the dose was excreted in urine between 0 and 12 h, from Table 3.2, the peak at 38.1 min would represent 56.7% of the 20% excreted (i.e., 11.3%) of the administered dose. To get the total percentage of each metabolite excreted, excreta over a sufficiently long time (accounting for approximately 95% of the dose) have to be profiled.

With plasma profiles, percentages of administered dose cannot be readily calculated, as the proportion of the dose represented in a given plasma sample is unknown. Metabolites in plasma are therefore usually expressed in terms of their relative proportions, and sometimes in terms of their proportion to the AUC.

It is sometimes necessary to estimate the actual amount of a metabolite (w/v) present in an HPLC peak. For example, it is necessary to know if sufficient amounts are present to conduct metabolite identification work with MS or NMR (Sections 3.5.12 and 3.5.13). The usual way of doing this is by knowing the radioactive concentration of the sample injected onto the HPLC, and then calculating the amount in any one peak by proportion. For example, let us say that a sample contained 20,000 dpm/mL and 100 µL was injected onto the HPLC (2000 dpm injected). Let us take the peak at 34.8 min (0 to 12 h) in Table 3.2 at 18% of the chromatogram. Thus, the amount in this peak is 18% of 2000 dpm, which is 360 dpm. If the specific activity of the radiolabeled drug administered was 1 MBq/mmol, then the 360 dpm would be equivalent to around 6 nmol (see Section 2.5 for the conversion factors; 1 MBq = 6×10^7 dpm). If the structure, and hence molecular weight, of the metabolite was known, the amount in micrograms can be calculated. (Sometimes the molecular

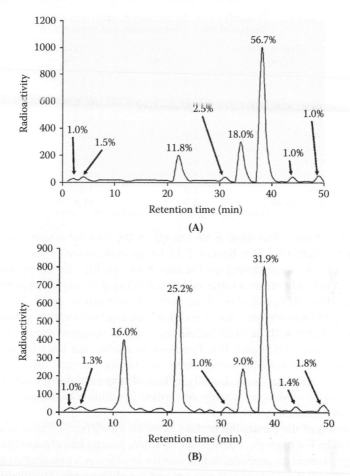

Figure 3.16 Radiochromatographic profile of urine collected over (A) 0 to 12 h and (B) 12 to 24 h. Each radiochromatographic peak is expressed as the percentage of the radioactivity recovered.

weight is known from mass spectrometry without necessarily knowing the full structure of the metabolite.)

If there was no information on the molecular weight of the metabolite, then an estimate can be made by assuming the metabolite is either half or twice the molecular weight of the parent drug. If we assume that the molecular weight of the parent drug was 350, then 6 nmol of metabolite would be equivalent to around 2.1 μg equiv. Thus, we would have somewhere in the region of 1 to 4 μg of metabolite. Mass spectrometry would be capable of obtaining a spectrum with this amount of metabolite, but it may be borderline for NMR. The above calculation does assume there is a high HPLC column recovery, but such calculations often only have to be approximate in order to gauge whether metabolite identification is feasible.

Table 3.2   Proportions of the Various Metabolites as
            Shown in the Chromatograms in Figure 3.16

Retention Time (min)	0–12 h %	12–24 h %
2.2	1.0	1.0
4.1	1.5	1.3
12.4	Not detected	16.0
22.2	11.8	25.2
31.5	2.5	1.0
34.8	18.0	9.0
38.1	56.7	31.9
44.0	1.0	1.4
48.6	1.0	1.8
Remainder	6.5	11.4

This also assumes that there is no change in the specific activity between the parent and the metabolite (see Section 2.11 for an explanation).

The effects of repeat dosing on the metabolite profile can be examined. The usual method is to administer a series of nonradiolabeled doses, followed by a single radiolabeled dose. Repeat dosing of radiolabeled drug can be given, but this complicates the quantitation somewhat. In addition, repeat administration of radiolabeled drug is not possible with humans (unless the study is designed around accelerator mass spectrometry — Chapter 10). Repeat-dose studies are intended to examine whether additional metabolites might arise due to, for example, the saturation of particular elimination pathways. Equally, effects of enzyme induction are also examined. Repeat-dose studies are usually performed in addition to, rather than instead of, single-dose studies.

Comparison of the metabolite profiles between the different routes of excretion should be made. For example, take a situation where plasma and urine only contained parent drug, whereas the predominant metabolite in bile was a glucuronide conjugate and feces contained a mixture of the parent and the glucuronide. The likelihood was therefore that the drug was conjugated in the liver, excreted as the glucuronide in bile, hydrolyzed back to the parent drug in the GI tract, and reabsorbed, to go back to the liver. A proportion of the parent at each pass exited from the liver into the systemic circulation, to be filtered by the kidney and end up in urine. Parent in the feces could be unabsorbed drug or the remnant of hydrolyzed glucuronide. If the drug exhibited a long plasma half-life, then enterohepatic recirculation could be a contributing factor.

A more complex example might be where plasma only contained parent drug, which exhibited a long plasma half-life. The predominant metabolite in urine was a hydroxylated metabolite and its glucuronide, but with no parent drug present. One explanation here could be that the drug itself was not cleared from systemic circulation, but the hydroxylated metabolite was. Thus, the rate of elimination from plasma was dependent upon the rate of formation of the hydroxylated metabolite. Once formed, the hydroxylated metabolite might be rapidly cleared, but it may also form a glucuronide in the liver. A bile duct cannulation experiment might reveal if the glucuronide underwent enterohepatic recirculation. If the hydroxylation was mediated specifically by a polymorphic CYP P450, then alarm bells would ring, as this example is then analogous to the debrisoquine situation (Section 3.4.15).

There is a regulatory expectation that at the very least, the structures of the major metabolites are elucidated, not least because of possible structural alerts (Section 3.7). The important issue, however, is to compare human metabolites with those from the toxicology species. The FDA guidelines* define major metabolites as those identified in human plasma that account for greater than 10% of the drug-related material (administered dose or systemic exposure, whichever is the less) and that were not present at sufficient levels to permit adequate evaluation during standard nonclinical animal studies. This definition leaves a lot of flexibility, which is not surprising, as this area is very difficult to describe precisely. For example, let us assume a metabolite identified in the human consists of 15% of the plasma radio-activity, and that it was not seen in the toxicology species (assume rat). Samples from the rat study are reanalyzed, and one of the small radio-HPLC peaks, previously ignored because it represented less than 1%, is now identified as the same metabolite seen in human. The metabolite in human is no longer human specific, but was exposure in the rat sufficient compared to human? In this example, probably not, but such issues have to be taken in context of all the data. Perhaps, for example, the human metabolite is a conjugate of a major metabolite in the rat. An argument could be made, therefore, that if the conjugate is present, then the aglycone had to be present at some point. Conjugates, however, are recognized today as not necessarily being as benign as they were once thought to be (Appendix 1).

If major human-related metabolite(s) are identified, then this may lead to specific toxicity testing. These tests would depend upon the nature of the metabolite but could include general toxicity, carcinogenicity, embryo-fetal development, and geno-toxicity. It is even possible that ADME or pharmacokinetic studies on the metabolite might be necessary.

Finally, there are practical difficulties with the above arguments. A situation where the plasma contains parent and one or two metabolites is very different from a situation where the drug is metabolized to a plethora of metabolites, any one of which constitutes only a small percentage of the dose. In addition, while the thera-peutic dose of a drug like acetaminophen (paracetamol) is measured in the hundreds of milligrams, more modern drugs can exhibit far greater potency. Identifying metab-olites in plasma from a drug where the dose is 1 mg or less is far more of a challenge.

3.6.9 Deconjugation

If the presence of glucuronide or sulfate conjugates is suspected, then samples of urine, plasma, feces, or bile can be treated with a suitable enzyme to hydrolyze the conjugate from the aglycone. The chromatographic profiles before and after enzyme treatment are then compared to determine if hydrolysis occurred. The definitive identification of conjugates, given modern analytical methods, should be conducted using mass spectroscopy or NMR, rather than purely relying on the results of enzyme deconjugation methods. Nevertheless, enzyme deconjugation is useful,

* At the time of writing (June 2005), the guidelines were under revision.

and it is a commonly used method for at least a preliminary investigation. For example, conjugates, being polar compounds, often appear as early eluting HPLC peaks in a region of the chromatogram that is poorly resolved. There may therefore be more than one conjugate appearing as an ill-resolved single peak in the chromatogram. The resulting aglycones from an enzyme digestion might appear in a later region of the chromatogram where they can be separated.

The most commonly used deconjugation enzyme is β-glucuronidase from *Helix pomatia*, which contains both β-glucuronidase and sulfatase activity. Being a non-specific enzyme, it has wide activity on a range of glucuronides and sulfates. Enzymes with higher specificities can be used for more targeted investigations. Glucuronidase from *Escherichia coli* is effective at hydrolyzing steroid glucuronides. Sulfatases can also be obtained, for example, from *Aerobacter aerogens* or *Patella vulgate*. Around 2000 Fishman units of β-glucuronidase (ex. *Helix pomatia*) in 0.2 *M* ammonium acetate buffer (pH 5.6) incubated for 4 to 6 h with 1 mL of sample is usually sufficient for putative conjugate hydrolysis. Enzymes from different sources have different pH optima, and these should be confirmed with the supplier. For β-glucuronidase, a positive control of phenolphthalein glucuronic acid is included to demonstrate the activity of the enzyme. As phenolphthalein is released during enzyme hydrolysis, a small amount of base will turn the solution pink. For sulfatase, the positive control is ρ-nitrophenol sulfate.

Not all glucuronides will necessarily be susceptible to enzyme hydrolysis for a variety of reasons. Acyl-glucuronides are usually susceptible, but O-glucuronides are not always. N-glucuronides vary in their susceptibility to enzyme hydrolysis, and S-glucuronides tend to be generally unstable. There is also the possibility of steric hindrance in the reaction. If a suspected conjugate is not hydrolyzed with β-glucuronidase, this does not necessarily rule out the possibility that it is a glucuronide.

False positives are sometimes seen resulting from the facile hydrolysis of a metabolite that is not a glucuronide or sulfate conjugate, but which simply occurs under the incubation conditions. Such false positives can be identified by conducting an incubation in the presence of D-saccharic acid 1,4-lactone, an inhibitor of β-glucuronidase. β-glucuronidase is incubated with the sample and the phenolphthalein glucuronic acid control, both with and without the inhibitor. The phenolphthalein glucuronic acid without the inhibitor should give a pink color on the addition of base, showing that the enzyme is active. The phenolphthalein glucuronic acid with the inhibitor should not produce any color change on the addition of base, showing the conditions for inhibition were appropriate. If the suspect conjugate is a glucuronide (and susceptible to enzyme hydrolysis), then the sample without inhibitor should show hydrolysis of the putative conjugate and the sample with the inhibitor should show no change. If the latter does hydrolyze, then this does not rule out the presence of a glucuronide; it only means that it is labile and the result is ambiguous. D-saccharic acid 1,4-lactone is a competitive inhibitor, and therefore excess is required to fully inhibit enzyme hydrolysis, typically 10-fold the amount of substrate.

An example of a β-glucuronidase experiment is shown in Figure 3.17, where the peak eluting at approximately 6 min in Figure 3.17A was suspected of being a glucuronide conjugate. Following incubation with β-glucuronidase, the peak at 6

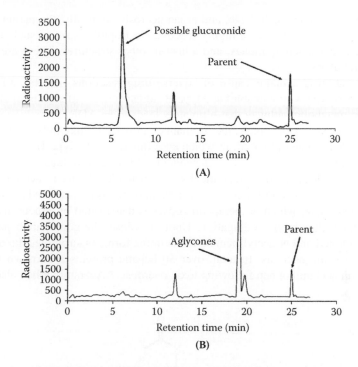

Figure 3.17 (A) A metabolic profile before β-glucuronidase treatment. (B) The profile after β-glucuronidase treatment.

min has virtually disappeared and two new peaks are seen eluting closely at approximately 18 and 19 min. The conclusion, therefore, is that the peak at 6 min consisted of two coeluting glucuronide conjugates, which upon hydrolysis to the aglycones were resolved on the chromatogram.

As a slight aside, assume that the two glucuronides were formed from the conjugation of phenols, each with the hydroxyl group in a different position on an aromatic ring. The molecular weight of the glucuronides would therefore be the same, so mass spectrometry would not be able to determine the precise position of conjugation. Metabolite standards are sometimes available (they are required if the metabolite is being monitored by bioanalysis in the clinical trials; Section 3.5.10). If the two phenolic metabolites were available as standards and they chromatographically coeluted with the aglycones, then the structures of the conjugates would also be confirmed.

3.7 STRUCTURAL ALERTS

On occasion, the products of metabolism may be more reactive than the parent compound, in a process known as metabolic activation or bioactivation.[28] The active metabolites may then form adducts with macromolecules such as protein and DNA, leading to cell damage, cell death, and organ necrosis. Typically, the parent drug is activated by the formation of a highly reactive electrophilic species such as nitrosamines, epoxides, semiquinones, and a host of other structures. These are known as structural alerts.

Bioactivation is a major cause of adverse drug reactions (ADRs). ADRs are categorized as type A (predicable) and type B (idiosyncratic). If structural alerts are seen in the metabolic pathway that ultimately leads to an ADR, then this would be classified as type A. Conversely, the mechanism of toxicity may only be elucidated after an ADR has been reported, in which case this would be type B.

Many ADRs are, however, dose dependent, and doses that lead to toxicity can be well above those used therapeutically. An example of this is acetaminophen (paracetamol), as shown in Figure 3.18. Acetaminophen is bioactivated to N-acetyl-benzoquinoneimine, which at therapeutic doses is deactivated by glucuronide, sulfate, and then glutathione conjugation. Upon overdose, the conjugation pathways become saturated and N-acetyl-benzoquinoneimine forms macromolecular adducts, leading to hepatic necrosis. In total, over 30 hepatic proteins are known to form adducts with acetaminophen following toxic overdose.[28] Acetaminophen also forms

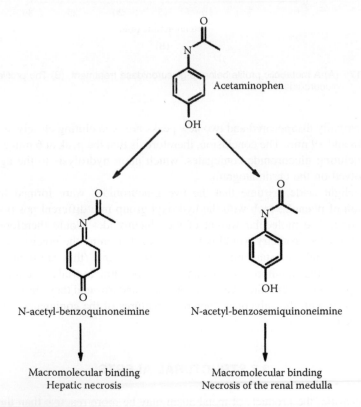

Figure 3.18 Bioactivation of acetaminophen (paracetamol).

N-acetyl-benzosemiquinoneimine, which binds to renal protein, leading to damage to the renal medulla.

To understand the possible chemical mechanism of toxicity, the elucidation of as complete a metabolic pathway as possible is important. For reasons previously discussed, radiotracers are an essential element in this process. The story is unfortunately not quite as simple as that. Structural alerts by their very nature are reactive, and therefore, by the process of binding, they may not actually be detected in the free form. Considerable expertise is necessary to identify downstream products that may have resulted from reactive and potentially toxic metabolites. Indeed, there has been much effort to automate the process using computer programs. Going back to acetaminophen, the presence of the glutathione conjugate is revealed by detection of the mercapturic acid in urine as the dose increases, the structure of which is remote from the original N-acetyl-benzoquinoneimine-reactive species. Acetaminophen remains a useful and widely used analgesic, as the therapeutic dose is safely below the toxic dose. When developing new pharmaceuticals, however, the relationship between the dose and any effects resulting from a structural alert are not necessarily understood. Simply rejecting a drug on the basis that it has a potential structural alert is therefore not necessarily appropriate.

APPENDIX 1: AN OVERVIEW OF XENOBIOTIC
BIOTRANSFORMATIONS

Introduction

A clarification is first required for the terms *biotransformation* and *metabolism*. Biotransformation refers to a chemical change brought about by a biological system. The term *metabolism* is the process by which that change is brought about. Sometimes biotransformation is used in the context of a single step, the addition of a single oxygen atom, for example. Metabolism, on the other hand, refers to the whole process, a series of biotransformations from the original drug (termed the parent) to the final metabolites seen, for example, in excreta. These differences, however, are minor and the two terms are generally synonymous.

Metabolic pathways are interpreted as a series of distinct chemical reactions, each catalyzed by an individual enzyme. Perhaps this interpretation is a consequence of the use of radiotracers in the elucidation of the pathway, as the intention is to isolate the reaction from the complexity of its surroundings. In reality, however, xenobiotics are metabolized by semispecific enzymes, and therefore pathways are better represented as multidimensional matrices rather than a series of linear steps. Furthermore, xenobiotics are subject to active transport mechanisms. All these effects within the cell will be interrelated in respect to the final metabolic products.[29] Here, like in the vast majority of other publications, metabolic pathways are shown as flat, two-dimensional depictions; to do otherwise would only confuse. Bear in mind, however, the reality is infinitely more complicated.

Although there are a bewildering array of xenobiotic biotransformations, it is possible to classify the most common ones into two major categories: the so-called phase I and phase II reactions. Phase I biotransformations consist principally of oxidation, reduction, hydrolysis and rearrangements. Phase II reactions involve the conjugation of xenobiotics with sugars, amino acids, sulfate, or glutathione. It is following phase II that a significant increase in water solubility occurs, facilitating excretion.

Figure 3.19 shows a stylized scheme where a xenobiotic already contains a functional group, or where phase I metabolism introduces a functional group into the molecule. The xenobiotic, following phase I metabolism, is likely to be more water soluble than the parent, but not necessarily significantly so. Depending upon the lipophilicity of the parent or the metabolite following phase I metabolism, a proportion may be excreted at this stage. It is possible that the functional group is highly reactive, which might lead to cellular damage or death. Reactive centers, such as strong electrophiles, are often targets for conjugating enzymes and phase II biotransformation. In the example shown in Figure 3.19, the original functional group is conjugated as well as the second functional group introduced by phase I metabolism. Phase II metabolism leads to a significant shift in the water solubility of the xenobiotic, and at this stage excretion is usually extensive. On occasions, both functional groups might be conjugated (i.e., a double conjugate), but such cases are quite rare.

Figure 3.19 is a simplification, as further biotransformations may occur with the conjugate, particularly in the case of glutathione, in what is known as phase III

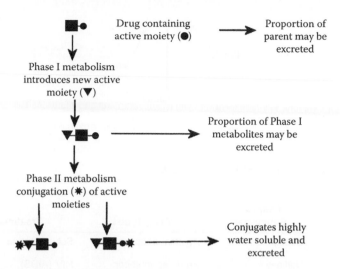

Figure 3.19 Schematic of phase I and phase II metabolism.

metabolism. There are many exceptions to the scheme shown in Figure 3.19. For example, in some cases phase I metabolites are extensively excreted without the formation of conjugates. Metabolites can be less polar than their precursors, due to the addition of alkyl groups.

What follows is a cursory review of xenobiotic metabolism. For a wider and deeper understanding of xenobiotic metabolism, see Parkinson (2001),[30] Gibson and Skett (2001),[31] and Evans (2004).[2]

Phase I Biotransformations

Oxidation, reduction, hydrolysis and rearrangements are common phase I biotransformations seen in animals and plants. These reactions are catalyzed by a wide array of enzymes, including the highly versatile cytochrome P450s (although by no means exclusively so). The cytochrome P450s (CYP P450) are central to drug metabolism and therefore deserve special mention.

CYP P450s get their name from the absorbance wavelength of the carbon monoxide-bound derivative at 450 nm (the P stands for protein). Cytochromes are heme-thiolate proteins containing an atom of iron at the center. Their very name reflects how little was known about them just a few years ago, and they were originally classified, like most other enzymes, by substrate specificity. This was very confusing, as there is a great deal of overlap between the enzymes. The modern classification of CYP P450s is based on the amino acid sequence and organization of the genes.[32,33]

CYP is followed by a number representing the family (generally groups of proteins with more than 40% amino acid sequence identity), a letter for subfamilies (greater than 55% identity), and a number for the gene (Figure 3.20). Some examples of CYP P450s are shown in Table 3.3.

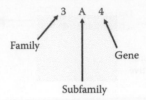

Figure 3.20   The modern nomenclature for cytochrome P450 enzymes.

Table 3.3   Examples of P450s and Their Substrates

Example CYP P450	Example Substrates	Drug Type	Treatment
1A2	Clozapine	Atypical antipsychotic	Schizophrenia
2C19	Nelfinavir	Protease inhibitor	HIV (AIDS)
2C9	Propafenone	Antiarrhythmic	Irregular heartbeat
2D6	Tamoxifen	Antiestrogen	Breast cancer
2E1	Carvedilol	Beta-blocker	Congestive heart failure
3A4	Erythromycin	Antibiotic	Infection

CYP P450s are known as mono-oxygenases, and as their name implies, they add a single oxygen to their substrate. There are many other enzymes involved in xenobiotic metabolism, some of which catalyze oxidations. For example, there are 12 types of aldehyde dehydrogenase (ALDH1 to ALDH8, γ-ABHD, FALDH, SSDH, and MMSDH), all involved in the oxidation of aldehydes to the corresponding carboxylic acid. It is difficult, therefore, purely from knowledge of substrate and reaction products, to assign a particular biotransformation to any particular enzyme. (*In vitro* systems can be used to examine the enzymology; Section 3.4.8). Other enzymes commonly implicated in xenobiotic metabolism are esterases, epoxide hydrolases, alcohol dehydrogenase, monoamine oxidases, and many more. Table 3.4 provides a summary of typical phase I biotransformations.

Phase II Biotransformations

Conjugations with sugars, amino acids, sulfate, or glutathione are all common phase II biotransformations. In mammalian systems, glucuronic acid is the conjugating sugar. Glucuronidation often occurs in parallel with sulfate conjugation.

The mechanism of glucuronide conjugation warrants some mention. Glucuronic acid is attached to the nucleotide sugar transporter, uridine diphosphate (UDP), forming a glucuronic acid–UDP carrier. Conjugation onto the xenobiotic is then catalyzed by UDP–glucuronyl transferase. The enzyme, which is only found in mammals, consists of a number of isoforms.

Table 3.4 Summary of typical Phase I biotransformations seen in mammals

Reaction type	Examples
Hydrolysis	Ester to carboxylic acid + alcohol
	Amides to carboxylic acid + amine
	Thioester to sulphide and carboxylic acid
	Phosphoric acid esters
	Epoxides to diol
Reduction	Ketone to alcohol
	Reductive dehalogenation (R1 can be aliphatic or aromatic)
	R1 — Cl ⟶ R1 — H
	Azo to amines
	R1 — N≡N — R2 ⟶ R1 — NH$_2$ + H$_2$N — R2
	Nitro to amine
	Sulfoxides and N-oxides
Oxidation	Aldehyde to carboxylic acid
	Amine oxidation
	R1 — C — NH$_2$ ⟶ R1 — CHO
	H$_2$
	Sulfide to sulfoxide and sulfone
	R1 — S — R2 ⟶ R1 — S — R2 ⟶ R1 — S — R2

Table 3.4   (continued)

Reaction type	Examples
Oxidation continued	Aliphatic oxidation to alcohol Aromatic oxidation to phenol More commonly hydroxylation on electrophilic carbon (e.g. para to the chlorine):
Oxidation continued	N-oxidation (primary amines to hydroxylamines and oximes, secondary amines to hydroxylamines and nitrones and tertiary amines to the N-oxide) Phospine to phosphine oxide Expoxidation

Table 3.4   (continued)

Reaction type	Examples
Oxidation continued	O, S or N dealkylation (R1 = O, S or N) $R1-CH_3 \longrightarrow \quad\quad\quad H_3C-OH$ $\quad\quad\quad\quad\quad\quad R1-H \quad +$ $R1-\overset{H_2}{\underset{CH_3}{C}} \longrightarrow \quad H_3C-\underset{H_2}{C}-OH$ Oxidative desulfuration $P\equiv S \longrightarrow P\equiv O$
Rearrangements	NIH-shift (named after the National Institute of Health, where it was discovered)

Glucuronide conjugates, once formed, can be further metabolized by so-called acyl migration, where the acyl group (COOH) moves around the glucuronide ring. In certain positions, the glucuronide can become reactive and binds to macromolecules. At one time glucuronides were considered completely benign, but this has had to be reassessed in more recent years.[34]

Sulfate conjugation is catalyzed by sulfotransferases, which exist as a large multigene family of enzymes. The sulfate moiety is derived from 3'-phosphoadenosine-5'-phosphosulfate (known as PAPS).

Conjugation with a number of amino acids may occur, but glycine and perhaps taurine are probably the most common. The mechanism for amino acid conjugation is quite complex (indeed more than one mechanism exists). One mechanism is *via* the acetyl–coenzyme A (CoA) activation of the xenobiotic. As an example, activation of benzoic acid to acetyl-CoA is catalyzed by acetyl-CoA synthetase, as shown in Figure 3.21. The formation of the glycine conjugate is catalyzed by acetyl-CoA amino acid N-acetyltransferase. Glycine conjugates are also known as hippuric acids.

An interesting example arises at this point — the conjugation of the fluoromethyl benzoic acids (Figure 3.22).[35,36] Whilst 2- and 3-fluoromethyl benzoic acids conjugate with glycine, 4-fluoromethyl benzoic acid is conjugated with glucuronide acid.

Glutathione is a tripeptide and conjugates to electrophilic species. There are a series of enzymes called the glutathione-S-transferases (GSTs) that catalyze glutathione conjugation. There are a range of GSTs, which consist of two subunits, with the active site formed at the junction.

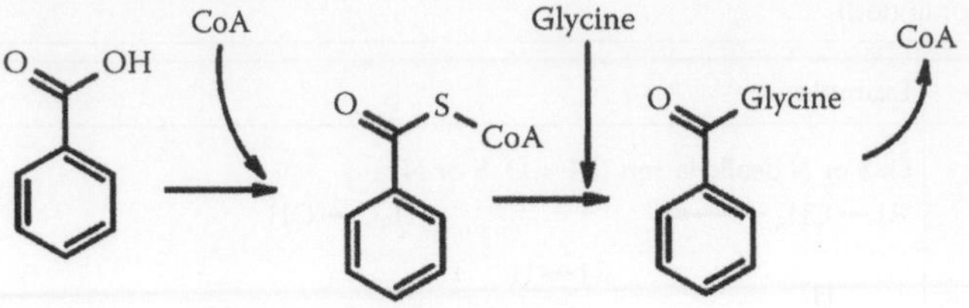

Figure 3.21   Conjugation of benzoic acid with glycine.

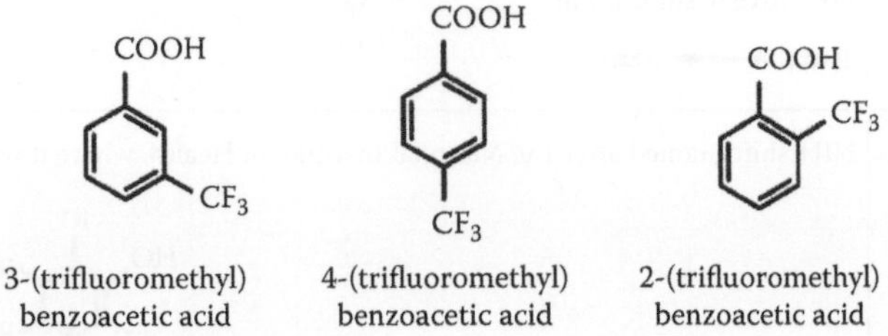

3-(trifluoromethyl)   4-(trifluoromethyl)   2-(trifluoromethyl)
benzoacetic acid   benzoacetic acid   benzoacetic acid

Figure 3.22   Trifluoromethyl benzoic acids.

Glutathione conjugation can also occur with epoxides. The enzyme responsible for this reaction is glutathione peroxidase, which interestingly contains selenium. Selenium was once thought to be entirely toxic, until selenium deficiency was observed in cattle. A little selenium is required for good health (50 to 200 µg/day for an adult) — too much and toxic symptoms will occur. A dose in excess of about 5 mg/day will result in toxicity.

Once the glutathione conjugate is formed, it can undergo extensive further metabolism forming a range of metabolites (Figure 3.23). Often the only sign of glutathione metabolism is the appearance of the N-acetyl cysteine in urine (which somewhat understates the complexity of its formation). ^{35}S-labeled glutathione or sulfate can be used to study the formation and metabolism of conjugates, in place of using a radiolabeled xenobiotic. A summary of typical phase II biotransformations is shown in Table 3.5.

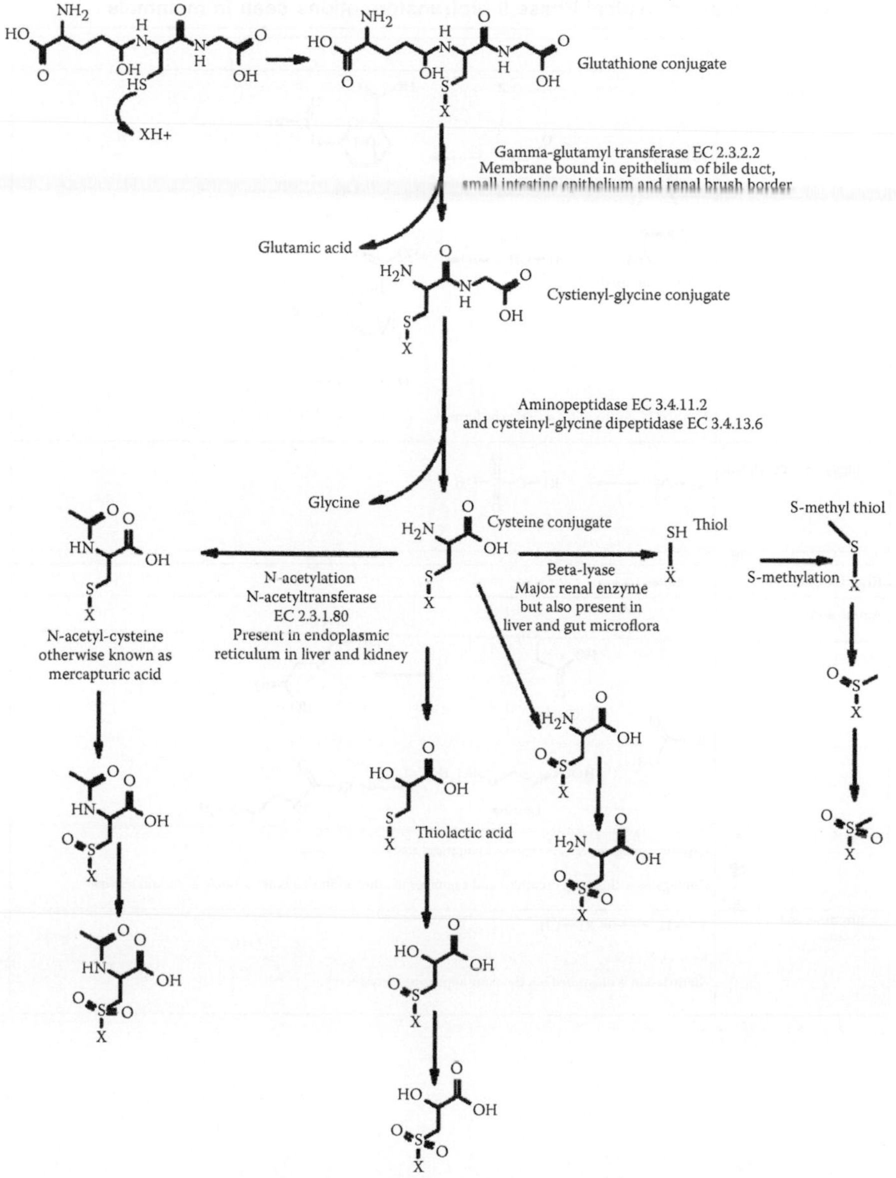

Figure 3.23 The glutathione pathway. The schematic shows the options available for phase III metabolism of a glutathione conjugate. Not all of the metabolites shown will necessarily be formed in all cases.

Table 3.5   Summary of typical Phase II biotransformations seen in mammals

Reaction type	Examples
Conjugation with glucuronic acid	Glucuronic acid + acyl → **Acyl-glucuronide** and R1—OH → **O-glucuronide** N, S and C glucuronides may also be formed
Conjugation with sulphate	$R1{-}OH \longrightarrow R1{-}O{-}\overset{\displaystyle O}{\underset{\displaystyle O}{\overset{\|}{\underset{\|}{S}}}}{-}OH$

Reaction type	Examples
Amino acids	**Glycine**, **Taurine** Glycine conjugates are also known as hippuric acids Conjugates with serine, ornathine and a number of other amino acids are possible in certain species
Methylation and acetylation	$R1{-}H \longrightarrow R1{-}CH_3$ R1 = O, N or S Methylation is illustrated but the same applies to acetylation

Table 3.5 (continued)

Reaction type	Examples
Glutathione	

Glutathione is often abbreviated to GS

Glutathione conjugation of epoxides

APPENDIX 2: EXAMPLES OF XENOBIOTIC METABOLISM STUDIES FROM THE LITERATURE

Introduction

There are a huge number of papers on the metabolism of xenobiotics, and so rather than trying to provide a comprehensive review, I have instead chosen examples in an attempt to put Chapter 3 into context. The intention is not to provide examples of complex biotransformations (indeed, the pathways in the examples have been simplified). Instead, the examples are intended to illustrate how radiotracers were used in the experiments. The purpose of the papers, on the other hand, were not focused on radiotracers, which were merely used as a means to an end. Some interpretation of the results was therefore necessary in the examples presented here.

Example 1

The metabolism of 8-OH DPAT, used experimentally as a serotonin 1A receptor agonist, was studied in the rat.[37] ^{3}H-8-OH DPAT was administered intraperitoneally, intravenously, or orally to male rats. 8-OH DPAT was tritium labeled in the propyl moiety (Figure 3.24), which, on the face of it, might be considered metabolically unstable, due to possible N-dealkylation (comment was made on this possibility in the paper). Indeed, some N-dealkylation did occur, and this is discussed below. Tritium exchange was assessed by freeze drying and was only around 5%, and

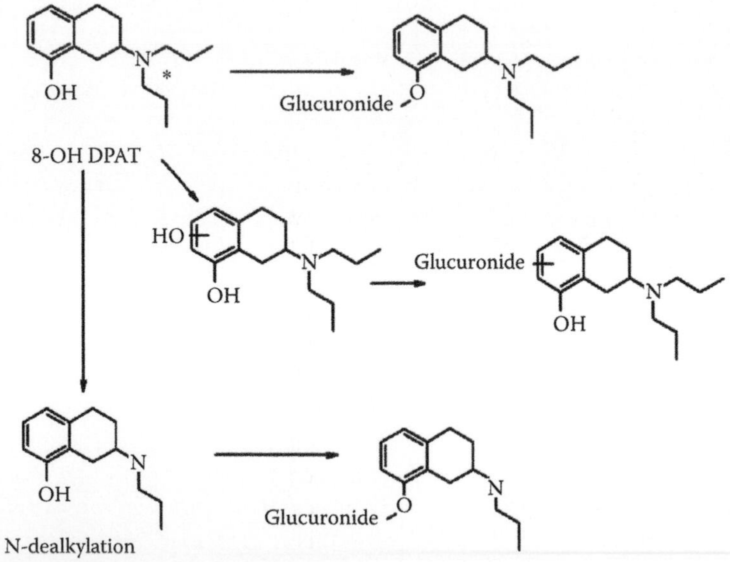

Figure 3.24 The metabolism of 8-OH DPAT. The asterisk (*) denotes the position of the ^{3}H label. (The pathway has been abbreviated for clarity.)

therefore could be ignored. The specific activity of the radiolabel was 219 mCi/mmol (8.1 GBq/mmol).

Urine was the principal route of excretion, with 80% of the dose being excreted in 24 h. Metabolites of 8-OH DPAT were identified with HPLC and LC-MS, and the pathway is shown in Figure 3.24. The phenolic hydroxyl group of 8-OH DPAT conjugated with glucuronic acid, forming O-glucuronide. 8-OH DPAT was hydroxylated on the aromatic ring, which formed a further O-glucuronide. In addition, a single N-dealkylation occurred, which is interesting from the radiotracer perspective. There are two propyl moieties attached to the nitrogen, which makes this part of the molecule symmetrical. One of the propyl moieties was reported as being cleaved from the molecule, leaving the other portion, which still contained the ^{3}H label. The specific activity of the N-dealkylated product was therefore half that of the parent compound, and thus the change in specific activity would have to be taken into account for the quantification of that metabolite (see Section 2.11). No specific mention was made of this in the paper, but since the relative amounts of each metabolite were not quantified, it was unimportant to the experiment. It does, nevertheless, serve as an example of how the specific activity of the metabolites can differ from that of the parent. Furthermore, it was possible that both the propyl moieties were cleaved from the nitrogen, but then, of course, the remaining portion of the molecule would not be labeled, and therefore would not be detected.

The position of aromatic hydroxylation could not be established using mass spectrometry and is therefore represented by a bond going through the aromatic ring in Figure 3.24.

Example 2

[^{14}C]-mazapertine succinate salt (an antipsychotic agent) was orally administered to beagle dogs.[38] Radioactivity was excreted in urine (30%) and feces (62%) over 7 days, with the majority of the radioactivity being excreted in the first 48 h (25 and 58% excreted in urine and feces, respectively). Urine was pooled over 0 to 24 h by combining 10% of the urine excreted at each time point for each animal. Pools of feces were prepared in a similar fashion. Feces were extracted with methanol. Urine and feces extracts were analyzed by TLC, HPLC, and mass spectroscopy. The metabolic pathway is illustrated in Figure 3.25.

Mazapertine was hydrolyzed into two products, with only one product containing the label. The [^{14}C]-product could be detected by radiochromatography, but elucidating further metabolism of the unlabeled product would be severely hampered by the lack of the ^{14}C label. If the metabolism of that part of the molecule was considered important, then a second labeled form of mazapertine would be required, perhaps labeled in the aromatic ring. Also note the opening of the aliphatic ring. Although not seen in this example, such ring opening can lead to the loss of small carbon fragments. If the compound was labeled in this ring structure, then this could lead to the loss of the label. The example of mazapertine illustrates the importance of placing the label in the right position and how this can be a difficult decision, without knowledge of the metabolism of the drug.

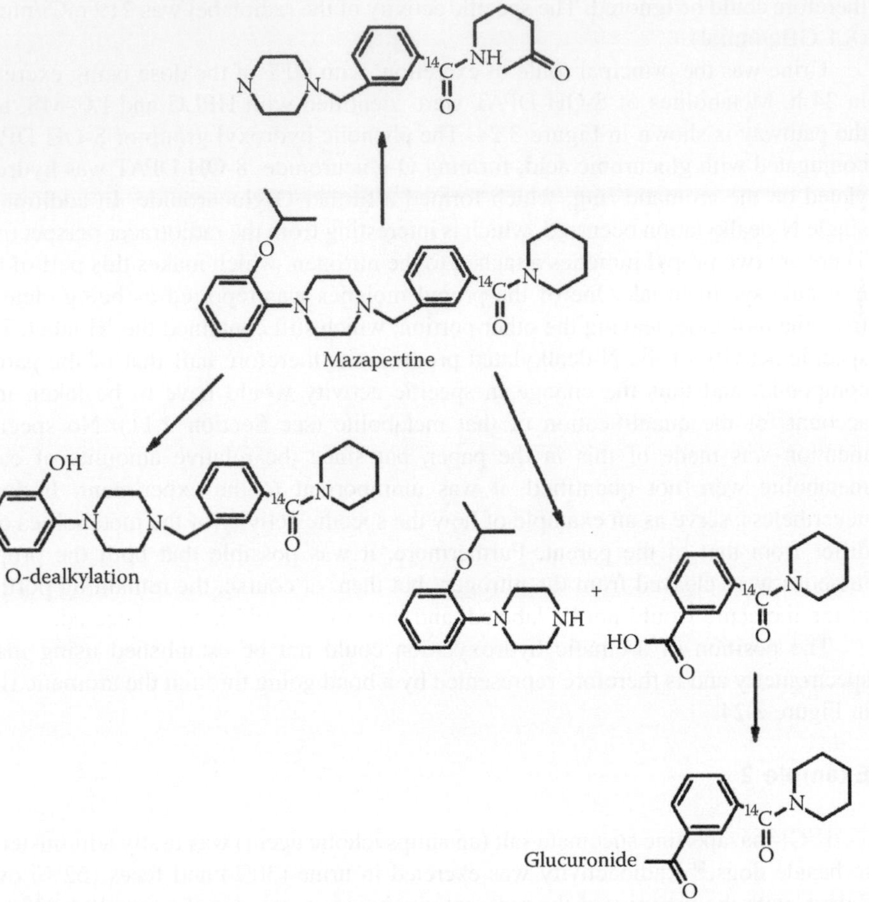

Figure 3.25 The metabolism of mazapertine. (The pathway has been abbreviated for clarity.)

Example 3

The metabolism of [^{14}C]-zolmitriptan (brand name Zomig®) (a 5HT receptor agonist used for the treatment of migraine) was investigated *in vitro*, and the CYP P450 enzyme involved in its metabolism was identified.[39] [^{14}C]-Zomig was administered to human hepatocytes (cryopreserved from male and female donors) at a concentration of 1 µm in the presence or absence of selected CYP P450 inhibitors. Figure 3.26 shows the metabolic pathway in the absence of inhibitor. The N-demethylated and N-oxide products were, however, absent in cultures incubated in the presence of furafylline, a selective inhibitor of CYP1A2, thus demonstrating the role of this enzyme in the metabolism of zolmitriptan.

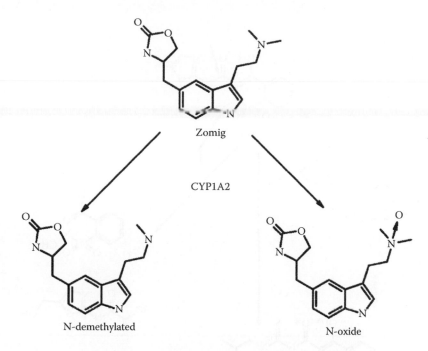

Figure 3.26 The metabolism of zomig. (The pathway has been abbreviated for clarity.)

Example 4

Meloxicam (brand name Mobic®) (an anti-inflammatory used in osteoarthritis and rheumatoid arthritis) labeled with ^{14}C in the ketone group (position 1, Figure 3.27) and in the N-methyl moiety (position 2, Figure 3.27) was orally dosed to normal and bile duct-cannulated rats.[40] Urine, feces, and, where appropriate, bile and exhaled CO_2 were collected and analyzed for total radioactivity. Samples were analyzed by HPLC and semipreparative HPLC and metabolites identified with mass spectrometry and NMR.

Following administration of labeled form 1, the recovery of radioactivity was 98%, with approximately 76% in urine and 22% in feces. The CO_2 traps did not contain detectable amounts of radioactivity. Only 9% of the dose was excreted in bile, so this did not represent a major route of excretion.

Following administration of labeled form 2, the recovery of radioactivity was 75%, with approximately 51% in urine and 24% in feces over 96 h. The carcass contained no detectable levels of radioactivity. For the animals where CO_2 traps were included, the recovery was approximately 99%, with 38% in urine, 19% in feces, 15% in the CO_2 traps, and 26% in the carcass over 48 h.

When animal systems are set up for the collection of volatiles, there is a practical limit to the length of the study, and this is the likely reason for the 48-h duration. The shorter experimental time led to high concentrations of radioactivity in the carcass, showing that after 48 h, radioactivity had not been completely eliminated from the animals. Although the label in the ketone moiety (position 1)

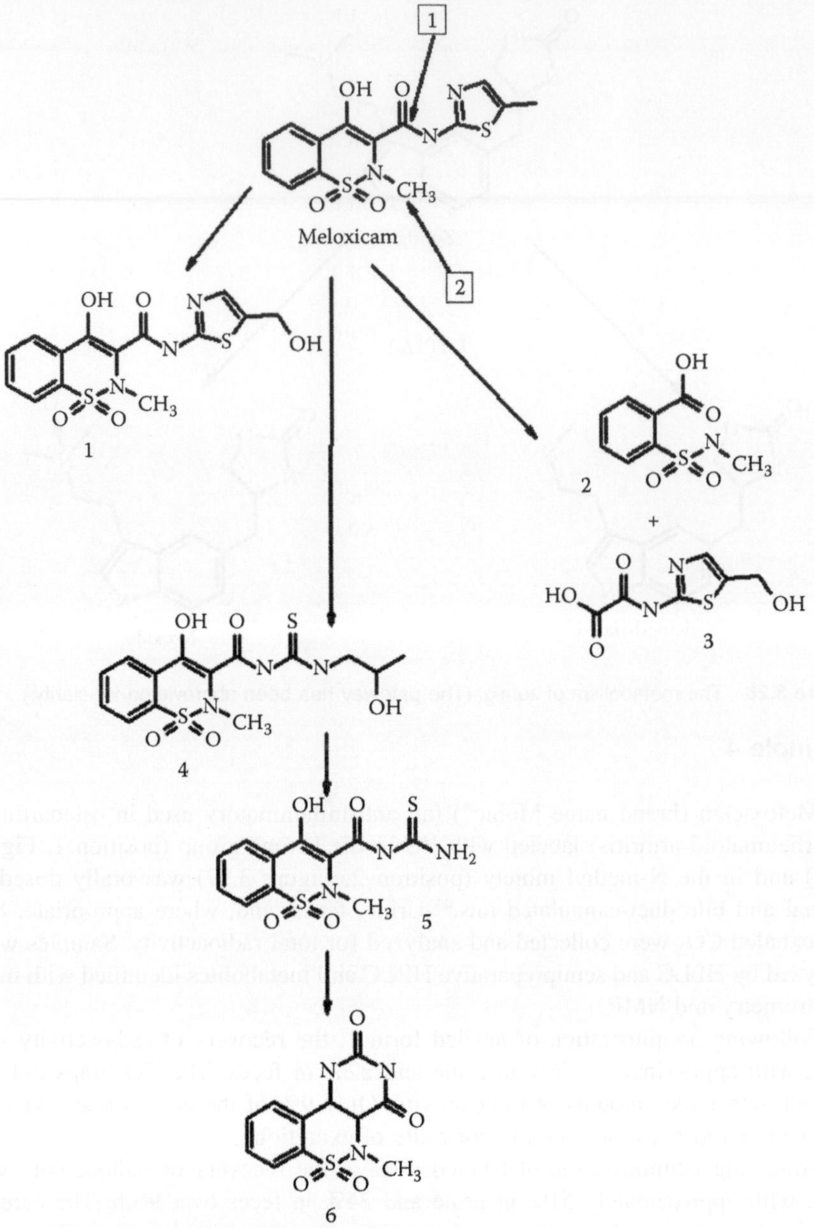

Figure 3.27 The metabolism of meloxicam. Two radiolabeled forms were used; the positions of the ^{14}C label are denoted by 1 and 2 in the boxes. (The pathway has been abbreviated for clarity.)

was in a metabolically stable position, the N-methyl label (position 2) was not and serves as a good example of the importance of the position of the radiolabel within the molecule.

Metabolites 1 and 3 (Figure 3.27) were the major metabolites in urine, with virtually no parent drug detected. Metabolite 3 was absent from bile. As would be expected from the position of the labels, metabolite 3 could not be detected when the N-methyl-labeled form of meloxicam was administered.

The metabolism of meloxicam was somewhat unusual, and apart from metabolite 1, the reaction types are not listed in Table 3.4. In particular, ring opening (metabolites 2, 4, and 5) and then a recyclization (metabolite 6) are not obvious and would be difficult to predict from the structure of the parent drug alone. Indeed, it is likely that MS analysis would be insufficient for the structural elucidation of these metabolites, and this is the likely reason the authors turned to NMR. This serves as a good illustration of how radiotracers are used to "home in" on metabolites that otherwise would be very difficult to predict.

Example 5

[^{14}C]-delmopinol (Decapinol®, a surface-active agent used to prevent colonization of bacteria in the mouth) was administered to six male human volunteers orally and as a mouthwash.[41,42]

Following dosing, urine feces and plasma samples were taken. For the mouthwash, 72% of the dose was expectorated (i.e., spat out) and the remainder was absorbed. The principle route of elimination was in the urine (92% of the dose after oral administration). Metabolites in plasma and urine were identified by separation on HPLC, followed by LC-MS and gas chromatography–mass spectrometry (GC-MS). Plasma samples were analyzed for each time point in order to study the pharmacokinetics of the parent compound and each of the major metabolites. The $t_{1/2}$ of all of the metabolites was similar for the rinse dose (1 to 2 h). Interestingly, for the oral dose, the $t_{1/2}$ for the same metabolites was shorter (0.5 to 1 h). Parent compound was detected in the plasma after the rinse dose, but very little was detected after the oral dose (although the data suggested the rinse dose had a low bioavailability, comparing the AUCs for the oral and rinse doses). The most likely explanation was that first-pass metabolism occurred following the oral dose, whereas the rinse dose was absorbed directly through the lining of the mouth, thus bypassing the liver in the first instance.

The metabolism of delmopinol is shown in Figure 3.28. The radiolabel was placed in the morpholine ring, as at the outset it would have no doubt seemed inappropriate to label propyl moieties, as there was the possibility of metabolic cleavage. In the event, however, a label anywhere in the molecule would have sufficed. From previous examples, the possibility of ring opening could not be ruled out, and so, with delmopinol, the position of the radiolabel in the absence of any metabolism data is a difficult choice. It is perhaps under these circumstances that tritium labels and *in vitro* experiments can yield useful information on the metabolic stability of a compound prior to the synthesis of the more expensive ^{14}C label.

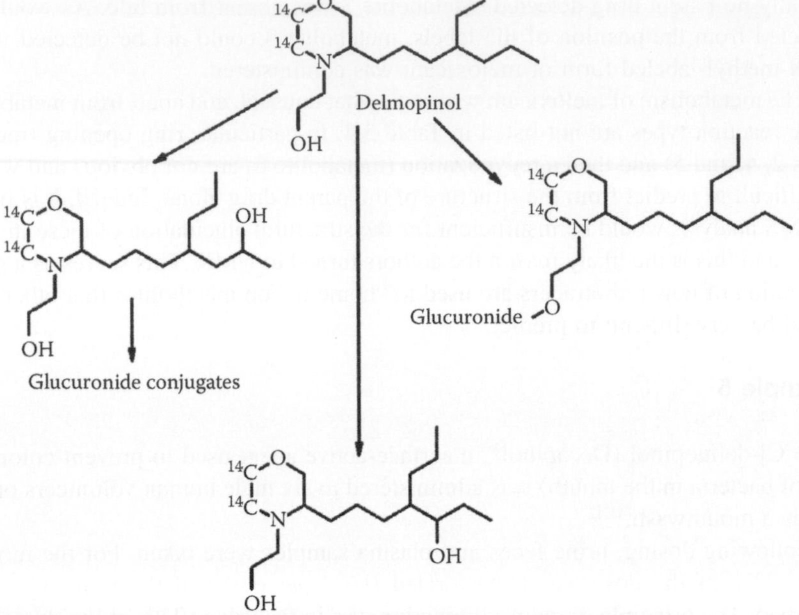

Delmopinol

OH

OH

Glucuronide

OH

Glucuronide conjugates

OH

OH

Figure 3.28 The metabolism of delmopinol. (The pathway has been abbreviated for clarity.)

Example 6

[14C]-levormeloxifene (a partial estrogen agonist, used as an alternative to estro-gen replacement therapy) was administered to the rat, Cynomolgus monkey, and postmenopausal women.[43,44] The position of the 14C label was not stated. The six human volunteers were orally dosed 25 μCi (approximately 1 MBq) of radioactivity. Although not specifically stated, dosimetry studies would have been necessary to justify this dose in humans (Chapter 5, Appendix 1). The dose was administered as a 20-mL drinking solution. Oral administrations were also given to normal and bile duct-cannulated male and female rats, by gavage. One female rat was dosed into the stomach, with bile collected from another animal administered [14C]-levormelox-ifene. Male and female Cynomolgus monkeys were administered [14C]-levormelox-ifene by stomach tube. In all species, blood, urine and feces were collected (plus bile from bile duct-cannulated rats). All excreta were analyzed for total radioactivity by liquid scintillation counting.

Excreta samples for metabolite profiling were pooled by collection time. Plasma and feces were extracted using solid-phase columns (extraction efficiencies were not stated). Urine, bile and extracts of plasma and feces were analyzed with HPLC and LC-MS/MS.

The principal route of excretion in all species was *via* feces (>90%), with very little in the urine (approximately 1% for animal species and <5% for human). Elimination of radioactivity was more rapid in the male rat, with 84% excreted in the male over 48 h and 53% in the female over the same time. No sex difference

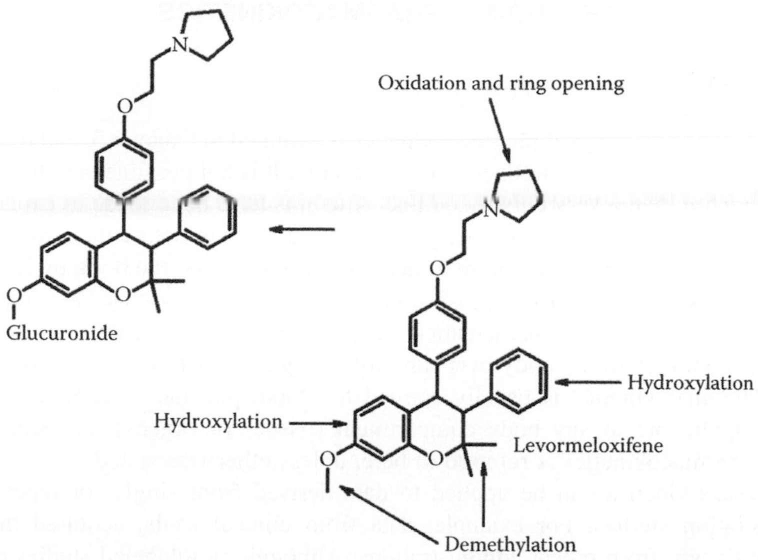

Figure 3.29 The metabolism of levormeloxifene. (The pathway has been abbreviated for clarity.)

in the rate of excretion was seen in the monkey, with 90% of the dose eliminated within 72 h.

Elimination of radioactivity in postmenopausal women was significantly slower than in the animal species, with 50% of the dose excreted after 15 days. Recoveries of radioactivity in the animal species were 92 to 100%. In the human volunteer study, however, the recovery was lower, at approximately 83%, probably due to the much longer collection periods (animals, 7 days; humans, up to 71 days).

In the bile duct-cannulated rat, between 16 and 35% of the administered dose was excreted in bile. Results from the rat administered bile from another animal dosed with [^{14}C]-levormeloxifene showed some uptake, and hence there may have been some enterohepatic recirculation, but the extent was not quantified.

The metabolic pathway for levormeloxifene is shown in Figure 3.29. Rat plasma contained mostly unchanged parent drug, whereas feces contained demethylated and ring hydroxylated products. Bile contained the glucuronide conjugate, which suggests that the glucuronide was hydrolyzed from the molecule in the GI tract, leaving the aglycones in feces. Some of the aglycones may have been reabsorbed to be reconjugated back to the glucuronide, which was the major component in the rat administered bile from a [^{14}C]-levormeloxifene dosed animal. Metabolism of levormeloxifene was similar in all three species, and the human, like the rat, contained mostly parent drug in the plasma. There is a statement in the paper that says, "The choice of the rat as a preclinical model for the clinical situation was fortuitous given the similarity of the metabolite profiles seen in the rat and the postmenopausal woman." Although, interestingly, the rat and monkey predicted the metabolism of levormeloxifene in the human, it did not predict the extended half-life (219 h) seen in the human volunteers.

APPENDIX 3: PHARMACOKINETICS

Introduction

A limited knowledge of pharmacokinetics is assumed in Chapter 3, and therefore some of the principles are outlined in this appendix. It is not possible here to provide anything more than a very cursory outline. Attempts have been made to explain the concepts of certain pharmacokinetic parameters rather than define them mathematically. If the reader requires a more in-depth knowledge, then the book by Rowland and Tozer[45] is an excellent source of information, as is the book by Dowden.[46]

Pharmacokinetics is a mathematical description of the concentration of a drug and its metabolites in the body over time following administration by a given dose route. Pharmacokinetics is usually applied to blood, plasma, or serum, but it is equally applicable to any body compartment (tissues or organs). For simplicity, plasma pharmacokinetics is referred to here, unless otherwise stated.

Pharmacokinetics can be applied to data derived from single- or repeat-dose administration studies. For example, data from clinical trials, acquired through bioanalysis, are from repeat administrations. Although radiolabeled studies can be performed using repeat-dose administrations, typically this is not for the study of pharmacokinetics *per se*. Here, therefore, we are only concerned with single-dose administrations. In addition, for simplicity, only oral and intravenous routes of administration are considered.

Figure 3.30 shows typical pharmacokinetic curves, where drug concentration on the y-axis is plotted against time on the x-axis. The oral dose shows an initial phase, where the drug is being absorbed, followed by an elimination phase. The intravenous dose, being introduced directly into the bloodstream, does not exhibit an absorption phase.

The subject of pharmacodynamics must not be forgotten. Pharmacodynamics is the study of the physiological or symptomatic effects of a drug over time. As an example, take a drug that inhibits a particular plasma enzyme. After dosing, the enzyme activity could be monitored in plasma over time and the degree of inhibition measured. Sometimes, however, it is more difficult to pin down a biochemical assay that is known to be mechanistically linked, and preferably unique, to the action of the drug. Monitoring symptoms is another way of measuring pharmacodynamic effects. An example might be a pain test vs. time after the administration of an analgesic. A pharmacodynamic effect that can be linked to the pharmacokinetics is obviously of great value. To use an example, consider an individual drinking alcohol at a party. The level of alcohol in the blood increasing as the evening continues and decreasing after bedtime is a measure of pharmacokinetics. Slurred speech and loss of balance would be a measure of pharmacodynamics. A relationship between the blood alcohol level and a symptomatic measure of inebriation would show that the absorption of alcohol was the likely cause of the physiological changes. Indeed, this is why law enforcement agencies are able to set limits for the concentration of blood alcohol for drivers.

The reader should be reminded that when pharmacokinetic calculations are applied to total radioactivity measurements, no distinction is being made between

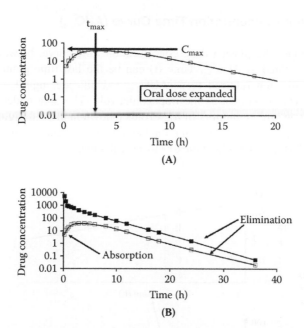

Figure 3.30 The bottom graph shows classical pharmacokinetic plots originating from an intravenous (■) and oral (□) dose. The upper graph is an expansion of the oral pharmacokinetic plot, demonstrating C_{max} and t_{max}.

drug and metabolites, and therefore interpretation of the data is limited. Pharmacokinetic calculations should be made based on a single compound, often the parent drug.

Time to Peak Maximum (t_{max})

The time at which the peak drug concentration in plasma (C_{max}) is reached is termed t_{max}. Strictly, t_{max} applies to an extravascular dose. Units of t_{max} are time, usually in hours.

Concentration at Peak Maximum (C_{max})

The maximum concentration in plasma a drug attains (i.e., the concentration at the t_{max}) is termed the C_{max}. Units are those of concentration, usually mg/L (= ng/mL).

Figure 3.30 illustrates t_{max} and C_{max}. Note that the x-axis (time) is linear and the y-axis (concentration) is logarithmic. Such log-linear or semi-log plots are the convention for pharmacokinetic plots. (The reason for this is that many drugs exhibit first-order kinetics, and therefore produce a straight line on a semi-log plot for the elimination phase.)

Area under the Concentration Time Curve (AUC$_{0-t}$)

The area under the plasma drug concentration time curve, between time zero and time t, is defined as AUC$_{0-t}$. Time (t) can be the last time point sampled (in which case it is often referred to as AUC$_{0-last}$). Units are mg·h/L. The AUC is calculated by what is known as the trapezoidal rule. The area under the curve is divided up into an infinite number of trapezoids (shown in gray in Figure 3.31). The sum of all the trapezoids then gives the total area under the curve (Figure 3.32). The calculation is performed mathematically using calculus.

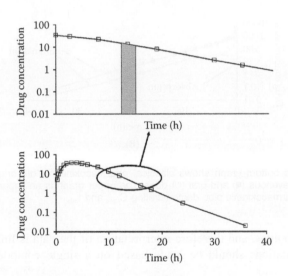

Figure 3.31 Calculation of AUC by the trapezoidal rule.

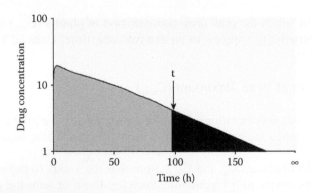

Figure 3.32 AUC$_{0-t}$ is defined by the gray area. AUC$_{0-\infty}$ is defined by the gray area + the black area. The black area expressed as a percentage of the black area + the gray area is the percent extrapolation.

Area under Curve, from Zero to Infinity ($AUC_{0-\infty}$)

$AUC_{0-\infty}$ is the area under the plasma drug concentration time curve, from time zero, extrapolated to infinity. As with AUC_{0-t}, units are mg·h/L.

Figure 3.32 illustrates AUC. The light gray area between 0 and time t represents AUC_{0-t}. The dark area represents $AUC_{t-\infty}$, so the sum of the light and dark gray areas represents $AUC_{0-\infty}$. The AUC is a measure of elimination and represents the total body burden of the drug. With an intravenous dose, it is assumed that the AUC (total amount eliminated) is equal to the amount administered.

Percentage Extrapolation

The percentage extrapolation is that necessary to derive $AUC_{0-\infty}$ from AUC_{0-t}. In Figure 3.32, it is the black area expressed as a percentage of the gray area plus the black area. The greater the extrapolation, the more questionable the $AUC_{0-\infty}$ value becomes. The ideal experiment will be conducted for a sufficient length of time so that the AUC_{0-t} is very close to the $AUC_{0-\infty}$. As a general rule, the degree of extrapolation should not be more than about 20%.

Calculation of the percentage extrapolation for the AUC based on total radioactivity can be used to assess how much of the drug and its metabolites have been eliminated during a metabolism study. For example, if the extrapolation is 5 to 10%, then the duration of the experiment was adequate. If the extrapolation is 20 to 30%, then the study perhaps should have been carried on for longer.

Absolute Bioavailability (F)

By definition, an intravenous dose introduces the drug directly into the bloodstream, and therefore there is no absorption phase. The AUC derived from an intravenous dose thus represents 100% of the dose. An extravascular dose, such as oral administration, however, may have a convoluted route before getting into systemic circulation. Indeed, not all of the dose may be absorbed, and a proportion of that part that is absorbed may be eliminated by first-pass metabolism (Sections 3.6.5 and 3.6.6). The AUC derived from the extravascular dose therefore represents that portion of the parent drug administered that reaches the systemic circulation. The amount of drug administered intravenously and extravascularly may not necessarily be the same, and so F is calculated from Equation 3.2, where iv is intravenous and ev is extravascular.

$$F = \left(\frac{AUC_{iv}}{AUC_{ev}} \right) \times \left(\frac{Dose_{ev}}{Dose_{iv}} \right) \tag{3.2}$$

Elimination Half-Life ($t_{1/2}$)

The elimination half-life is the time taken for the drug concentration in plasma to fall by one half. Elimination half-life is defined by the slope of the curve for the

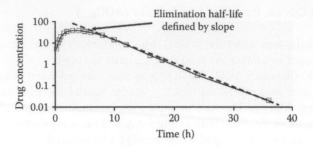

Figure 3.33 Half-life.

elimination phase (Figure 3.33). There are certain assumptions in this definition, in that the elimination phase is assumed to have first-order kinetics (i.e., the line is linear when displayed semi-logarithmically, as shown in Figure 3.33). This is not necessarily always the case, but this is outside the scope of this book.

Volume of Distribution (V)

The volume of distribution (V) is defined as the apparent volume of plasma required to account for a given concentration of drug once a distribution equilibrium has been achieved. Volume of distribution only applies to an intravenous dose. Volume of distribution is illustrated in Figure 3.34. In Figure 3.34A, 1 mg of a solute is dissolved in an unknown amount of solvent. A sample of the solution is taken, assayed, and found to have a concentration of 1 mg/L. Thus, the volume of the solvent was 1 L. In Figure 3.34B, the same situation occurs, except that the solvent contains an absorbing substance (represented by the black area) with an affinity for the solute. A proportion of the solute therefore binds to the absorbing substance and is removed from the solution. A sample of the solution is taken, assayed, and this time found to have a lower concentration of 0.1 mg/L. The apparent volume of distribution is therefore 10 L.

The volume of distribution is thus defined as the amount of drug in the body divided by the plasma drug concentration. For an intravenous dose, the amount in the body is the amount injected. The concentration of a drug in systemic circulation is heavily dependent upon how the drug is distributed in the body. If the drug is sequestered in a deep body compartment (e.g., fat), then the plasma concentration will diminish and the volume of distribution will rise. If the volume of distribution for a given drug is known, then the plasma concentration can be predicted from a given intravenous dose.

Clearance (Cl)

The clearance (Cl) of a drug is the volume of plasma from which the drug is completely and irreversibly removed per unit time. This parameter is calculated for an intravenous dose only.

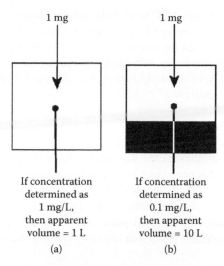

If concentration
determined as
1 mg/L,
then apparent
volume = 1 L

(a)

If concentration
determined as
0.1 mg/L,
then apparent
volume = 10 L

(b)

Figure 3.34   Schematic demonstrating the principle of volume of distribution.

The rate of elimination of a drug is the amount of drug removed per unit time. For example, if 1 mg of drug is removed per hour, then the elimination rate is 1 mg/h.

Clearance is the elimination rate divided by the plasma concentration. If the plasma concentration is expressed as mg/L, then mg/h (elimination) divided by mg/L (concentration) gives L/h, which are the units of clearance.

As an illustration, assume the blood flow through the liver is 90 L/h. If the liver contained a drug, one third of which was irreversibly removed by the 90 L of blood over 1 h, then the clearance would be 30 L/h.

Half-life, volume of distribution, and clearance are related as shown in Equation 3.3:

$$t_{1/2} = \frac{0.693 \times V}{Cl} \tag{3.3}$$

where $t_{1/2}$ is the half-life, V is the volume of distribution, and Cl is clearance.

Thus, a drug with a half-life of 2 h and a volume of distribution of 100 L will have the same clearance as a drug exhibiting a half-life of 4 h and a volume of distribution of 200 L, namely, 34.65 L/h.

Renal Clearance (Cl$_R$)

Renal clearance (Cl$_R$) is calculated from Equation 3.4:

$$CL_R = \text{amount of parent excreted in urine/plasma AUC} \tag{3.4}$$

All urine is collected for a specific period of time (typically five or six elimination half-lives for the drug). The total amount of parent drug is measured in the urine.

This is divided by the plasma AUC to give the renal clearance. There can be certain practical difficulties in measuring Cl_R, not least of which is the volume of urine that has to be collected to account for five or six elimination half-lives. In theory, biliary clearance can be calculated in the same way, except the parent drug is measured in bile rather than urine. Experimentally, however, collecting bile for a sufficient period of time is likely to be restrictive.

Mean Residence Time (MRT)

MRT, as its name implies, is the mean time that a drug resides in the body. A dose of drug consists of a very large number of molecules; for every millimole of drug, there are 6.03×10^{20} molecules (from Avogadro's number). Statistically, some of these molecules will be eliminated very rapidly, some will remain for a period of time and then will be eliminated, and some may remain for a lifetime. The average time a molecule resides in the body defines the MRT. It is calculated from Equation 3.5:

$$MRT = \frac{AUMC}{AUC} \tag{3.5}$$

The AUMC is the area under the first moment curve, which is the area under the concentration × time vs. time curve (Figure 3.35).

Allometric Scaling

Extrapolation of data from animals to man is not simply a matter of proportionality. A dose of 1 mg/Kg in a 250-g rat is not necessarily equivalent to a dose of 280 mg in a 70-Kg human. Extrapolation is carried out by a process known as allometric scaling. In a typical allometric scaling exercise, the body weight of the species is plotted against the pharmacokinetic parameter on a log-log scale. Some schools of thought believe that surface area is a better parameter than body weight. A typical example of allometric scaling is shown in Figure 3.36.

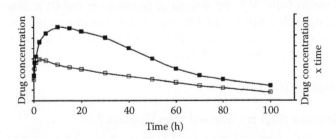

Figure 3.35   Drug concentration × time (■) and drug concentration (□) vs. time. The area under the drug concentration × time curve (AUMC) divided by the area under the drug concentration curve (AUC) gives the mean residence time (MRT).

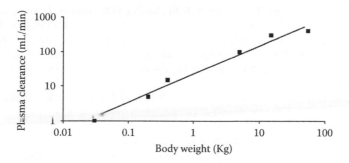

Figure 3.36 Pharmacokinetic parameter of clearance vs. body weight as an example of allometric scaling. Each datum point (■) represents a different species from, say, mouse at the far left to human at the far right.

ACKNOWLEDGMENTS

I thank Natasha Dow, Paul Dow, and Trevor Hardwick for their input and suggestions, and Sheila Nicholson for her proofreading.

REFERENCES

1. Raunio, H., Taavitsainen, P., Honkakoski, P., Juvonen, R., and Pelkonen, O., *In vitro* methods in the prediction of kinetics of drugs: focus on drug metabolism, *Altern. Lab. Anim.*, 32, 425–430, 2004.
2. Evans, G., *A Handbook of Bioanalysis and Drug Metabolism*, CRC Press, Boca Raton, FL, 2004.
3. Karyekar, C.S., Eddington, N.D., Garimella, T.S., Gubbins, P.O., and Dowling, T.C., Evaluation of P-glycoprotein-mediated renal drug interactions in an MDR1-MDCK model, *Pharmacotherapy*, 23, 436–442, 2003.
4. Le Ferrec, E., Chesne, C., Artusson, P., Brayden, D., Fabre, G., Gires, P., Guillou, F., Rousset, M., Rubas, W., and Scarino, M.L., *In vitro* models of the intestinal barrier. The report and recommendations of ECVAM Workshop 46. European Centre for the Validation of Alternative methods, *Altern. Lab. Anim.*, 296, 649–668, 2001.
5. Elsinga, P.H., Franssen, E.J., Hendrikse, N.H., Fluks, L., Weemaes, A.M., van der Graaf, W.T., de Vries, E.G., Visser, G.M., and Vaalburg, W., Carbon-11-labeled daunorubicin and verapamil for probing P-glycoprotein in tumors with PET, *J. Nucl. Med.*, 37, 1571–1575, 1996.
6. Petri, N., Tannergren, C., Rungstad, D., and Lennernas, H., Transport characteristics of fexofenadine in the Caco-2 cell model, *Pharm. Res.*, 21, 1398–1404, 2004.
7. Scott, R.C.A.C. and H.M., *In vitro* percutaneous absorption experiments: a guide to the technique for use in toxicology assessments, *Toxicol. Methods*, 2, 113–123, 1992.
8. Dierks, E.A., Stams, K.R., Lim, H.K., Cornelius, G., Zhang, H., and Ball, S.E., A method for the simultaneous evaluation of the activities of seven major human drug-metabolizing cytochrome P450s using an *in vitro* cocktail of probe substrates and fast gradient liquid chromatography tandem mass spectrometry, *Drug Metab. Dispos.*, 29, 23–29, 2001.

9. Madan, A., Graham, R.A., Carroll, K.M., Mudra, D.R., Burton, L.A., Krueger, L.A., Downey, A.D., Czerwinski, M., Forster, J., Ribadeneira, M.D., Gan, L.S., LeCluyse, E.L., Zech, K., Robertson, P., Jr., Koch, P., Antonian, L., Wagner, G., Yu, L., and Parkinson, A., Effects of prototypical microsomal enzyme inducers on cytochrome P450 expression in cultured human hepatocytes, *Drug Metab. Dispos.*, 31, 421–431, 2003.

10. Wang, E.J., Casciano, C.N., Clement, R.P., and Johnson, W.W., Inhibition of P-glycoprotein transport function by grapefruit juice psoralen, *Pharm. Res.*, 18, 432–438, 2001.

11. Mills, E., Montori, V.M., Wu, P., Gallicano, K., Clarke, M., and Guyatt, G., Interaction of St. John's wort with conventional drugs: systematic review of clinical trials, *BMJ*, 329, 27–30, 2004.

12. Lightfoot, T., Ellis, S.W., Mahling, J., Ackland, M.J., Blaney, F.E., Bijloo, G.J., De Groot, M.J., Vermeulen, N.P.E., Blackburn, G.M., Lennard, M.S., and Tucker, G.T., Regioselective hydroxylation of debrisoquine by cytochrome P4502D6: implications for active site modelling, *Xenobiotica*, 30, 219–233, 2000.

13. Sorgel, F., Naber, K.G., Kinzig, M., Mahr, G., and Muth, P., Comparative pharmacokinetics of ciprofloxacin and temafloxacin in humans: a review, *Am. J. Med.*, 91, 51S–66S, 1991.

14. Gurney, H., Defining the starting dose: should it be based on mg/kg, mg/m² or fixed?, in *Handbook of Anticancer Pharmacokinetics and Pharmacodynamics*, Figg, D.W. and McLeod, H.L., Eds., Humana Press, NJ, 2004.

15. Diehl, K.H., Hull, R., Morton, D., Pfister, R., Rabemampianina, Y., Smith, D., Vidal, J.M., and van de Vorstenbosch, C., A good practice guide to the administration of substances and removal of blood, including routes and volumes, *J. Appl. Toxicol.*, 21, 15–23, 2001.

16. Renton, K.W., Cytochrome P450 regulation and drug biotransformation during inflammation and infection, *Curr. Drug Metab.*, 5, 235–243, 2004.

17. Diehl, K.H., Hull, R., Morton, D., Pfister, R., Rabemampianina, Y., Smith, D., Vidal, J.M., and van de Vorstenbosch, C., A good practice guide to the administration of substances and removal of blood, including routes and volumes, *J. Appl. Toxicol.*, 21, 15–23, 2001.

18. Lehmann, W.D., Fischer, R., Heinrich, H.C., Clemens, P., and Gruttner, R., Metabolic conversion of L-[U-14C]phenylalanine to respiratory 14CO2 in healthy subjects, phenylketonuria heterozygotes and classic phenylketonurics, *Clin. Chim. Acta*, 157, 253–266, 1986.

19. Scarfe, G.B., Wright, B., Clayton, E., Taylor, S., Wilson, I.D., Lindon, J.C., and Nicholson, J.K., 19F-NMR and directly coupled HPLC-NMR-MS investigations into the metabolism of 2-bromo-4-trifluoromethylaniline in rat: a urinary excretion balance study without the use of radiolabelling, *Xenobiotica*, 28, 373–388, 1998.

20. Dear, G.J., Ismail, I.M., Mutch, P.J., Plumb, R.S., Davies, L.H., and Sweatman, B.C., Urinary metabolites of a novel xuinoxaline non-nucleoside reverse transcriptase inhibitor in rabbit, mouse and human: identification of fluorine NIH shift metabolites using NMR and tandem MS, *Xenobiotica*, 30, 407–426, 2000.

21. Lindon, J.C., Bailey, N.J.C., Nicholson, K., and Wilson, I.D., Biomedical applications of directly coupled chromatography-nuclear magnetic resonance (NMR) spectroscopy and mass spectroscopy (MS), in *Handbook of Analytical Separations*, Wilson, I.D., Ed., Elsevier Sciences, Amsterdam, 2003, pp. 293–329.

22. Caster, W.O., Poncelet, J., Simon, A.B., and Armstrong, W.D., Tissue weights of the rat. I. Normal values determined by dissection and chemical methods, *Proc. Soc. Exp. Med.*, 91, 122–126, 1956.

23. Miranda, J.J., Highly reactive cysteine residues in rodent hemoglobins, *Biochem. Biophys. Res. Commun.*, 275, 517–523, 2000.

24. Clark, A.G., Hirom, P.C., Millburn, P., Smith, R.L., and Williams, R.T., Reabsorption from the biliary system as a factor influencing the biliary excretion of organic anions, *Biochem. J.*, 115, 62P, 1969.

25. Hirom, P.C., Millburn, P., Smith, R.L., and Williams, R.T., Species variations in the threshold molecular-weight factor for the biliary excretion of organic anions, *Biochem. J.*, 129, 1071–1077, 1972.

26. Colburn, W.A., Hirom, P.C., Parker, R.J., and Milburn, P., A pharmacokinetic model for enterohepatic recirculation in the rat: phenolphthalein, a model drug, *Drug Metab. Dispos.*, 7, 100–102, 1979.

27. Ouellet, D.M. and Pollack, G.M., Biliary excretion and enterohepatic recirculation of morphine-3-glucuronide in rats, *Drug Metab. Dispos.*, 23, 478–484, 1995.

28. Kalgutkar, A.S. and Soglia, J.R., Minimising the potential for metabolite activation in drug discovery, *Expert Opin. Drug Metab. Toxicol.*, 1, 91–142, 2005.

29. Cornish-Bowden, A., Cardenas, M.L., Letelier, J.C., Soto-Andrade, J., and Abarzua, F.G., Understanding the parts in terms of the whole, *Biol. Cell*, 96, 713–717, 2004.

30. Parkinson, A., Biotransformation of xenobiotics, in *Casarett and Doull's Toxicology: The Basic Science of Poisons*, 6 ed., Klaassen, C.D., Ed., McGraw-Hill, New York, 2001.

31. Gibson, G.A. and Skett, P., *Introduction to Drug Metabolism*, 3rd ed., Nelsom Thornes, 2001.

32. Nelson, D.R., Koymans, L., Kamataki, T., Stegeman, J.J., Feyereisen, R., Waxman, D.J., Waterman, M.R., Gotoh, O., Coon, M.J., Estabrook, R.W., Gunsalus, I.C., and Nebert, D.W., P450 superfamily: update on new sequences, gene mapping, accession numbers and nomenclature, *Pharmacogenetics*, 6, 1–42, 1996.

33. Denisov, I.G., Makris, T.M., Sligar, S.G., and Schlichting, I., Structure and chemistry of cytochrome P450, *Chem. Rev.*, 105, 2253–2277, 2005.

34. Huskey, S.W., Doss, G.A., Miller, R.R., Schoen, W.R., and Chiu, S.H., N-glucuronidation reactions. II. Relative N-glucuronidation reactivity of methylbiphenyl tetrazole, methylbiphenyl triazole, and methylbiphenyl imidazole in rat, monkey, and human hepatic microsomes, *Drug Metab. Dispos.*, 22, 651–658, 1994.

35. Cupid, B.C., Beddell, C.R., Lindon, J.C., Wilson, I.D., and Nicholson, J.K., Quantitative structure-metabolism relationships for substituted benzoic acids in the rabbit: prediction of urinary excretion of glycine and glucuronide conjugates, *Xenobiotica*, 26, 157–176, 1996.

36. Cupid, B.C., Holmes, E., Wilson, I.D., Lindon, J.C., and Nicholson, J.K., Quantitative structure-metabolism relationships (QSMR) using computational chemistry: pattern recognition analysis and statistical prediction of phase II conjugation reactions of substituted benzoic acids in the rat, *Xenobiotica*, 29, 27–42, 1999.

37. Mason, J.P., Caldwell, J., and Dring, L.G., Metabolism of [propyl-3H]-8-hydroxy-2-(N,N-di-n-propylamino)tetralin in the rat, *Xenobiotica*, 25, 71–80, 1995.

38. Wu, W.N., McKown, L.A., Takacs, A.R., Jones, W.J., and Reitz, A.B., Biotransformation of the antipsychotic agent, mazapertine, in dog: mass spectral characterization and identification of metabolites, *Xenobiotica*, 29, 453–466, 1999.

39. Wild, M.J., McKillop, D., and Butters, C.J., Determination of the human cytochrome P450 isoforms involved in the metabolism of zolmitriptan, *Xenobiotica*, 29, 847–857, 1999.
40. Schmid, J., Busch, U., Trummlitz, G., Prox, A., Kaschke, S., and Wachsmuth, H., Meloxicam: metabolic profile and biotransformation products in the rat, *Xenobiotica*, 25, 1219–1236, 1995.
41. Eriksson, B., Hallstrom, G., Ottersgard Brorsson, A.K., Svensson, L., and Gunnarsson, P.O., Metabolic fate of delmopinol in man after mouth rinsing and after oral administration, *Xenobiotica*, 30, 179–192, 2000.
42. Eriksson, B., Ottersgard Brorsson, A.K., Hallstrom, G., Sjodin, T., and Gunnarsson, P.O., Pharmacokinetics of 14C-delmopinol in the healthy male volunteer, *Xenobiotica*, 28, 1075–1081, 1998.
43. Mountfield, R.J., Kiehr, B., and John, B.A., Metabolism, disposition, excretion, and pharmacokinetics of levormeloxifene, a selective estrogen receptor modulator, in the rat, *Drug Metab. Dispos.*, 28, 503–513, 2000.
44. Mountfield, R.J., Panduro, A.M., Wassmann, O., Thompson, M., John, B., and van der Merbel, N., Metabolism of levormeloxifene, a selective oestrogen receptor modulator, in the Sprague-Dawley rat, Cynomolgus monkey and postmenopausal woman, *Xenobiotica*, 30, 201–217, 2000.
45. Rowland, M. and Tozer, T.N., *Clinical Pharmacokinetics, Concepts and Applications*, Lippincott, Williams & Wilkins, Philadelphia, 1995.
46. Dowden, J.S., *Pharmacokinetics Made Easy*, McGraw-Hill, New South Wales, Australia, 2004.

CHAPTER 4

DNA Binding, Isotope Dilution, and Other Uses of Radiotracers

Graham Lappin

CONTENTS

4.1 INTRODUCTION

The majority of pharmaceuticals will have a least some metabolism and pharmacokinetic data submitted as part of the regulatory submission. The ADME studies (Chapter 3) are routine for new chemical entities (NCEs), and they are very likely to utilize radiotracers. The registration of biologicals also requires some pharmacokinetic data, but the use of radiotracers may not necessarily be routine. There are a number of other areas where radiotracers might be employed; these investigations are not conducted with every drug and may only be carried out if absolutely neces-sary. This chapter discusses these occasional study types, which consist primarily of DNA binding and metabolic turnover.

4.2 DNA BINDING

Some drugs, such as those used to treat cancer, are designed to be cytotoxic and may well exert their action by binding to DNA. For other drugs, cytotoxicity is an undesirable property and macromolecular binding, particularly to DNA, is unwanted. Suspicion that a drug may bind to DNA is usually raised from the results of toxicity tests, but standard toxicity studies are more concerned with symptomatic endpoints, rather than mechanisms of action. If a drug is suspected of binding to DNA, then a specific DNA binding study may be required.

The basic protocol of a DNA binding study is to administer the radiolabeled drug to a test system, allow time for binding to occur, extract and purify the DNA, and analyze for radioactivity. The test system can be an animal model, an *in vitro* system (Section 3.4.3), or isolated DNA. It has even been possible to conduct DNA binding studies in humans (Section 10.7). DNA binding studies are generally unpop-ular with the pharmaceuticals industry, as it is difficult to prove a negative result. Usually at best "no evidence for DNA binding" can be found. A positive result may well be fatal to the further development of the compound.

4.2.1　Radiotracer

In theory there is no restriction on the choice of radioisotope (Section 3.2). Tritium can be used *in vitro*, but any degree of tritium exchange *in vivo* makes quantification difficult (Section 3.2.1). For *in vivo* studies, the highest possible specific activity should be used, as there are potentially huge dilution effects from dosing to analysis of the purified DNA. The ability to detect what may be small amounts of radioactivity in the DNA is one of the limiting factors in the design of DNA binding studies, and ultrasensitive analytical methods such as accelerator mass spectrometry (AMS; Chapter 10) may be necessary.

Radioisotopes with relatively short half-lives have the advantage of higher spe-cific activities at the start of the experiment, but DNA binding studies can be prolonged and isotopes with short half-lives may have undergone significant decay by the end of the experiment. ^{14}C remains the most popular isotope for DNA binding studies, although the possibility of natural incorporation into DNA has to be con-sidered. The use of ^{35}S, where possible, may seem a better choice because of the high maximum specific activity and the fact that DNA does not contain sulfur, and therefore there is no danger of natural incorporation. The half-life of ^{35}S, however, is only 85 days (also see Section 4.2.3).

4.2.2 Dose Administration and Test System

Doses are administered to the test system in the same way as described for drug metabolism studies (Section 3.4.2 and Section 3.5.2 to Section 3.5.4). *In vitro* systems can be isolated DNA, often used as a general screen. Incubations with isolated DNA should be carried out in both the absence and presence of S9 (Section 3.4.4), as it may be a metabolite of the drug that binds. The most commonly used animal model for DNA binding studies is the mouse, although other species have been used, depending upon the specific circumstances of the drug. DNA binding studies have also been conducted with humans, but these types of studies, at least currently, are somewhat specialized (Section 10.7).

For *in vivo* studies in particular, there are two variables in the study design that have to be considered carefully: the choice of tissues for analysis and the time from dosing to sample collection. Tissues usually include liver and any susceptible organs, identified in the pathology. The optimum sample collection time is a balance between allowing enough time for the compound to bind to DNA and not allowing sufficient time for DNA repair processes to remove potential adducts. Moreover, the optimum time may be different for different organs, depending upon the time it takes for the drug to penetrate (for example, liver compared to bone marrow). Usually, therefore, a range of sampling times are taken, typically 2, 6, 12, and 24 h. It is important to consider any other data in the choice of sampling times, such as quantitative whole-body autoradiography (Chapter 5), which may give information on the rate of organ penetration.

4.2.3 DNA Extraction and Purification

There are a number of methods for the extraction and purification of DNA. The traditional methods go back more than 40 years and involve phenol extraction[1–3] and are still used today.[4] More modern methods use more benign reagents, such as Tris-EDTA (TE), PrepMan Ultra, sodium dodecyl sulfate (SDS) buffers, and Qiagen systems.[5] Irrespective of the extraction method, the DNA is typically treated with proteinase-K to remove protein and RNase to remove RNA. The isolated DNA is further purified using proprietary systems (e.g., Qiagen), hydroxyapatite chromatography,[6] or buoyant density centrifugation.[7,8] As can be seen from the references sited, some of these methods were first developed a number of years ago.

The purity of the DNA is very important, as impure DNA may lead to artifacts in the interpretation. The biggest concern is contamination with protein. The drug may well bind heavily to protein but not to DNA, and so any protein contamination may be incorrectly interpreted as DNA binding. The problem of protein contamination is exemplified in a study where ^{35}S was used as the radioisotope. DNA does not contain sulfur, but the DNA in this study, even though purified on cesium chloride density gradients, contained sufficient amounts of contaminating protein to produce a false positive result.[9] If radioactivity is found to be associated with DNA, then the DNA should be hydrolyzed to individual bases and analyzed chromatographically in an attempt to identify the adduct (Section 4.2.6).

4.2.4 DNA Analysis

The isolated DNA should be assayed for protein using a suitably sensitive technique such as Coomasie Blue.[10] It should be borne in mind that any amount of contaminating protein may lead to a false positive at levels well below the capabilities of most protein assays. If *any* protein is detected, then the DNA requires repurification. If possible, the DNA should be continuously purified to a constant specific activity, but this is rarely possible due to the small amounts of sample. The purity of the DNA can be assayed by measuring the ultraviolet (UV) spectrum and determining the absorbance at 260, 280, and 325 nm. An absorbance ratio ($A_{260/280nm}$) between 1.7 and 1.9 is indicative of pure DNA. Measuring the absorbance at 325 nm is useful, as absorbance at this wavelength is indicative of particulates. An absorbance of 1 AU is equal to a concentration of 50 μg DNA/mL.

The purified DNA is then analyzed for radioactivity using either liquid scintillation counting (Chapter 6) or AMS (Chapter 10). Bear in mind that although the UV assay is not destructive, the addition of Coomasie Blue and liquid scintillation fluid are, and so the limits of the assay may be determined by the amount of DNA available.

4.2.5 Calculation of DNA Binding

Assuming radioactivity is detected in the DNA, then the degree of binding is expressed in terms of the number of adducts per number of DNA bases (usually the number of adducts per 10^6 nucleotides*). The covalent binding index (CBI) is also sometimes used, which is defined as the number of adducts per 10^6 nucleotides based on a theoretical dose of 1 mmol/Kg.[11] The degree of binding is calculated from the number of moles of adduct bound to the number of moles of DNA. The number of moles of adduct is calculated from the amount of radioactivity and the specific activity of the compound dosed. For example, assume that a ^{14}C-labeled compound with a specific activity of 2 GBq/mmol was administered (equivalent to 1.2×10^{11} dpm/mmol; see Section 2.8) and a sample of 1 mg of DNA was analyzed and found to contain 500 dpm. Then 1 mg of DNA would contain $500/(1.2 \times 10^{11})$ mmol of adduct ($= 4.2 \times 10^{-9}$ mmol adduct per 1 mg of DNA). The 1 mg of DNA has to be expressed in millimoles, but what is the molecular weight of DNA? Figure 4.1 shows the structure of single-stranded DNA, containing a single residue of each of the four nucleotides. The molecular weight of the molecule shown in Figure 4.1 is 1236. Since there are four nucleotides, then the average molecular weight of a nucleotide is 309. Since binding is based upon the number of adducts per nucleotide, 309 is used as the molecular weight in the calculations. (A value of 309 g to 1 mol of DNA is also used by Lutz in the original paper describing CBI.[11]) In our example, 1 mg of DNA will therefore

---

* The nomenclature can be a little confusing. A *nucleotide* is a base with a sugar (ribose or deoxyribose) and phosphoric acid. The nucleotides are adenine, guanine, cytosine, uracil, and thymine. A *nucleoside* is a base with a sugar (ribose or deoxyribose) but without the phosphoric acid. The nucleosides are adenosine, guanosine, cytidine, and uridine (RNA, containing ribose); and deoxyadenosine, deoxyguanosine, deoxycytidine, and thymidine (DNA, containing deoxyribose).

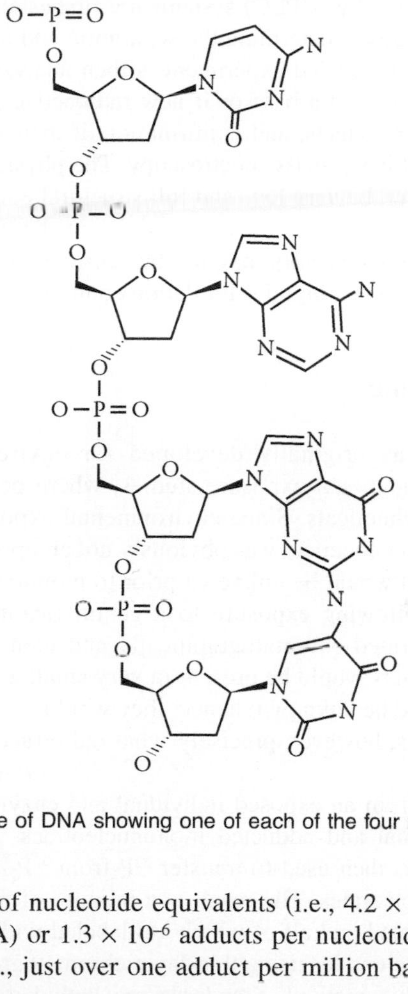

Figure 4.1   The structure of DNA showing one of each of the four nucleotides.

contain 0.0032 mmol of nucleotide equivalents (i.e., 4.2×10^{-9} mmol of adducts per 0.0032 mmol DNA) or 1.3×10^{-6} adducts per nucleotide (7.7×10^{-5} adducts per 10^6 nucleotides i.e., just over one adduct per million bases).

4.2.6   Identification of Adducts

If radioactivity is detected in the isolated DNA, there is always the possibility that it is due to an artifact such as contamination with protein. As was explained in Section 3.6.3, detection of radioactivity only confirms the presence of the radioisotope introduced into the experiment; it gives no intrinsic information as to its chemical nature. There is also the possibility that the radiolabel from the compound under study entered the general metabolism of the organism and was incorporated into the structure of DNA itself. Such natural incorporation then leads to the labeling of the DNA, although no adducts are formed.

Further information can be obtained by hydrolyzing the DNA (with acid or enzymically) and analyzing the nucleotides, nucleosides, or individual bases with radiochromatography (individual bases are more common). Suitable high-perfor-

mance liquid chromatography (HPLC) systems are first established using commercially available DNA bases to determine the separation and retention times. Hydrolyzed DNA from the radiolabeled experiment is then analyzed to see either if any
radioactive peaks coelute with a base or if new radioactive peaks are seen.[12] New
peaks are candidates for adducts, and confirmation of their structural identity can,
in theory, be carried out using mass spectroscopy. The physical amount of base per
HPLC peak can, however, be very low, and full structural elucidation is likely to be
challenging. In addition, the levels of radioactivity in the chromatographic peaks
can be very low, and flow detectors may not be sensitive enough, therefore necessitating fraction collection and liquid scintillation counting (Section 6.14.1) or AMS
analysis (Chapter 10).

4.2.7 ^{32}P-Postlabeling

^{32}P-postlabeling was originally developed for environmental monitoring,
mainly as part of occupational exposure studies, where people were exposed to
potentially genotoxic chemicals. Since environmental exposure was the concern,
radiolabeling the suspect chemical was obviously not an option (indeed, the nature
of the suspect chemical would be unknown prior to monitoring). If covalent DNA
adducts are formed following exposure to a genotoxicant, then in theory such
adducts could be separated chromatographically and identified. The problem is,
of course, that the adducts would be present in very small amounts and the precise
chemical identity would be unknown; hence, they would be very difficult to locate.
This type of problem is, however, precisely what radiotracer techniques are good
at solving.

DNA is extracted from an exposed individual and enzymically digested to the
3'-phosphorylated normal and adducted mononucleotides. An enzyme called T4
polynucleotide kinase is then used to transfer ^{32}P from ^{32}P-ATP to the 5'-hydroxyl
groups of the mononucleotides. The result is a mixture of mononucleotides, some
of which may be adducted and all of which are labeled with ^{32}P. The next stage is
to separate the mononucleotides using thin-layer chromatography (TLC) or another
suitable chromatographic method. Standards are included to locate the normal,
unadducted nucleotides. Areas on the chromatographic separation that are labeled
with ^{32}P but do not match the naturally occurring mononucleotide are candidates
for DNA adducts.[13,14]

The same method can be used by administering to animals the suspect genotoxicant, extracting DNA, and conducting the ^{32}P-postlabeling assay. This has the
advantage that the suspect genotoxicant does not have to be radiolabeled. ^{32}P-
postlabeling is sensitive and can measure to about one adduct in 10^9 bases. Once
located, adducts have been identified using mass spectrometry,[15] but on the whole,
this can be very difficult. The assay has been criticized for both false positives
and false negatives, but it nevertheless remains a useful research tool. Moreover,
it suffers from the same dilemma as any DNA binding study in that a negative is
difficult to prove.[16]

4.3 RADIOIMMUNOASSAY

Radioimmunoassays (RIAs) are an analytical method for quantifying an amount of drug in a biological matrix, typically serum. They are normally applicable to the measurement of therapeutic proteins (i.e., large molecules such as proteins). RIAs have mostly been replaced with enzyme-linked immunosorbent assay (ELISA), and so they will only be covered briefly.

The analyte can be any substance with antigenic properties; that is, it will illicit an immune response, stimulating the production of an antibody. The antibody is typically raised in an animal (e.g., rabbit) exposed to the analyte (antigen). In the RIA, samples containing the analyte are mixed with the antibody and binding occurs. Assuming the antibody is added in excess, then in theory all of the analyte will bind and a number of binding sites in the antibody will remain unbound. The analyte, suitably labeled, is then added and the remainder of the binding sites on the antibody are filled. By measuring the bound radioactivity, the amount of analyte can be quantified.

Because antigen–antibody binding may not be complete, standard curves have to be generated and the analyte quantified from them. The usual method of labeling the analyte is by iodination (Section 2.12.3).

As with any immunoassay, there is the possibility of cross talk, where the antibody binds ligands other than the one of interest.

4.4 GEL BLOTTING

Gel blotting is a technique for visualizing particular macromolecules, such as DNA, RNA, or protein. There are three types of blot: Western, Northern, and Southern (there is no Eastern blot). The technique was developed by E.M. Southern in the 1970s, and hence the Southern blot was named after him. In the Southern blot technique, DNA is first separated, typically by gel electrophoresis. A membrane made of nylon or nitrocellulose is laid over the gel, which has the property of binding to the DNA fragments. The membrane is washed and the DNA fragments fixed by exposure to UV light. DNA fragments are synthesized as a complementary sequence to the one of interest. These synthetic fragments are then labeled and used as probes. The label can be a radiolabel, but it can also be fluorescent, etc. If the membrane contains the target DNA sequence, then the probe will bind and can be visualized.

If RNA is detected instead of DNA, this then becomes the Northern blot. The technique was modified for the detection of protein (Western blot) using an antibody, as opposed to a DNA probe.

4.5 ISOTOPE DILUTION

The amount of body water in animals can be measured by isotopic dilution methods. The technique uses water, which can be labeled with ^3H or a stable isotope such as ^2H or ^{18}O, although radioactive isotopes make the measurement easier. If

tritium is used, then a given number of moles of ^3H water, at a defined specific
activity, are administered. A short time later (to allow for distribution in the body),
a blood sample is taken and (1) the number of moles of water are measured (e.g.,
comparison of wet and dry weight) and (2) the level of radioactivity is measured.
The amount of water in the body is then calculated by Equation 4.1:

$$B = M \times \frac{S_d}{S_s} \tag{4.1}$$

where B is the amount of water in the body (in mol), M is the number of moles
administered, S_d is the specific activity of ^3H_2O dosed, and S_s is the specific activity
of the water in the sample.

The same basic principles can be used to determine the amount of any endogenous substance in the body. Certain drugs are found naturally in the body. For
example, some monoclonal proteins are genetically engineered from human origins.
When such drugs are administered, they mix with the constitutive pools within the
body.

Mammalian homeostasis is remarkably efficient at maintaining the systemic
concentrations of certain constitutive compounds. For example, normal blood glucose levels are tightly maintained around 4 to 8 mmol/L. Maintenance of the normal
blood glucose concentration is a result of an equilibrium between the amount made
by the body (input) and the amount used by the body (output). This is illustrated in
Figure 4.2A, where the input equals the output, and so the body pool (represented
by the square) remains constant. In Figure 4.2B, the body pool is the same as in
case A, but the input has increased, which is balanced by an equivalent increase in
output. In other words, the metabolic turnover illustrated in Figure 4.2B is higher
than that in Figure 4.2A. This would not, however, be apparent from merely measuring the concentrations of A and B.

In some cases of metabolic disease, the levels of constitute metabolites can rise
or fall markedly. Figure 4.2C illustrates a situation where the input to a metabolic
pool has dropped and the output has increased. The size of the pool has therefore
diminished. The converse is also possible, as shown in Figure 4.2D, where the pool
size has increased due to a higher input than output. By simply measuring the pool
size of C and D, however, one cannot tell if an increase or decrease is caused by a
change in input or a change in output (or indeed, a shift in equilibrium due to a
change in both).

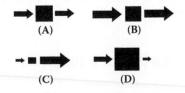

Figure 4.2   An illustration of metabolic turnover. For A to D, see text.

Turnover can be measured using radiotracers. A known amount of radiotracer, with a certain specific activity, is administered. Samples are taken over time. As the tracer enters the pool, it becomes isoptopically diluted (in the same way as described above for water). The degree of dilution over time is a measure of turnover.

There are three main parameters used to describe turnover: turnover rate, fractional turnover rate and turnover time.

The turnover rate is measured in terms of mass of drug per time (e.g., mg/h). This does imply that the input and output are in equilibrium (i.e., the substance being measured is in the steady state).

The fractional turnover rate relates the turnover rate to the size of the pool and is calculated from Equation 4.2:

$$K_t = \frac{R_t}{A_{ss}} \qquad (4.2)$$

where K_t is the fractional turnover time, R_t is the turnover rate, and A_{ss} is the amount of drug in the body at steady state. K_t is measured in units of time.

Another measure of turnover is the turnover time (t_t), which is the time taken to theoretically renew the entire metabolic pool. It is calculated using Equation 4.3:

$$t_t = \frac{A_{ss}}{R_t} \qquad (4.3)$$

where A_{ss} is the amount of drug in the body at steady state and R_t is the rate of turnover (mg/h).

Providing certain conditions are met, then the turnover time equals the mean residence time (MRT; see Chapter 3, Appendix 3). MRT is measured by the administration of a bolus intravenous dose. When a bolus dose is administered, the volume in which the drug distributes is known as the initial dilution volume. For MRT to be the same as the turnover time, it is assumed that both the input and output from the pool occur in the initial dilution volume.

4.6 MISCELLANEOUS USES

Radiotracers can be used in any situation where there is a need to follow the fate of, or track, a molecule in a biological system. Radiotracers have been used in enzyme assays, investigation into cell uptake, cell transporters, and a host of other applications. The author conducted experiments, for example, where following the administration of a $[^{14}C]$-drug, white blood cells were separated into individual cell types with an automated cell sorter and the levels of radioactive uptake in each cell type were then measured. A variety of isotopes are available, for example, ^{59}Fe for erythrocyte labeling.[17] Radioisotopes have a diversity of applications and their use is limited only by the imagination.

REFERENCES

1. Kirby, K.S., Isolation of deoxyribonucleic acid and ribosomal ribonucleic acid from *Escherichia coli*, *Biochem. J.*, 93, 5C–6C, 1964.
2. Kirby, K.S. and Cook, E.A., Isolation of deoxyribonucleic acid from mammalian tissues, *Biochem. J.*, 104, 254–257, 1967.
3. Kirby, K.S., Fox-Carter, E., and Guest, M., Isolation of deoxyribonucleic acid and ribosomal ribonucleic acid from bacteria, *Biochem. J.*, 104, 258–262, 1967.
4. Shimelis, O., Zhou, X., Li, G., and Giese, R.W., Phenolic extraction of DNA from mammalian tissues and conversion to deoxyribonucleoside-5'-monophosphates devoid of ribonucleotides, *J. Chromatogr. A*, 1053, 143–149, 2004.
5. Aldous, W.K., Pounder, J.I., Cloud, J.L., and Woods, G.L., Comparison of six methods of extracting *Mycobacterium tuberculosis* DNA from processed sputum for testing by quantitative real-time PCR, *J. Clin. Microbiol.*, 43, 2471–2473, 2005.
6. Markov, G.G. and Ivanov, I.G., Hydroxyapatite column chromatography in procedures for isolation of purified DNA, *Anal. Biochem.*, 59, 555–563, 1974.
7. Luk, D.C. and Bick, M.D., Determination of 5'-bromodeoxyuridine in DNA by buoyant density, *Anal. Biochem.*, 77, 346–349, 1977.
8. Tatti, K.M., Hudspeth, M.E., Johnson, P.H., and Grossman, L.I., Enhancement of buoyant separations between DNA's in preparative CsCl gradients containing distamycin A or netropsin, *Anal. Biochem.*, 89, 561–571, 1978.
9. Provan, W.M., Eyton-Jones, H., Lappin, G., Pritchard, D., Moore, R.B., and Green, T., The incorporation of radiolabelled sulphur from captan into protein and its impact on a DNA binding study, *Chem. Biol. Interact.*, 96, 173–184, 1995.
10. Bradford, M.M., A rapid and sensitive method for the quantitation of microgram quantities of protein utilizing the principle of protein-dye binding, *Anal. Biochem.*, 72, 248–254, 1976.
11. Lutz, W.K., *In vivo* covalent binding of organic chemicals to DNA as a quantitative indicator in the process of chemical carcinogenesis, *Mutat. Res.*, 65, 289–356, 1979.
12. Bolt, H.M. and Jelitto, B., Biological formation of the 1,3-butadiene DNA adducts 7-N-(2-hydroxy-3-buten-1-yl)guanine, 7-N-(1-hydroxy-3-buten-2-yl)guanine and 7-N-(2,3,4-trihydroxy-butyl)guanine, *Toxicology*, 113, 328–330, 1996.
13. Randerath, K., Reddy, M.V., and Gupta, R.C., 32P-labeling test for DNA damage, *Proc. Natl. Acad. Sci. U.S.A.*, 78, 6126–6129, 1981.
14. Reddy, M.V. and Randerath, K., Nuclease P1-mediated enhancement of sensitivity of 32P-postlabeling test for structurally diverse DNA adducts, *Carcinogenesis*, 7, 1543–1551, 1986.
15. Singh, R., Sweetman, G.M., Farmer, P.B., Shuker, D.E., and Rich, K.J., Detection and characterization of two major ethylated deoxyguanosine adducts by high performance liquid chromatography, electrospray mass spectrometry, and 32P-postlabeling. Development of an approach for detection of phosphotriesters, *Chem. Res. Toxicol.*, 10, 70–77, 1997.
16. Carmichael, P.L., Sardar, S., Crooks, N., Neven, P., Van Hoof, I., Ugwumadu, A., Bourne, T., Tomas, E., Hellberg, P., Hewer, A.J., and Phillips, D.H., Lack of evidence from HPLC 32P-post-labelling for tamoxifen-DNA adducts in the human endometrium, *Carcinogenesis*, 20, 339–342, 1999.
17. Edelson, J. and Douglas, J.F., Measurement of gastrointestinal blood loss in the rat: the effect of aspirin, phenylbutazone and seclazone, *J. Pharmacol. Exp. Ther.*, 184, 449–452, 1973.

CHAPTER 5

Quantitative Whole-Body Autoradiography (QWBA)

Brian Whitby

CONTENTS

5.1 INTRODUCTION

Part of the regulatory process in the safety testing and development of a new pharmaceutical requires the study of the distribution of the drug and its metabolites into the tissues of experimental animals. The experimental methods employed generally utilize radiolabeled test substances, which can be accurately traced and measured. Quantitative whole-body autoradiography (QWBA) is one such powerful analytical tool, and over the last few years, the QWBA technique has become the preferred research instrument for studying such distribution. Earlier and alternative methods relied upon dissection of tissues and subsequent radioanalysis of the samples. These methods are very labor-intensive and only allow measurement of radioactivity in whole organs. In addition, the processing of many tissues is required, as there is no indication of their radioactive content until analysis is complete, even though a large proportion of them may contain little or no drug-related material.

The QWBA technique relies on the preparation of images showing the distribution of radioactivity in the whole animal, followed by accurate measurement using computer-based image analysis techniques. Not only can relevant tissues be selected for measurement by this technique, but the distribution of drug-related material can be studied at the sub-organ level. On a cautionary note, it must be remembered that it is the distribution of radioactivity that is being studied in these experiments, and not the fate of the drug, as administered. Although the parent drug may constitute some of the radioactivity measured, it is probable that radiolabeled metabolites will also be present, in unknown amounts. Separation and evaluation of this possibly complex mix of parent compound and metabolites can only be performed by other analytical means (e.g., extraction followed by high-performance liquid chromatography or mass spectrometry).

5.2 PRINCIPLES AND HISTORY OF QWBA

In its most basic form, autoradiography refers to the localization within a solid specimen of radioactivity, by placing the specimen against a detection matrix. In practice, this relates to the capture of radiation energy emanating from a specimen by the detection matrix and the conversion of this stored (or latent) energy into a visible image. Historically, photographic emulsions or films were extensively used, whereby the radiation changes the nature of silver halides in the emulsion to metallic silver (the latent image). The latent image can then be amplified by development, and unexposed crystals are removed by dissolution in the fixer. Film technology was used for many decades in the production of autoradiograms, but has now been largely superseded by phosphor screen technologies, sometimes known as radioluminography. The latter will be dealt with in more detail later in this chapter.

The first records relating to the use of autoradiography date back to the late 19th century when Niepce de St. Victor[1] and Becquerel[2–5] showed that uranium salts were capable of affecting photographic plates (1867 and 1896, respectively). It is believed that the first direct application of this phenomenon involving biological material is attributable to London[6] in 1904. He produced the first whole-body autoradiograms from a frog following exposure to radium salts. Further methods were developed throughout the first few decades of the 20th century by, among others, Lacassagne and Lattes,[7] Lomholt,[8] Leblond,[9] and Libby[10] (1924, 1930, 1943, and 1947, respectively). However, it was not until 1954 that Ullberg[11] developed the basis of the modern technique of whole-body autoradiography. Ullberg's method was to administer a radioactive test material to small rodents, kill them, and plunge them into a freezing bath. The frozen carcasses were then attached to the stage of a hand-driven sledge microtome mounted on a bench inside a refrigerated room, maintained at about −15°C. Sections were cut onto Scotch cellulose tape and allowed to freeze-dry in the refrigerated room for several days, after which they were placed in contact with photographic films for several weeks of exposure. After the exposure period, the sections were removed and the films photographically processed. The resulting images gave excellent detail of the distribution of radioactivity in the tissues and, at the time, allowed a good, subjective, semi-quantitative analysis to be made.

5.3 THE MODERN TECHNIQUE OF WHOLE-BODY AUTORADIOGRAPHY

5.3.1 Commonly Used Radioisotopes

The most commonly used isotopes include ^{14}C, ^{3}H, ^{35}S, and ^{32}P. The gamma-emitting ^{125}I may also be used for WBA studies, but the radiation is much more penetrating, so additional personal safety measures need to be put in place over and above those used for studies involving β-emitters (see Sections 2.3 and 2.4). Additional and expensive shielding is also required in order to ensure that the gamma rays do not fog adjacent detection devices. The above-mentioned radioisotopes are commonly used, but many alternatives have also been used to great effect in the past, the only limitation being the ability of the detection matrix to capture energy from the source.

5.3.2 Preparation of Materials for Dose Administration

The selected radioisotope is integrated into the test substance under investigation at synthesis. The chosen drug dose levels will, of course, be dependent on the potency and efficacy of the material. Radioactive dose levels will often need to be tailored to requirements based on the energy of the isotope, dose route, sampling time, and anticipated distribution within tissues. For β-energy isotopes such as ^{14}C, ^{35}S, and ^{32}P, radioactive dose levels will normally be in the range of 2.5 to 7.4 MBq/Kg body weight (70 to 200 μCi/Kg). For tritium (a lower-energy β-emitter) the radioactive dose levels required are typically somewhat higher, i.e., doses in the range of 37 to 74 KBq/Kg body weight (1 to 2 mCi/Kg). Radioactive doses for ^{125}I are very much dependent on the detection matrix used. When using film technology for registering the radiation energy, relatively high levels of radioactivity need to be administered to the test animals, normally in the region of 7.4 MBq/Kg body weight (about 200 μC/Kg body weight). If phosphor imaging plates are used, the radioactive dose levels can be reduced to safer and more easily manageable levels, i.e., about 1 MBq/Kg body weight (30 μCi/Kg).

Once the test substance has been radiolabeled, it needs to be formulated in a vehicle suitable for dose administration. If the material is water soluble, this will not cause a problem, as it may be dissolved in water for oral administration or isotonic saline for intravenous dosing. However, many newly developed drugs are insoluble in water. This may not be a problem in the case of oral administration, as suspensions can be dosed, but for intravenous administration, quite exotic vehicles are sometimes used, in order that the test material can be kept in solution. Such vehicles may have a detrimental effect on the animal or can aid or even prevent the distribution of the test substance. Indeed, it is not unknown for test substances to precipitate either before or after dose administration. This will result in microscopic-size crystals in the systemic circulation that may collect and accumulate in blood capillaries (e.g., the capillary system of the lungs). This may cause the test animal pain or suffering and is also likely to provide a depot of test substance leading to protracted release back into the blood supply. Whichever of the above, the scientific integrity of the experiment will be compromised. Dose vehicles must therefore be selected with great care.

In addition to oral and intravenous administration, all commonly used dose routes may be used. These include, but are not be limited to, intramuscular, intraperitoneal, dermal, inhalation, intranasal, intratracheal, and intrabladder.

5.3.3 In-Life Phase

The in-life phase of a WBA study is similar to in-life phases of most radiolabeled studies involving animals. Many animal species can be used for WBA investigations. They include most types of small rodents (most commonly rats and mice) as well as rabbits (preferably small varieties, such as the Dutch Belted strain) and primates (including marmosets, squirrel monkeys, and Cynomolgus monkeys; the latter up to a maximum of about 4 Kg). The only constraint with specimen size is that it must fit onto the largest microtome stage used in the microtome (normally about 150 × 400 mm). A vast variety of less commonly used specimens can also be considered for autoradiographic use. These include (but are by no means limited to) fish, birds, plant material and tissues, and limbs and body organs that are removed from animals post-mortem.

Following dose administration, a series of animals will normally be processed at different times in order to study the distribution of drug-related materials into tissues over time. The time points are usually chosen based on available information, such as blood or plasma pharmacokinetic data following administration of the radiolabeled or nonradiolabeled test material to separate animals. For a typical rat single-oral dose experiment, sampling times might be 2, 6, and 24 h, 3 and 7 d after dosing. Due to rapid distribution via the systemic circulation after intravenous dosing, additional, earlier sampling times are often required. These may include 5, 15, 30 and 60 min after dosing.

At the allotted time, the animal needs to be killed by an appropriate and humane method and rapidly frozen. Sacrifice methods may range from asphyxiation in a rising concentration of CO_2 gas to deep inhalation anesthesia, followed by immersion in the freezing bath (death by cold shock) and intravenous or intramuscular overdose of a barbiturate.

5.3.4 Preparing the Animals for Cryosectioning

From a theoretical point of view, whole animals should be frozen as quickly as possible once death is confirmed, in order to ensure tissue integrity. Rapid and complete freezing is required in order to prevent the growth of ice crystals within the tissues, which may degrade the biological matrix by breaking down cell and tissue membranes. The objective is to lock drug-related radioactivity into place, by freezing, as soon as possible after death, and then to keep the tissues frozen throughout the remaining processes. Any subsequent melting will potentially allow relocation/translocation of radioactive material within the biological material and could yield a false result as a consequence. There are two standard methods of freezing the whole animals. The entire freshly killed animal can be placed on its side on a microtome stage, which is surrounded by a frame. Embedding fluid (2% aqueous (w/v) carboxy methylcellulose (CMC), or a suitable alternative) is poured around the animal, and the whole apparatus is immersed in a suitable freezing mixture (e.g., dry ice/hexane or dry ice/petroleum ether at about −70°C). The second and more versatile method is to first plunge the freshly killed or deeply anesthetized animal (suitably positioned) into the freezing mixture. It is advantageous to first place a drop of the CMC embedding fluid over each eye, prior to freezing, in order to reduce the potential for freeze-drying of these exposed tissues. It should be noted that organic fluids other than hexane or petroleum ether can be used, provided they do not unduly affect the tissue, e.g., by defatting the skin. This is particularly important for this second method, as the carcass comes into direct contact with the freezing mixture and is not protected by the embedding fluid. After freezing the carcass can be stored frozen and then later placed in an individual metal mould surrounded by the 2% CMC and freeze-embedded by immersion in the freezing mixture. The frozen block can then be removed from the mould and fixed to a pre-cooled microtome stage (using CMC as glue) as required. The second method has a number of advantages. Importantly, the freezing will be far more efficient. Using dry ice/hexane, in direct contact with the animals, it normally takes about 10 to 12 min for the center of a 250-g rat to become frozen and about 30 min for the core temperature to drop to about −20°C. A minimum period of about 30 min in the freezing mixture is therefore recommended for this species. The use of the first method introduces a buffer against rapid freezing; i.e., the warm animal is surrounded by CMC before being placed in the freezing mixture. The time taken for the core of the animal to reach −20°C will be much extended. Another advantage of the second method is that it will allow a stock of frozen, blocked animals to be prepared and stored in the freezer.

On a cautionary note, liquid nitrogen alone, which might appear to be a better freezing agent because of its lower temperature (about −196°C), is actually far too cold for freezing whole animals. It is likely to cause them to split open due to contracting of the skin relative to the internal organs.

5.3.5 The Cryomicrotome and Preparation of Sections

The first microtomes used for the WBA technique were the standard, hand-operated, base sledge type that were abundant in histology departments at the time. As described previously, these were placed on the bench in a freezer room for use — not a very hospitable environment for the scientist! However, over the intervening years, the modern cryomicrotome has developed. Bright Refrigerator Services, Ltd. in London (later to become the Bright Instrument Company, Ltd.) pioneered the earliest models. In the very first machine, a commercially available Cambridge microtome was modified and placed in a purpose-built thermostatically controlled freezer chamber (not unlike a domestic freezer) with a power drive to the microtome itself. Although the basic principle has not changed in the intervening years, the technology has evolved. This has culminated in purpose-designed machines that are extremely robust and capable of sectioning specimens up to 3 or 4 Kg in weight. Much lower cryocabinet temperatures are also achievable with the modern refrigerants. Most of these modern, purpose-built machines are manufactured by Leica Microsystems, Germany, or the Bright Instrument Company, Ltd., U.K.

For the sectioning process itself, the animal is attached to the microtome stage and allowed to equilibrate to the cryocabinet temperature (normally between about −20 and −30°C). A suitable knife (steel, tungsten carbide, or, more often these days, a purpose-manufactured disposable steel blade) is clamped into the microtome and tissue is trimmed from the surface of the block. Most modern cryomicrotomes operate with the specimen holder (plus specimen) passing backward and forward under a knife support column that cranks down a preset distance at the end of each stroke. For trimming purposes, sections can be cut at any thickness from about 10 to 100 μm. When a level of interest is reached, the section thickness control is turned to between 20 and 40 μm (thickness depending on personal preferences), the block face is carefully cleaned, and a length of transparent tape is applied to the exposed surface. A piece of Perspex or the bristles of a stiff brush are placed at the interface of the knife, and the tape and the microtome is slowly driven forward. The tissue adheres to the support matrix and a full-length animal section can be obtained (Figure 5.1). Many types of tapes are now available for the sectioning process, although they all have two major properties in common: (1), they must have the ability to

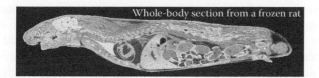

Figure 5.1   **(See color insert following page 178.)** A 30-μm-thick section obtained from a male rat.

adhere strongly to frozen surfaces, and (2) they must remain relatively flexible at the low temperatures encountered.

Once taken, the section must be prevented from melting prior to and during autoradiographic exposure. There are two ways to do this. First, the detection matrix (film or imaging plate) needs to be precooled in the cryocabinet. The frozen section can then be placed against the cooled matrix and left at −20°C to expose. This can be a useful technique, particularly if volatile radiolabeled materials or metabolites are likely to be present. However, from a logistical point of view, it is less than ideal, as exposure equipment may become contaminated with radioactive tissue debris, which will inevitably collect in the cabinet. Also, exposure cassettes will take up a great deal of valuable space in the cabinet. The more common approach is to freeze-dry the sections so that subsequent procedures may be carried out on the bench, at room temperature. There are two ways to achieve this. The easiest method is to leave the sections, mounted on frames, in the cryocabinet for several days. During this time, the water in the sections will relocate and condense on the coldest surfaces in the cabinet, usually the freezer condenser coils or the inside of the cabinet itself. Depending on the thickness of the sections, number of samples in the cabinet, and ambient humidity, this will normally take anywhere between 2 and 5 days. However, just like exposure cassettes, the sections will be exposed to potential contamination. A more efficient and controlled method is to transfer the sections, in a cold box, to the dome of a conventional bench-top freeze-dryer. Under vacuum, sublimation will occur and water will relocate to the freeze-dryer's condenser chamber. Melting does not occur during the sublimation process, and most whole-body sections can be dried perfectly within 30 or 40 min. This latter method is very efficient and also ensures that the drying process is standardized.

5.3.6   Preparation of Autoradiograms

As previously mentioned, there are currently two commonly used matrices employed for the production of whole-body autoradiograms. The first, and these days least used, is photographic film technology. Purpose-made, large-grain fast films and x-ray plates are the most commonly used film detectors. The simple chemistry involved in producing a latent image, followed by subsequent development, has been described earlier in this chapter, but as with all autoradiography detection matrices, it is important to ensure that the sample is in very close contact with the matrix. A common way of doing this with films is to apply the sections (tissue side downward) and place a stiff card on each side of the film. This package is then enclosed in a paper envelope, which in turn is enclosed in a light-tight cassette.

All of the above processes need to take place under darkroom conditions. Groups of cassettes can then be stacked together, and to ensure good contact between sections and films, the whole bundle can be either vacuum packed or placed in a press. Exposure is best carried out at about −20°C, as these lower temperatures reduce the formation of unwanted background noise, while not overly affecting the accumulation of the autoradiographic signal.

More commonly used now is the image plate or phosphor screen technology, often referred to as radioluminography (Section 8.10). Sections are placed against these screens in a fashion similar to that of film and enclosed in purpose-designed cassettes, which ensure good contact between specimen and detection matrix. However, while these plates are sensitive to beta and gamma radiation, they are not particularly sensitive to daylight. The procedures can therefore be carried out under normal or slightly subdued room lighting conditions. Imaging plates are very sensitive to cosmic radiation, so they have to be carefully screened during the exposure period in order to minimize cosmic strikes. The recommended screen is a box of 50-mm-thick, post-Second World War (low-background) lead, sandwiched between oxygen-free copper (on the inside) and iron plate (on the outside). The box can also be refrigerated to about +4°C to reduce background noise even further.

The structure and function of the imaging plate were well described by Hamaoka[12] in 1990. The imaging plate itself consists of a layer of photostimulable phosphors sandwiched between a protective (antiscratch) layer and a base support material. Radiation emanating from the sample source will affect the phosphors and elevate them to a higher-energy state, the level of excitation being directly proportional to the amount of radiation captured. This stored energy can be compared to the latent image formed in the photographic matrix after exposure to radiation. To develop, or visualize, this latent image, the imaging plate is scanned by a He-Ne laser. A bluish purple luminescence (known as photostimulated luminescence, PSL) is released by the laser excitation, detected by a photomultiplier tube, and converted to an analog electrical signal. This can be viewed on a computer screen as an electronic autoradiogram (Figure 5.2).

5.3.7 Radioluminography vs. Film Autoradiography

There is little doubt that the advent of the imaging plate and radioluminography technology has revolutionized the production of whole-body autoradiograms. Probably the main advantage with using radioluminography is the reduction in exposure periods required in order to acquire the autoradiogram. When using film technology, exposure time of the specimen to the detection matrix is often measured in weeks.

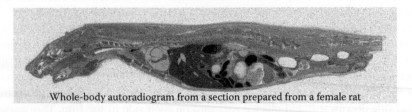

Whole-body autoradiogram from a section prepared from a female rat

Figure 5.2   An autoradiogram prepared from a section of a female rat using radioluminography.

Indeed, exposures of 10 to 15 weeks are not uncommon when dealing with the ^{14}C and ^{3}H isotopes. Imaging plates allow similar intensity autoradiograms to be acquired in a fraction of the time needed for film. Exposure periods are regularly reduced to a few days, or perhaps 14 days in the case of the ^{3}H isotope, but this advantage does have its cost. Sensitivity (speed or rate of detection) is directly linked to resolution. The higher the sensitivity, the lower the resolution is likely to be, and this is the case when comparing the two methods. The very mechanics of current radioluminography systems limit the spatial resolution of the autoradiogram to between about 25 and 200 μm (depending on the equipment available). Film technology has a spatial resolution of a few microns for autoradiography. Notwithstanding this, radioluminography is certainly suitable for most whole-body autoradiography needs, but it is certainly sensible to develop and retain the skills needed to produce film autoradiograms.

The resolution issue aside, radioluminography has many other advantages over film autoradiography. While expensive to purchase in the first place, the detection plates have the advantage of being reusable. After use they can be cleared by exposure to light of a specific wavelength and reused time and again. Indeed, some of the author's plates have been used more than 100 times for ^{14}C studies with no detectable deterioration in sensitivity. The only exception to the rule is when very low β-emitting isotopes (such as tritium) are used. In these cases, the radiation energy is so low that it can barely penetrate the antiscratch layer of the plate, and consequently, for these experiments, special plates, lacking the protective layer, need to be used. These plates are very prone to permanent physical damage and can only be reused a very few times. An obvious advantage of the imaging plate technology is that expensive darkroom facilities are not required.

Another of the disadvantages of film technology is the limited dynamic range of this matrix. It has only a short linear range, the response being sigmoidal. Once the film becomes blackened by radioactivity, it can become no blacker, so the response quickly plateaus at higher levels of radiation. While the same argument holds true for the imaging plate technology, the linear response is many orders of magnitude greater (five orders of magnitude for imaging plates).

A final and major advantage of the radioluminogram (or electronic autoradiogram) is that it is naturally in a format that readily lends itself to analysis using computer-based image analysis programs, being itself a computer image file. Manipulation and analysis of film-based autoradiograms, while not impossible, are difficult skills to acquire. Films are placed on a light box and either analyses using an optical density light pen device (as described by Cross et al.[13] in 1974) or the autoradiogram image is captured using a charge-coupled device (CCD) camera, digitized, and then analyzed by computer image analysis software.

5.3.8 Quantification of Autoradiograms

For many decades, autoradiograms (film derived) were looked upon as qualitative data, at best, with the potential for subjective, semiquantification only. Early attempts at quantification were quite successful (the method of Cross et al.[13] and technologies for capturing images using CCD cameras, so that digitized images could be analyzed, were dealt with earlier), but quantification is now almost exclusively carried out on electronic autoradiograms (radioluminograms). Methods of quantification vary widely, although the basic principle is to include standards of known concentrations of radioactivity with the samples during exposure, so that calibration lines can later be constructed using image analysis software. A typical method (for ^{14}C studies) would be to spike a number of fresh blood samples with [^{14}C]-glucose and freeze the samples into a separate block or even in the same block containing the animal specimen. Before freezing, portions of the blood samples can be submitted to scintillation counting, so that accurate radioactive concentrations per unit weight (KBq/g, for instance) can be determined. The frozen blood samples are processed as for the specimen, and all sections are exposed in the same cassette. When the radioluminogram is scanned, the blood standards will appear in differing shades of gray, according to radioactivity content.

The gray levels (PSL values) can be plotted against the predetermined concentrations of radioactivity in order to construct a calibration line (Figure 5.3 and Figure 5.4).

Image analysis software will then allow the scientist to highlight organs on the computer screen, and the software will calculate the average PSL value in the defined area. This can be referenced to the calibration line and a true concentration, in terms of radioactivity per unit weight, derived. There are now a number of software packages available that allow this quantification to be carried out under the strictly controlled conditions recommended by international guidelines for good laboratory practice. These include SeeScan Densitometry (Lablogic Systems, Ltd.), Aida (Raytest Isotopenmessgeraete GmbH), and MCID (Imaging Research, Inc.).

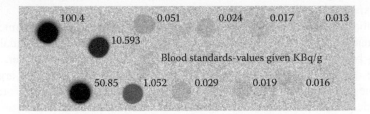

Figure 5.3   Autoradiogram obtained from blood standards spiked with [^{14}C]-glucose.

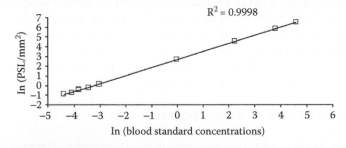

Figure 5.4   A typical calibration line prepared from an autoradiogram obtained from blood standards, such as those shown in Figure 5.3.

5.4 SOME SPECIFIC USES OF THE QWBA TECHNIQUE

5.4.1   Melanin Binding

Much of the work carried out in the safety testing of new pharmaceuticals utilizes the albino rat (or mouse) as the main rodent species. The use of these animals is historical, the standard albino laboratory rat and mouse being easy to breed, house, and maintain. Consequently, a large database of background information exists for these species. However, many pharmaceuticals and their metabolites, produced *in vivo*, are chemically basic in nature and will bind to melanin, to a greater or lesser degree. Although such binding is normally reversible, the half-life of depuration can be extensive (often measured in days or even weeks). Hence, information gathered from albino animals will not necessarily reveal the full picture. Lindquist (1973)[14] and Ings (1984)[15] have collated and published a great deal of data on this subject, covering a wide variety of test substances capable of binding to melanin. Notwithstanding the above, one should not overreact to this potential issue. Although basic chemicals will bind to melanin, particularly in such structures as the uveal tract (choroid, ciliary body, and iris of the eye), the skin, and meninges, it has been shown that toxicity (as a direct result of such binding) is quite rare (Figure 5.5 and Figure 5.6).

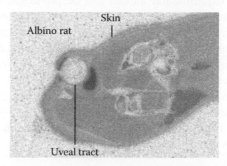

Figure 5.5   The eye region of an Albino rat, following administration of a radiolabeled drug. The Albino rat lacks the pigment melanin, and therefore no binding is observed.

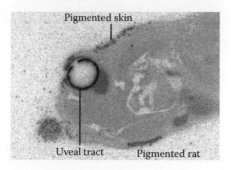

Figure 5.6   The same situation as shown in Figure 5.5, but this time with a pigmented rat, and melanin binding can be clearly seen around the eye.

Similar doses of the same radiolabeled test substance were administered to albino and pigmented rats. Animals of each strain were then processed for whole-body autoradiography at predetermined time points. Figure 5.5 is part of an autoradiogram showing the distribution of drug-related material into the head and neck region of an albino animal. Figure 5.6, on the other hand, illustrates the distribution into the pigmented rat at the same time point. It is evident that very high levels of radioactivity are associated with the uveal tract and the skin in the pigmented animal.

5.4.2   Blood–Brain Barrier

The membranes surrounding the brain are quite efficient at excluding drugs and their metabolites from the brain, particularly by means of the P-glycoprotein (P-gp) efflux pump mechanism. Unfortunately, certain drugs may act as P-gp inhibitors and allow penetration into some or all parts of the nervous system. Co-administration of two or more drugs is common, and it is quite feasible that one of the pharmaceuticals administered may act as a P-gp inhibitor, and thus allow some or all of the other drugs to penetrate the blood–brain barrier. The issue of potential penetration of the blood–brain barrier during co-administration of a new drug with a P-gp inhibitor can be investigated in two ways using the WBA technique. First, the experimental animal can be pre-dosed with a known P-gp inhibitor and then dosed with the radiolabeled test drug once the blood–brain barrier is compromised (Figure 5.7). Indeed, in this particular experiment, levels of drug-related (radioactive) material in the blood of the systemic circulation were almost non-detectable, even though relatively high levels were apparent in the brain. Second, a genetically modified strain of animal can be used (e.g., a transgenic strain of mouse that does not express P-gp), with the radiolabeled test substance administered on its own. In each case, the extent of penetration of the blood–brain barrier can be studied by direct comparison to animals whose blood–brain barrier is not compromised.

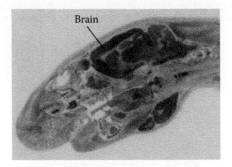

Figure 5.7   Shows an enlargement of an autoradiogram depicting the brain of a male animal after intravenous dosing with radiolabeled drug. Penetration into the brain can be clearly seen.

5.4.3   Studies in Pregnant and Suckling Animals

It is important to gain some idea of the potential for distribution of drug-related material into fetuses and into suckling neonates via the mothers milk. The rat serves as an excellent model in each case. The gestation period of the laboratory rat is 21 to 22 days, and placental penetration studies are often conducted where the radio-labeled test substance is administered to the dam anywhere from day 16 to day 19 of gestation. Figure 5.8 shows an example where radioactive material from the dam's systemic circulation has penetrated the placenta and is widely distributed into fetal tissues. Of additional interest are the high levels of radioactivity associated with the fetal eyes. In this illustration, the pregnant rat is pigmented and the radiation present in the eyes of the dam and fetuses is due to melanin binding.

Figure 5.9 illustrates the potential for the transport of drug-related material to neonates via the mother's milk. In this example, a pregnant rat was allowed to produce a litter. Ten days later the mother was administered a radiolabeled test substance and a neonate was humanely killed at 4 hours after the dam was dosed. The neonate was then subjected to WBA processing. The autoradiogram shows the

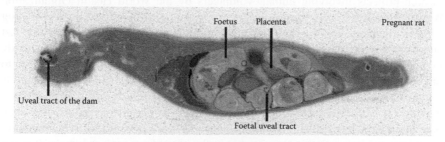

Figure 5.8   An example where radioactive material from the dam's systemic circulation has penetrated the placenta and is widely distributed into fetal tissues.

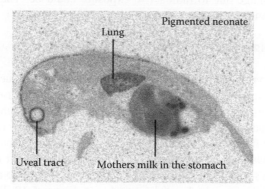

Figure 5.9   Illustration of the potential for transport of drug-related material to neonates via the mother's milk.

presence of radioactivity in the milk in the stomach as well as the liver, lung, skin, eye and other tissues. The radioactivity in the eye and skin are, once again, attributable to melanin binding, as the animal strain used was pigmented.

5.4.4   Determination of Human Exposure from QWBA Data

At some stage in the development of a new drug, radiolabeled test material is likely to be administered to human volunteers in order to determine rates and routes of excretion. The use of QWBA is invaluable in helping to calculate the safe level of radioactivity that can be given. Quantitative tissue distribution data and excretion information obtained from the rat (or other animal test species) are used in a complex algorithm in order to calculate this value.[21] The assumption is made that the level of uptake in the human volunteers will be similar to that seen in the animal tissues. In the U.K., the committed equivalent doses to tissues and organs and committed effective dose (CED) are calculated according to the 1990 Recommendations of the International Commission on Radiological Protection (ICRP)[16] as implemented in the *Ionising Radiations Regulations* (1999)[17] in response to EU Council Directive 96/29/EURATOM.[18] The CED is compared with the dose categories proposed for research projects involving human volunteers by the World Health Organization (WHO)[19] and ICRP.[20] Of particular concern is the potential of a radiolabeled drug to bind to melanin. Indeed, data reflecting strong melanin binding have in the past caused the acceptable human dose to be so low that the human radiotracer study has not been viable by conventional means. Notwithstanding this, it is feasible to perform such studies using accelerator mass spectrometry, where much lower levels of radioactivity can be detected. The potential for melanin binding highlights the necessity for performing the tissue distribution work in a pigmented strain of animal. As indicated previously, the retention of high levels of radioactivity in the melanin-rich tissues rarely implicates toxicity, but in the case of a human volunteer, it is not desirable to have high levels of radioactivity in a small mass of tissue (i.e., the pigmented region of the eye, for instance) for long periods. Toxicity is not the issue, but biological damage due to radioactive exposure could be. The calculations are discussed in Appendix 1 to this chapter.

5.4.5   Autoradiography of Chromatography Plates

Although the visualization of radioactivity in biological tissues by autoradiography has been described above, radioluminography can also be used in conjunction with thin-layer chromatography, paper chromatography, or gel chromatography to show profiles of radiometabolites. A thin layer of Mylar foil may be used to protect the imaging plate from direct contact with the above matrices, but the principle is the same as for whole-body autoradiography. After development of the chromatogram in a suitable solvent, the matrix may be dried and applied to the imaging plate for exposure, and then scanned in the normal way. Figure 5.10 illustrates an autoradiogram prepared from a thin-layer chromatography plate showing the profile of radiolabeled metabolites derived from the urine of an animal after administration of an ^{125}I test compound. A number of clearly defined metabolites can be seen in each

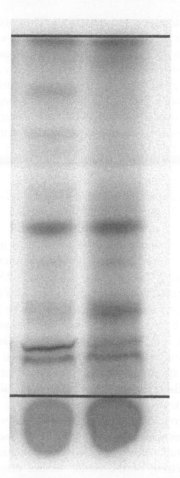

Figure 5.10 Autoradiogram prepared from a thin-layer chromatography plate showing the profile of radiolabeled metabolites derived from the urine of an animal after administration of an ^{125}I test compound.

track, and calculation of the PSL in each band can furnish the scientist with quantitative data.

5.5 MICROAUTORADIOGRAPHY

The techniques discussed in this chapter thus far describe the use of macroautoradiography. Whether using film or imaging plate equipment, the derived images are all relatively large in size and the scientists' interest is drawn to major differences in distribution levels of radioactivity. There is another powerful tool available that will allow investigation of biologically bound radioactivity, at the cellular or subcellular level. This technique is known as microautoradiography. The technique is normally used in a qualitative capacity rather than quantitative and, due to the requirement of high-resolution images, requires the use of photographic emulsions.

The preferred radioisotope for this work is ^{3}H. The energy of the radiation from ^{3}H is much lower than for most other commonly used β-emitters, e.g., almost 10-fold lower than that from ^{14}C. This results in higher-resolution autoradiograms. Paradoxically, it is also possible to work with much higher specific activity material when dealing with ^{3}H, which will increase the rate of formation of the autoradiogram. The radiolabeled test substance is dosed to the animals as required, and after sacrifice the target organs are removed by dissection. These tissues are cut into pieces no more than about 7.5 mm^3 and rapidly frozen by immersion in a cooling bath. Because the distribution of radioactivity is to be studied at the microscopic level, it is important to freeze the sample rapidly and then maintain it at low temperatures prior to further processing. The recommended way of freezing is to drop the tissue sample into a solvent such as isopentane, pre-cooled to about –120°C with liquid nitrogen. The specimen is then retained either in a low-temperature freezer at about –80°C or, ideally, in a liquid nitrogen storage facility.

For sectioning, the specimen should be attached to the mounting chuck of a biopsy type microtome mounted in a cryocabinet and allowed to equilibrate to the cabinet temperature (normally between about –18 and –25°C).

Prior to sectioning, emulsion-coated microscope slides need to be prepared. This emulsion is fine grained and supplied in gel form. Once heated to about 40°C, it becomes liquid and may be further diluted with water before glass microscope slides are dipped in it. The slides are allowed to drain and then placed in lighttight cassettes ready for use. All of the above preparatory work is carried out in a darkroom under either dark red or brown safe-lighting conditions. The cassettes containing the slides can then be transferred to the microtome cryocabinet or retained at room temperature, depending on the subsequent method to be used.

Under safe-lighting conditions, thin sections or ribbons of tissue can be cut (section thicknesses between about 3 and 8 μm). These sections can then be picked up onto the emulsion-coated slides using one of two methods. For the first method, it is argued that any melting of the tissue section may result in relocation of radiolabeled material, and thus compromise the result. For this technique, the sections can be any thickness between about 3 and 8 μm. Frozen emulsion-coated slides are removed from their cassette and lightly touched onto the knife surface, where the sections are sitting. Assuming that conditions are ideal, the sections will transfer from knife to slide. However, humidity and the temperature differential between section and slide need to be perfect for the sections to transfer, and they may not adhere evenly to the emulsion on the slide. This can cause autoradiographic artifacts, but assuming that the picking up of the sections is successful, the slides can be returned to their cassettes and allowed to expose at low temperatures.

In the second method, the sections are normally cut at 3 or 4 μm, at most, and allowed to thaw-mount onto the emulsion-coated slides at room temperature. It has been argued (Stumpf, 2003[22]) that a 4-μm section will collapse to about 1 μm on transfer and will thaw and evaporate so quickly that relocation of radioactivity is not significant. This technique does allow excellent contact to the emulsion and makes the interpretation of subsequent results somewhat easier.

After the required exposure period (worked out empirically by processing replicate samples after different times of exposure), the slides are equilibrated to room

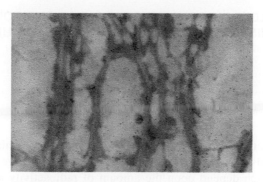

Figure 5.11 **(See color insert following page 178.)** Microautoradiogram of the fundic stomach region in a rat.

temperature (if required) under safe-lighting conditions and may be histologically
fixed in a weak (2 to 4% v/v) aqueous paraformaldehyde solution. The slides are
then processed through a suitable photographic developer and fixer baths before
being histologically stained and mounted.

At the end of processing, the slides can be viewed under a suitable microscope
and individual or clumps of silver grains (autoradiography) will be seen overlaying
specific cell or subcellular structures. Figure 5.11 shows a microautoradiogram of
the fundic stomach region in a rat. The animal was dosed with a test substance
intended to modulate hydrochloric acid secretion from the stomach mucosa. The
silver grains are present as discrete clumps in the region of the parietal cells of the
gastric pits, i.e., those cells responsible for HCl production.

5.6 SUMMARY

This chapter attempts to describe the development and use of autoradiography
in the laboratory. Using whole-body autoradiography, coupled with computer-
assisted image analysis, it is now possible to attain lower limits of quantification
similar to those possible using liquid scintillation techniques (but not as low as
attained using accelerator mass spectrometry). Autoradiography is an extremely
powerful tool in its own right and can give the scientist an invaluable insight into
the overall distribution of a radiolabeled drug and its radiolabeled metabolites.
Nevertheless, if data generated by this technique are to be submitted to international
regulators, then the hardware and software used need to be extensively validated in
order to prove their robustness and suitability for use.

As eluded to above, tissue distribution data can be gathered from liquid scintillation counting, whole-body autoradiography and accelerator mass spectrometry
techniques. Other methods also exist, including detectors that can capture radiation
directly from the source (whole-body section), e.g., the β- and Microimagers made
by Biospace Measures, France, and methods such as x-ray ablation coupled to mass
spectrometry, where radioisotopes are not required at all.

While measurement of drug-related materials in biological materials is required,
there is no doubt that technology will continue to develop.

APPENDIX 1: DOSIMETRY CALCULATIONS FOR THE ADMINISTRATION OF RADIOISOTOPES TO HUMANS

Graham Lappin

Introduction

The amounts of radioactivity that can be administered to humans are restricted by regulatory limits. The limits are defined in terms of radioactive dose equivalents (Section 2.6), which depend upon the amount of radioactivity administered and the duration of exposure. Since the duration of exposure is dependent upon the time the drug resides within the body, experiments have to be conducted on a compound-by-compound basis, to determine how much radioactivity can be safely administered. These experiments are known as dosimetry studies and largely utilize QWBA. Calculating the maximum dose is quite complex, and the terminology can be confusing. To add to the confusion, the terminology is going through some changes.

The reader should be familiar with units of dose (Section 2.5 and Section 2.6) and the regulatory guidelines (Section 1.7.3 and Section 5.4.4).

Regulations Dealing with Human Exposure to Radioactivity

Limits laid down by the World Health Organization (WHO)[16] and the International Commission on Radiological Protection (ICRP)[17] are shown in Table 5.1.

Background and Other Sources of Radiation

To put the values given in Table 5.1 into context, a chest x-ray results in an exposure of about 50 μSv, and a 1-h flight in an aircraft at 9000 m would result in

Table 5.1 Limit Doses Defined by WHO and ICRP

WHO Category	Dose (mSv)	WHO Level of Risk
I	Less than 0.5	Within variations of a natural background
II	More than 0.5	Within dose limits for members of the public
III	More than 5 but less than 50	Within dose limits for persons occupationally exposed to radiation

ICRP Category	Dose Range (mSv)	ICRP Level of Risk
I	<0.1	Trivial
IIa	0.1–1	Minor
IIb	1–10	Intermediate
III	>10	Moderate

a dose of about 5 μSv. There are a variety of natural sources of radiation, the most prominent being radon and thoron gases. The levels of these gases vary depending upon the geology of a particular geographic location. A reasonable average estimate for natural exposure, however, would be about 2.5 mSv per year, of which about 1.3 mSv per year originates from natural radioactive gas.

Factors Affecting Biological Damage

When a drug is absorbed into the body, its distribution is not uniform. It may, for example, accumulate in fat, or it may cross the blood–brain barrier (Section 5.4.2). It may be eliminated from the bloodstream rapidly, or it may circulate for some considerable time. Consequently, the level of radioactivity within any one tissue or organ and the time that it resides there varies, depending upon the physiological properties of the drug. Furthermore, different body organs or tissues exhibit a greater or lesser susceptibility to damage when exposed to radiation. For example, the gonads are more susceptible than, say, the skin; bone marrow is more susceptible than the surface of the bone. (Susceptibility may be a little oversimplified, but it is a convenient phrase to use in the present context. It is more a matter of the consequences of certain tissues becoming damaged by radioactivity.)

The calculation of dose (measured in Sv) therefore depends upon a combination of certain physical and biological effects.

The physical effects are:

1. The energy of the radiation
2. The duration of exposure*

The biological effects are:

3. The duration of exposure*
4. The extent to which various body organs are exposed
5. The susceptibility of the organs and tissues in which radioactivity is deposited

*The duration of exposure can be due to the residence time of the drug in the body (biological effect) or the half-life of the radionuclide (physical effect). For radionuclides such as ^{14}C with long half-lives (5730 years), only the residence time of the drug in the body is a factor. For radionuclides with very short half-lives (e.g., ^{11}C, ca. 20 min), the half-life of the radionuclide is likely to be the dominant factor.

Introduction to Dosimetry

A general overview of the dosimetry calculations are given below for the reader who just requires the basic principles, largely in nonmathematical terms. The equations are then covered. (It is poignant that these equations are largely based upon our knowledge of biological damage arising from the atomic bombs dropped on Japan during the Second World War.) These equations are a little complex, and the terminology can be confusing. Our concern here is exposure to radioactivity due to the deliberate administration of radiolabeled drugs to human volunteers. This is, however, only one instance of exposure to radioactivity. The regulations and equations can equally apply to, for example, workers at a nuclear power station. The regulations, the literature, and other textbooks may therefore contain terms and definitions that are not relevant to the current situation. Moreover, the technical language can sometimes have very similar terms for what are quite different definitions. To add to the confusion, at the time of writing (2005) the regulations are on the verge of being updated, and it is likely that some of the terminology might change.

It must be stressed that the information below is an overview so that the general principles can be understood. The specific regulations must be followed, depending upon in which country the human radiolabeled study is being performed. (As an example, the weighting factors given in Table 5.5 are different for WHO and ICRP.) Furthermore, expert advice should be sought if in doubt, as the regulations are often not specific and local practical knowledge may be necessary (the equations below are based upon those published by the ICRP). The principles apply to any radioisotope, but for simplicity, reference will be made to ^{14}C.

Dosimetry Calculations: An Overview

The limits summarized in Table 5.1 give the maximum doses of radioactivity in units of Sv. In conducting a radiolabeled study, however, the amount of radioactivity administered is expressed as dpm (or the equivalent units of MBq, µCi, etc.). What the researcher therefore needs to know is how much radioactivity (measured in dpm) can be administered to human volunteers so as not to exceed the national limits (expressed in Sv). This is done experimentally using an animal model, typically the pigmented rat. Pigmented animals are used in case the drug binds to melanin (Section 5.4.1). Since the radioactive dose (Sv) depends upon the physiological properties of the compound, studies have to be performed on a drug-specific basis.

Animals are administered a known amount of $[^{14}C]$-drug (typically 4 to 5 MBq/Kg) by the dose route intended for human administration. Two sets of data are then acquired: (1) By collection of excreta, the relative proportions of the dose in urine and feces are determined (Section 3.5.1). (2) At prescribed time points after dosing, animals are killed and the levels of radioactivity in the various tissues and organs are determined using QWBA. Typically, animals are killed at four time points, with one being equivalent to the expected peak blood level. The ICRP publication[17] specifies 12 tissues where measurements must be made (Table 5.2).

The concentrations of radioactivity in tissues and organs obtained for the several time points are used to calculate the number of transformations per Bq. This is calculated using essentially the same method of calculating area under the curve (AUC) as a pharmacokinetic parameter (Chapter 3, Appendix 3). The AUCs for dosimetry calculations, however, are based upon an assumed plasma half-life of 100 days (i.e., AUC_{0-t} is extrapolated to $AUC_{0-100 \text{ days}}$). If melanin binding occurs, then this is taken as a special case and may necessitate lengthy experiments to determine a more detailed pharmacokinetic profile.

Exposure from excreta is dealt with slightly differently than those from the tissues and organs, as a certain amount of radioactivity in excreta will be absorbed by the excreta itself. By collecting excreta, the proportion of the dose eliminated *via* urine

Table 5.2   Tissues Specified by ICRP

Gonads
Colon
Lung
Red bone marrow
Stomach
Bladder
Breast
Liver
Esophagus
Thyroid
Bone surface
Skin

and feces is determined. Radioactivity may also be eliminated in bile, and the amount eliminated by this route can be determined from bile duct cannulation experiments (Section 3.5.6) or from an estimation based on QWBA data. The time of exposure to radioactivity present in excreta is given in tables of mean residence times (MRTs) published by the regulatory authorities (MRT is a pharmacokinetic parameter described in Chapter 3, Appendix 3).

The potential for biological damage to each tissue and organ then depends upon:

- The energy of the radionuclide. (This is a constant for any given radionuclide.)
- The exposure of radioactivity to each tissue and organ based upon the number of transformations per Bq, as determined by QWBA.
- The exposure to radioactivity of the excretory organs based upon the proportion of radioactivity excreted by any given route of elimination and the mean residence time.
- The weight of each tissue and organ. (Remember, a Sv is defined as 1 J of energy absorbed by 1 Kg of matter; Section 2.6.)
- A weighting factor is used to correct for the different susceptibilities of each tissue or organ to biological damage.

The calculated value for each tissue and organ is known as the effective dose. The sum of the effective doses for all tissues and organs gives the committed effective dose. This is, in effect, the total body exposure, and this is the value stated in the regulations that must not be exceeded.

The Equations

The calculations can be divided into three sections:

1. Calculation of the dose equivalent: This is the energy absorbed per kilogram for each separate tissue or organ in the body.
2. Calculation of the effective dose equivalent: This is where the susceptibility of the various organs and tissues to radioactive damage is taken into account.
3. Calculation of the committed effective dose: This is the total body burden of radioactivity.

Calculation of Dose Equivalent

Dose equivalent is calculated from Equation 5.1:

$$H_T = \frac{U\varepsilon\phi A}{m} \tag{5.1}$$

where H_T is the dose equivalent for each target organ or tissue (in Sv); U is the transformations per Bq dose administered (Bq·sec) as determined by QWBA (U is calculated from its own equations; see below); ε is the dose constant for the radio-isotope (for ^3H, $\varepsilon = 9.12 \times 10^{-16}$ Kg Gy/Bq/sec; for ^{14}C, $\varepsilon = 79.4 \times 10^{-16}$ Kg Gy/Bq/sec); ϕ is the fraction of radioactive emissions absorbed (tissues = 1; excreta = 0.5); A is the number of Bq of radiolabel administered; and m is the mass of the organ or tissue in man (Kg) (see Table 5.3).

Calculation of U (Transformations per Bq)

For each tissue and organ U is calculated by the trapezoidal rule (Appendix 3, Chapter 3) and extrapolated using Equation 5.2:

$$U = \frac{A_0}{\lambda} + \frac{8640000}{e} \tag{5.2}$$

where A_0 is the peak concentration in organ or the value extrapolated to time zero, whichever is greater; λ is the elimination half-life of radioactivity from the tissue or organ; 8,640,000 = seconds in 100 days (as AUC_{0-t} extrapolated to AUC_{0-100} days); and e is the exponential constant (= 0.693).

Table 5.3   Examples of Organ Weights

Tissue/Organ	Weight (Kg)	Tissue/Organ	Weight (Kg)
Bladder	0.2	Adrenals	0.014
Red bone marrow	1.5	Brain	1.4
Bone surfaces	—	Eyes	0.0015
Breast	0.026	Gall bladder	0.062
Colon (LLI and ULI)	0.355	Heart	0.33
Esophagus	0.04	Kidneys	0.31
Liver	1.8	Muscle	28
Lung	1	Pancreas	0.1
Ovaries	0.011	Pituitary	0.0006
Skin	2.6	Prostate	0.016
Stomach	0.25	Small intestine	0.4
Testes	0.035	Spleen	0.18
Thyroid	0.02	Thymus	0.02

For excreta U is calculated from Equation 5.3:

$$U = F \times MRT \tag{5.3}$$

where F is the fraction of dose that passes through the given route (fraction of 1-Bq dose) and MRT is the mean residence time (Table 5.4).

Calculation of Effective Dose Equivalent

Once the dose equivalent (H_T) for each tissue, organ and excreta has been calculated, a weighting factor (W_T) is applied (Equation 5.4). The weighting factors are listed in Table 5.5.

$$H_T \times W_T = \text{the effective dose equivalent} \tag{5.4}$$

The ICRP is preparing new recommendations, and changes to some weighting factors are proposed based on the commission's new approach to the calculation of detriment. In an attempt to be as up to date as possible, the proposed new weighting

Table 5.4   Mean Residence Times in Minutes

Tissue/Organ	MRT
Stomach	1
Small intestine	4
Upper large intestine	13
Lower large intestine	24
Urine	10
Bile	2.53

Table 5.5   Selected Weighting Factors for Organs and Tissues as Given by the ICRP

Organ	W_T
Gonads	0.2
Red bone marrow	0.12
Colon	0.12
Lung	0.12
Stomach	0.12
Bladder	0.05
Breast	0.05
Liver	0.05
Esophagus	0.05
Thyroid	0.05
Bone surface	0.01
Skin	0.01
Remainder	0.05

Table 5.6   Proposed Weighting Factors for Organs and Tissues as Given
by the ICRP 2005 Recommendations

Organ	W_T
Red bone marrow	0.12
Breast	0.12
Colon	0.12
Lung	0.12
Stomach	0.12
Bladder	0.05
Esophagus	0.05
Gonads	0.05
Liver	0.05
Thyroid	0.05
Bone surface	0.01
Brain	0.01
Kidneys	0.01
Salivary glands	0.01
Skin	0.01
Remainder	0.10

Source: From International Commission on Radiological Protection (ICRP),
Draft recommendations of ICRP 2005, http://www.icrp.org/icrp_rec_june.asp.

factors are given in Table 5.6 (remember, at the time of writing, these are proposed,
not in use).

The Committed Effective Dose

The **committed effective dose** is the sum of the effective dose equivalents for
all the various tissues and organs.

The above equations will generate values for the effective dose equivalent (Sv)
for each tissue and organ and the committed effective dose (Sv), for whole-body
exposure, based on the administration of 1 Bq. Thus, if the maximum dose allowed
was 1 mSv and the equations showed that 1 Bq = 0.0003 Sv, then the administration
of 3.3 MBq would be the maximum amount of radioactivity that could be administered to humans for the particular drug in question.

ACKNOWLEDGMENT

I thank Dr. Michele Ellender, Radiation Effects Department, NRPB, U.K.

REFERENCES

1. Niepce de St. Victor, Sur une nouvelle action de la lumiere, *C.r. hebd. Séanc. Acad.
Sci., Paris*, 65, 505, 1867.
2. Becquerel, H., Sur les radiations émises par phosphorescence, *C.r. hebd. Séanc. Acad.
Sci., Paris*, 122, 420–421, 1896a.

3. Becquerel, H., Sur les radiations invisibles émises par les corps phosphorescents, *C.r. hebd. Séanc. Acad. Sci., Paris*, 122, 501, 1896b.
4. Becquerel, H., Sur les radiations invisibles émises par les sels d'uranium, *C.r. hebd. Séanc. Acad. Sci., Paris*, 122, 689, 1896c.
5. Becquerel, H., Émission de radiations nouvelles par l'uranium metallique, *C.r. hebd. Séanc. Acad. Sci., Paris*, 122, 1086, 1896d.
6. London, E.S., Étudessur la valeur physiolgique et pathologique de l'émanation du radium, *Arch. Élec. Méd.*, 12, 363–372, 1901.
7. Lacassagne, A. and Lattes, J., Répartition du polonium (injecté sous la peau) dans l'organisme de rats porteurs de greffes cancereuses, *C.r. Séanc Soc. Biol.*, 90, 352–353, 1924.
8. Lomholt, S., Investigation into the distribution of lead in the organism on the basis of a photographic (radiochemical) method, *J. Pharm. Exp. Ther.*, 40, 235-245, 1930.
9. Leblond, C.P., Localisation of newly administered Iodine in the thyroid gland as indicated by radio-iodine, *J. Anat.*, 77, 149–152, 1943.
10. Libby, R.L., Anon. trans., *N.Y. Acad. Sci.*, 9, 249, 1947.
11. Ullberg, S., Studies on the distribution and fate of [^{35}S]-labelled benzylpenicillin in the body, *Acta Radiol.*, Suppl. 118, 1–110, 1954.
12. Hamaoka, T., Autoradiography of new era replacing traditional x-ray film, *Cell Technol.*, 9, 456–462, 1990.
13. Cross, S.A.M., Groves, A.D., and Hesselbo, T., A quantitative method for measuring radioactivity in tissues sectioned for whole-body autoradiography, *Int. J. Appl. Radiat. Isotopes*, 25, 381–386, 1974.
14. Lindquist, N.G., Accumulations of drugs on melanin, *Acta Radiol.*, Suppl. 325, 1973.
15. Ings, R.M.J., Melanin binding of drugs and its implications, *Drug Metab. Rev.*, 15, 1183–1212, 1984.
16. International Commission on Radiological Protection (ICRP), *Recommendations of the International Commission on Radiological Protection*, ICRP Publication 60, ICRP, 1991.
17. *The Ionising Radiations Regulations*, U.K. Parliament Statuary Instruments, No. 3232, HMSO, London, 1999.
18. EURATOM, Council Directive 96/29/EURATOM of May 13, 1996, laying down basic safety standards for the protection of the health of workers and the general public against the dangers arising from ionizing radiation, *Off. J. Eur. Commun.*, 39, OJ L-159, 1996.
19. World Health Organization, *Use of Ionising Radiation and Radionuclides on Human Beings for Medical Purposes*, Technical Report Series, No. 611, WHO, Geneva, 1977.
20. International Commission on Radiological Protection (ICRP), *Radiological Protection in Biomedical Research*, ICRP Publication 62, ICRP, 1991.
21. Evans, G. et al., *A Handbook of Bioanalysis and Drug Metabolism*, CRC Press, Boca Raton, FL, 2004.
22. Stumpf, W.E., *Drug Localisation in Tissues and Cells*, IDDC Press, 2003.
23. International Commission on Radiological Protection (ICRP), Draft recommendations of ICRP 2005, http://www.icrp.org/icrp_rec_june.asp.

FURTHER READING

Young, G., Ayrton, J., and Pateman, T., Isotope drug studies in man, in *A Handbook of Bioanalysis and Drug Metabolism*, Evans, G., Ed., CRC Press, Boca Raton, FL, 2004, chap. 11.

CHAPTER 6

Scintillation Counting

Simon Temple

CONTENTS

6.1 INTRODUCTION

This chapter describes the theory and practice behind the detection and measurement of radioactivity using scintillation counting. Both positron emission tomography (PET) and γ-scintigraphy utilize scintillation effects but these are rather specialized techniques and so they are dealt with separately (Chapter 11 and Chapter 12, respectively). Scintillation counting is inextricably linked to the instrumentation, with different manufacturers developing their own technologies and methods of data processing. Indeed, many innovations have arisen in the field of scintillation counting as a result of fierce competition among the manufacturers. The present chapter however, as far as possible, deals with the general principles of scintillation counting. The development, history, and idiosyncrasies of the instrumentation are covered in Chapter 8. The reader should be familiar with Section 2.3, which describes modes of radioactive decay. Sample preparation is covered in Chapter 9 and the statistics behind scintillation counting are covered in Chapter 7.

Although there are differences in practice, β^-, β^+, α, and γ can all be analyzed using scintillation counting. In terms of drug development, the most commonly used radioisotopes are the β- and γ-emitters and this chapter will focus on those.

Irrespective of the isotope, the principle of scintillation counting is the same: decay energy is converted to photons of light by a scintillator and it is the photons that are detected and measured. (Radioactive decay also gives off heat but this is far too small to be measured with current instrumentation.) There are two types of scintillator: liquid and solid. With liquid scintillation counting, the sample is dissolved in a cocktail containing a solvent and a liquid scintillator, thus bringing the radionuclide into intimate contact with the scintillator. This is necessary, as liquid scintillation counting is the preferred method for analyzing relatively low energy emitters such as β-particles, which have very short path lengths before they are absorbed by surrounding matter. Higher-energy γ-radiation is measured using solid scintillation counting and so the sample tends to be farther away from the scintillator. It is possible to use solid scintillation counting for the measurement of β^--radiation, provided the sample is in close physical contact with the solid scintillator.

6.2 HOW DOES SCINTILLATION COUNTING WORK?

In liquid scintillation counting, energy from nuclear decay is transferred first to a solvent and then to a scintillator. As the scintillator receives the energy from the solvent it becomes excited and moves to a higher-energy state. Upon returning to the ground state, the energy is released as photons of light by fluorescence. The photons are detected by photomultiplier tubes and hence the light can be directly related to the energy of the nuclear decay (Figure 6.1). Very small energies can be detected in this way. The process of solid scintillation counting is similar to liquid scintillation counting, but since no solvent is involved, the energy from the nuclear decay is absorbed and trapped directly by the solid scintillator, which then emits photons.

The light intensity is proportional to the energy of the nuclear decay. Therefore, a strong emitter such as ^{32}P (1710 KeV; for a description of energy levels measured in KeV, see Section 2.3.2) will result in light 91 times the magnitude of that generated by ^{3}H (18.6 KeV).

6.3 PHOTOMULTIPLIERS AND ACCOMPANYING CIRCUITRY

Photons arising from fluorescence (solid and liquid scintillators) are detected and measured by photomultipliers. Light photons strike a photoemissive cathode (photocathode) on the exposed surface of the photomultiplier. Just behind this surface are focusing electrodes, an electron multiplier, and an electron collector (anode), which are all held under vacuum (Figure 6.2). When light strikes the photocathode, photoelectrons are emitted into the vacuum. These photoelectrons are directed by the focusing electrode voltages toward the electron multiplier, where electrons are multiplied by a cascade effect known as secondary emission. A series of dynodes

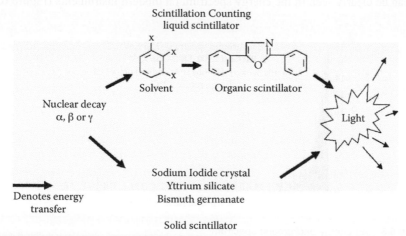

Figure 6.1 Principles of scintillation counting.

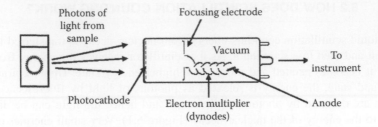

Figure 6.2   The photomultiplier tube.

are positioned with a sequentially increasing potential difference between them, thus accelerating the electrons as they proceed down the tube. Electrons striking the first dynode result in the release of a greater number of electrons, which then strike the next dynode and so on down the tube. The multiplied electrons are collected by the anode as an electronic output. It is the secondary emission multiplication that gives photomultiplier tubes their extremely high sensitivity coupled with fast response times.

They are able to detect radiant energy in the ultraviolet, visible and near-infrared regions, but they are most sensitive at 405 nm (in the visible blue range). The photomultiplier tube is a linear device, so the amplitude of the output is directly proportional to the number of photons striking the photocathode. Thus, each time a pulse of light is registered at the photocathode, it is a measurement of the scintillations that are occurring in the sample due to radioactive events.

As stated above, a photomultiplier tube is very sensitive to light and if a single photomultiplier tube is exposed to a scintillator, even in the absence of a radioactive sample, the background signal will be in the region of 10,000 counts per minute (cpm). The majority of this noise is electronic and thermal background from the instrument and the photomultiplier tubes themselves and is in the 0 to 10 KeV region; this can be clearly seen in the energy spectrum on modern instruments (Figure 6.3).

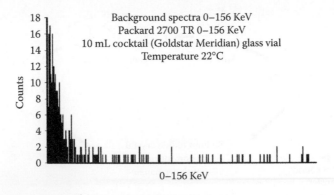

Figure 6.3   An energy background spectrum.

The lower limit of detection for any analytical instrument depends upon the ratio of the signal arising from the sample compared to the background noise. Background noise from a photomultiplier therefore restricts its limit of detection.

In the early 1950s, the problem of high background was alleviated by the introduction of two photomultipliers, instead of just one (i.e., coincidence counting). Photons produced during scintillation are emitted in all directions (i.e., they are isotropic). The radioactive event and the light produced have very fast decay times, in the region of 2 to 10 nsec. (There are approximately 10 photons of light produced per KeV of radioactive energy.) A coincidence counting photomultiplier assembly is designed so that a signal is only recorded if the photons are detected by both tubes within a short time frame (about 18 nsec). Thus, spurious events such as electronic noise detected in one photomultiplier but not in the other are rejected. Photons originating in the sample and detected by both photomultipliers, within the designated time window, are considered real, and these events are counted. A schematic shows this in Figure 6.4.

The introduction of coincidence counting reduced the level of background from thousands to about 60 cpm. Later developments in the design of photomultiplier tubes and the introduction of lead shielding further reduced the background noise, and the average background nowadays is in the region of 22 cpm for ^{14}C and 17 cpm for ^{3}H. The coincidence circuit is now standard in all standard liquid scintillation counters.

The next stage of instrument design was circuitry for the summing of the two photomultiplier signals. The summing of the two coincident signals allowed better optimization of the signal-to-noise ratio. In addition, there are circumstances where light produced from a radioactive event reaches the photomultipliers as two different intensities. For example, if the sample is colored and the decay event takes place nearer one photomultiplier than the other, the more distant of the signals will be attenuated. A schematic of a modern liquid scintillation counter is shown in Figure 6.5.

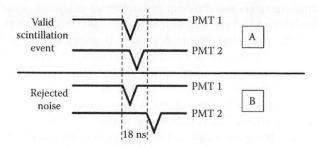

Figure 6.4   (A) The scintillation pulse reaches both photomultipliers within the 18-nsec time window and is therefore accepted as a valid event. (B) The photomultipliers detect the scintillation pulse but the pulse recorded by the second photomultiplier is outside the 18-nsec window and is therefore rejected (PMT = photomultiplier tube).

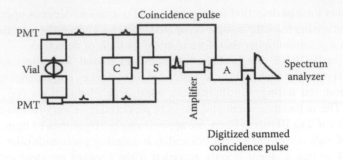

Figure 6.5 A schematic of the circuitry of a modern liquid scintillation counter. C, the coincidence circuit; S, summation circuit; A, analog-to-digital converter (ADC); PMT, photomultiplier tube.

6.4 SPECTRUM ANALYSIS AND THE INTRODUCTION OF THE MULTICHANNEL ANALYZER

As described in Section 2.3, β- particles and certain other nuclear decay processes are emitted with a range of energies, from zero to a maximum energy level known as E_{max}. Since the magnitude of the light registered by the photomultiplier is proportional to the energy of the decay event, a plot of pulse height vs. counts provides the energy spectrum.

Perhaps one of the most important advances in scintillation counting was the development of the multichannel analyzer, which allowed the energy spectrum of a given isotope to be visualized. The analog signal from the photomultiplier was digitized and digital pulses were placed in a range of storage bins or slots over a range of about 0 to 2000 KeV. The conversion process is linear and so during the counting of the sample the multichannel analyzer accumulates counts amounting to the complete energy spectrum of the radionuclide.

Different manufacturers use different multichannel analyzers, some with 4000 bins or slots available and others with as many as 32,000 (the more bins, the greater the resolution of the spectrum). Figure 6.6A and B shows spectra of ^3H and ^{14}C, respectively, obtained by the use of a multichannel analyzer. Table 6.1 (in Section 6.5) shows the range of energies for the principal isotopes used in ADME (absorption, distribution, metabolism, and excretion) studies.

The scintillation counter therefore records the number of photons (counts) and the energy of those photons. The counts are proportional to the amount of radioactivity (decay events) being measured and the energy is related to the specific radioisotope under analysis.

6.5 SCINTILLATORS

The use of solid scintillators is somewhat dependent upon the application and so they are dealt with separately (γ-measurement, Section 6.12; β-measurement,

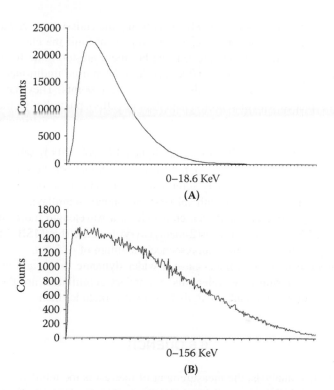

Figure 6.6   Energy spectra of (A) ³H and (B) ¹⁴C obtained by a multichannel analyzer.

Table 6.1   Energy Range and Counting Efficiencies of Some Isotopes

Isotope	E_{max}	Range of Expected % Efficiencies Using Liquid Scintillation Counting
³H	18.6 KeV	5–50
¹⁴C	156 KeV	70–95
³⁵S	167 KeV	70–95
³³P	249 KeV	70–95
³²P	1710 KeV	90–100
¹²⁵I	35 KeV	60–80

³²P is suitable for Cherenkov counting.

Section 6.13). In liquid scintillation counting, the sample is dissolved in a cocktail of solvent and liquid scintillator.

The average path length of a β⁻ particle from ³H is about 6×10^{-3} cm in water, and therefore its kinetic energy is easily absorbed and hence lost for detection. It is therefore important to minimize the path length from the point of emission to the point of energy capture. For this reason, the solvent is selected so that it not only dissolves the analyte but also is capable of capturing the emission energy and passing it on to the scintillator. This does, however, somewhat limit the choice of solvent. The first solvents were dioxane and benzene but these are too toxic for routine use in the modern laboratory. Toluene and xylene have been used traditionally but these also have toxicity issues and they also have low flash points. They have therefore been largely replaced with diisopropyl naphthalene (DIN), phenylxylylethane (PXE), dodecylbenzene, long-chain alkyl benzenes, and 1,2,3- and 1,2,4-trimethylbenzene (pseudocumines).[1,2]

At one time the only scintillator was 2,5-diphenyloxazole (PPO), which emits light at 370 nm (Figure 6.7A). This wavelength was not optimal for the photomultipliers of the time and therefore secondary scintillators were added (secondary scintillators are sometimes known as wavelength shifters). Secondary scintillators absorb energy from the primary scintillator and then emit light at a wavelength more suited to the photomultiplier. For example 1,4-bis(2-methylstyryl)benzene (bis-MSB; Figure 6.7B) is a secondary scintillator with a fluorescence maximum of 425 nm.

More modern photomultipliers have a wider dynamic range and are sensitive across a wider spectrum of wavelengths. Secondary scintillators are therefore less critical today, but commercial cocktails tend to still include them.

6.6 QUENCH

In radioactive analysis, the measurement of interest is the number of disintegration events per unit time (e.g., disintegrations per minute, dpm; see Section 2.5). A proportion of disintegration events occurring in a sample, however, will fail to generate photons that reach the photomultiplier. In other words, scintillation counting is subject to a given efficiency. The scintillation counter therefore measures counts per minute (cpm), and the efficiency has to be taken into account in order to convert cpm to dpm. Table 6.1 shows the energy range and typical counting efficiency for the principal isotopes used in ADME studies.

It should be noted that cpm are instrument dependent and a measurement in cpm on one instrument may not yield the same result as another instrument. This is because of differences in electronics, age of the photomultipliers, etc. Once counting efficiency is taken into account, the dpm values between different instruments should, in theory, be the same (or at least very close).

Anything that interferes with the conversion of the decay energy to the detection of photons is known as quench. By quantifying quench, the counting efficiency can

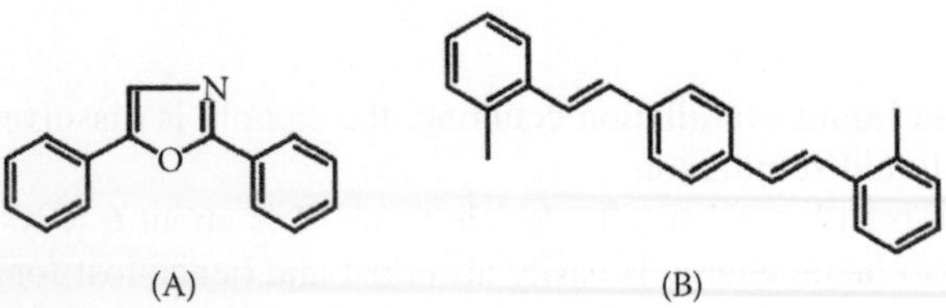

(A)   (B)

Figure 6.7   (A) Primary liquid scintillator, PPO. (B) Secondary scintillator, bis-MSB.

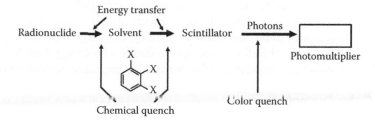

Figure 6.8 The process of quench.

be calculated and cpm can be converted to the required unit of dpm. To understand how quench is quantified, we must first understand how quench arises. In Figure 6.8 the process of quench is shown. The energy of the decay is first transferred to the solvent in the scintillation cocktail. The solvent then passes the energy onto the scintillator, which fluoresces as it returns to the ground state. The photons of light then have to travel through the scintillation cocktail, through the wall of the vial, and into the photomultiplier. Quench can therefore be divided into two broad categories. Quench that occurs during the transfer of the decay energy to the scintillator is known as chemical quench. Quench that occurs during the passage of the photons to the photomultiplier is known as color quench.

6.6.1 Chemical Quench

Energy may be quenched at any point of transfer. A β⁻ particle, for example, may collide with other sample material or particulates, thus losing its energy without transfer to the solvent. Even if the β⁻ particle passes its energy to the solvent, there is the possibility that there will be quenching between the solvent and the scintillator. Chemical quenching occurs in all liquid scintillation counting conditions. Even the smallest amount of chemical can cause quench. It is true to state that the more and varied the chemicals in the final solution, the greater the opportunity for quenching.

Chemical quench will cause the energy spectrum to shift toward its low-energy end (Figure 6.9). A measure of the spectral shift enables the degree of quench to be

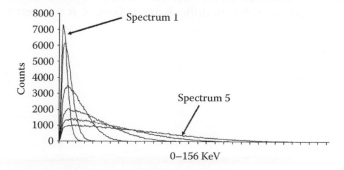

Figure 6.9 An example of an energy spectrum subject to increasing chemical quench. Spectrum 1 is heavily quenched, and it therefore concentrated at the lower-energy end of the spectrum. Spectrum 5 shows virtually no quench.

quantified and is known as the quench indicating parameter (QIP). It should be noted that with solid scintillation counters there is effectively no chemical quench. For low-energy detection by solid scintillation counting, the sample is placed directly on to the scintillator and therefore there are no issues with energy transfer. (Solid scintillation counting can, however, suffer from color quench, described below.)

6.6.2 Color Quench

Color quench occurs when photons are attenuated in the sample, thus restricting the light output.

To use an analogy, color quench is similar to the action of a colored filter: the darker the color, the less light that will get through. Highly colored samples will therefore lead to significant quench and although some correction can be made (Section 6.6.9), they are best avoided (see Sample Preparation, Chapter 9). In theory, color quench leads to an overall depression of the spectrum. In the author's experience, there is also a shift to the lower-energy region (Figure 6.10). Both solid and liquid scintillators potentially suffer from color quench.

6.6.3 Quench Correction

Different manufactures have developed a variety of methods, some quite sophisticated, for quench correction. The reader may well be working with one type of instrument and may wish to know how quench is corrected in his or her particular case. Chapter 8 covers the different quench correction systems used by different types of instruments. In the current chapter the general principles are considered.

6.6.4 Quench Correction Using an Internal Standard

Internal standardization is, in theory, the most accurate method of quench correction but it demands great technical skill. At one time, the internal standard method was the only method available for quench correction but things have moved on considerably nowadays and very few laboratories use this technique. The internal standard method is discussed here for historical interest but it is a technique that should not be forgotten. Although difficult and tedious, it is the most transparent

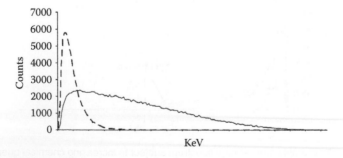

Figure 6.10 Example of color quench: (–)unquenched and (----) highly quenched.

method of quench correction, not relying on (invisible) computer algorithms. It does have uses, therefore, if there are problems with instrumentation or if the validity of quench curves (Section 6.6.10) is in doubt.

The process of the internal standards method is as follows:

1. The sample is analyzed to obtain a cpm value.
2. An exact and known amount of radioactivity, in the form of a standard, is added to the vial.
3. The vial is analyzed for a second time and the cpm value obtained.
4. The counting efficiency is determined from Equation 6.1:

$$\%E = \frac{C2 - C1}{D} \tag{6.1}$$

where C1 is the net cpm without the internal standard, C2 is the net cpm with the internal standard, and D is the amount of radioactivity (in dpm) added in the form of a standard. (Note that net cpm is cpm minus the background count.)

The following points are important when using the internal standards method:

1. The standard must be the same isotope as the one being analyzed.
2. The added internal standard radioactivity should be at least equal to and preferably greater than, the sample activity.
3. The internal standard activity should be accurately determined and if possible, traceable to a regulatory body.
4. The addition of the standard must be accurate. This is the most difficult aspect of the method and it cannot be overstated as to how much this method relies on accurate and precise procedures.

If the internal standard is a radioisotope dissolved in a solvent, then the solvent should not be volatile, as evaporation will cause a change in the specific activity. $[^{14}C]$-toluene can be used as a standard and although volatile, since the standard and solvent are the same, evaporation does not lead to a change in specific activity. Toluene can be difficult to pipette accurately and so the amount added can be calculated by the difference in weight before and after addition of the standard.

6.6.5 Quench Correction Using Sample Channels Ratio

This is a little used method of quench correction today, but it has seen extensive use in the past and so is covered here for historical interest. It relies on the relationship between two regions of the energy spectrum to detect the degree of spectral shift. The method does not rely on the instrument being able to produce a spectrum; it merely calculates the counts in each region and compares them.

As stated above, the energy distribution spectra shifts toward lower energy as quench increases. The signals attributable to two channels on the spectrum in a quenched and unquenched sample are measured (channels A and B in Figure 6.11). As quench increases, the number of events seen in channel A gets higher, while those

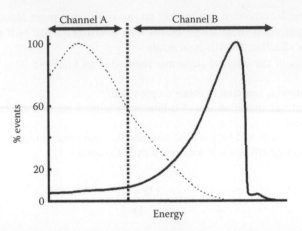

Figure 6.11 Quench correction using samples channel ratio.

in B become lower. The ratio of cpm in channel A to that in channel B therefore becomes a measure of quench. If a set of quenched standards is counted, the ratio of channel A to channel B is plotted against efficiency to produce a quench curve (Section 6.6.7). This method of determining quench only works for single isotopes. If two isotopes are present, the composite spectrum becomes complex and the shift is difficult to measure. This method is only accurate when relatively high levels of radioactivity are present and if the sample is very highly quenched, then the whole of the spectrum will move into channel A and it will be impossible to determine a ratio.

6.6.6 Quench Correction Using an External Standard

Modern counters use an external standard to measure quench. This method is common practice today and so will be covered in some detail. Before discussing the way that external standards work, however, the Compton scattering effect has to be explained. Arthur H. Compton was awarded the Nobel Prize in 1927 for the discovery of the effect named after him. Compton scattering is the scattering of photons of electromagnetic radiation from (quasi-)free electrons in matter. Upon absorption of γ irradiation, the solvent in a scintillation cocktail ejects electrons. These Compton electrons are ejected with a range of energies from zero to E_{max}, showing a characteristic Compton spectrum. The Compton electrons react with the scintillation cocktail, causing light to be emitted in a fashion analogous to the β-spectrum. Compton electrons and the resulting photons are subject to the same quench effects as the radionuclide in the sample. Thus, by measuring the shift in the Compton spectra, the amount of quench can be calculated.

In practice, the Compton spectrum is generated by bringing a γ source close to the vial containing sample dissolved in the scintillation cocktail. The spectral shift for the Compton spectrum is obtained as a measure of quench (QIP). The γ source is removed and the radioactivity in the sample counted in the normal way. The counting efficiency is calculated against a quench curve and is used to derive dpm from cpm. It should be made clear that the measurement of quench and the measurement of radioactivity in the sample are never conducted at the same time and have no effect on each other.

Different manufactures have developed different systems of handling data from the Compton spectrum and its use in quench correction. This is discussed further in Chapter 8.

6.6.7 The Quench Curve

A quench curve is constructed from a series of vials, each containing an equal, known and exact amount of radioactivity along with a scintillation cocktail. The series of vials contain differing amounts of quenching agent, from none to a sufficient amount to cause significant quench. These standards are known as quenched standard set (sometimes called quench correction standard set). A typical quenching agent is nitromethane in a concentration of around 25 to 30% for the most quenched standard. Compton spectra and hence spectral shift and QIP, are obtained for each sample, along with the cpm value. The efficiency of counting is determined by knowing the actual radioactivity level of the standard (dpm) and the measured level (cpm) (Equation 6.2). Efficiency is plotted on the y-axis, and the QIP is plotted on the x-axis. This constitutes the quench curve (Figure 6.12A and B).

$$\%E = \left(\frac{cpm}{dpm} \right) \times 100 \qquad (6.2)$$

where %E is the percentage efficiency, cpm is the cpm value obtained from the scintillation counter, and dpm is the known amount of radioactivity in the standard.

The liquid scintillation counter first determines the QIP from the Compton spectrum, then the cpm value from radioactivity in the sample. The counting efficiency (%E) is determined from the y-axis of the quench curve from the QIP on the x-axis (Figure 6.12). From the efficiency, cpm can be converted to dpm from Equation 6.3. Naturally, modern counters compute the dpm values automatically:

$$dpm = \frac{cpm}{\%E/100} \qquad (6.3)$$

There are usually 10 vials in a quenched standard set, although a quench curve may be constructed using a minimum of 2 vials. Quench sets are usually best purchased, as they are sold with traceable levels of radioactivity (e.g., National Institute of Science and Technology (NIST) standards) and it is very difficult for the average user to construct a quenched standard set to the level of statistical precision required. There are occasions, however, which require a quench standard set to be made by the user. For example, the radioisotope of interest may not be commercially available in quenched standard sets. Commercial standards typically contain 100,000 dpm (^{14}C) or 300,000 dpm (^{3}H), and if quench curves are required for low-level analysis, again this will require the user to construct a specific set of standards.

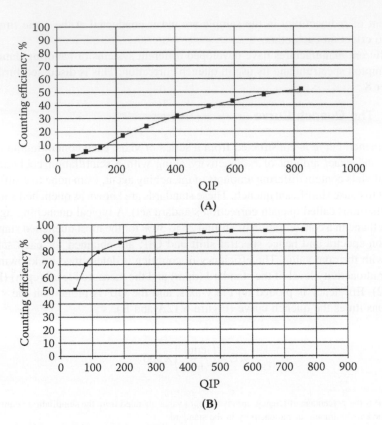

Figure 6.12   Typical quench curves for (A) ^{3}H and (B) ^{14}C. The QIP ranges from 0 (highly quenched) to 1000 (no quench).

6.6.8   Quench Curve Construction

The first vial in a quenched standard set is unquenched and the last vial is highly quenched. The intention is to build a curve that exceeds the limits of quench for any sample analyzed. If the quench standard set is made by the user, then it is imperative that each vial has exactly the same amount of radioactivity. (Wallac introduced a capsule with a standard amount of radioactivity. The capsule was dropped into a vial and then cocktail added.) Alternatively, improved precision can be obtained by preparing a single solution of cocktail and radioactive standard and then accurately pipetting from this into the vials. When the quench curve is constructed, any vial that deviates from the mean by more than 2% should be discarded. For the best accuracy it is recommended that standards are counted for 30 min or 0.5%2σ (Section 7.3).

6.6.9   When Is a Quench Curve Applicable?

Some laboratories will operate on very few quench curves, with perhaps one for each scintillation cocktail in use. Others will have a plethora of quench curves covering every scintillation cocktail, vial and sample type. When, therefore, are quench curves genuinely required? Clearly there should be different quench curves for each radioisotope. The other major factor is the scintillation cocktail, or to be more precise, the solvent in the cocktail. Is it necessary to construct quench curves for chemical and color quench? In general, scintillation counters will deal with the issues of color influence in quench correction. However, there are many documented instances of quench correction sets that contain both chemical and color quenchers. A common color quencher is methyl orange, which will account for both color and chemical quench. If colored samples are being analyzed, it is probably worthwhile to develop suitable quench curves, although it is better to avoid colored samples in the first place (see Chapter 9).

6.6.10 Maintenance of Quench Curves

Different laboratories will have different policies on the frequency of replacing existing quench curves. Some laboratories have used the same quench curves for years and others seem to regenerate quench curves so frequently that there is hardly time to analyze any samples.

Quite simply, a quench correction curve is a calibration device. The quench correction curve therefore needs to be replaced if the instrument goes out of calibration. In order to verify the performance of the quench correction curve, it is usual to count the quench standard set as if it were a sample set. If the result is significantly different from what it should be, then the quench curve needs maintenance (how significantly different will depend on the type of analysis, but typically 2 to 5% would seem appropriate). Of course, if ^{3}H is being used, its half-life has to be taken into account. For short-lived isotopes (e.g., ^{35}S and ^{32}P), quench curves will inevitably have to be established more frequently. Quench curves should be checked after instrument maintenance, installation of software, or major cleaning. If the scintillation counter has had reflectors or a photomultiplier tube replaced then the quench correction curves must be reinstalled as matter of necessity.

Figure 6.13 shows a faulty ^{14}C quench curve that needs replacing. First, looking at the percent counting efficiency, there is a discrepancy between the dpm values

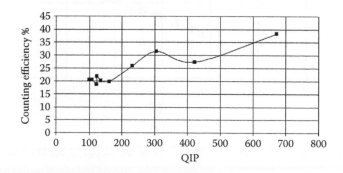

Figure 6.13 A poor ^{14}C quench curve.

intended and those measured. The likelihood is that an error was made in dispensing the standard into the quench standard set. Second, it appears the quenching agent is not in the correct progression (zero quench to high quench).

Figure 6.14A shows an unusable ³H quench curve, but with some attention this can be rescued. Because it is of lower energy, the counting efficiency of ³H is not as high as ¹⁴C (Table 6.1). Nevertheless, three of the least quenched standards fall outside the general shape of the curve. These can be edited out or replaced (Figure 6.14B), but the curve still has inadequacies, in that the upper and lower quench ranges are too small. Ideally, the upper range should go to 700 and the lower range should go to 100 on the QIP scale illustrated.

6.7 INTERFERENCES IN SCINTILLATION COUNTING

In addition to quench, there are a number of other factors that can adversely affect the results of scintillation counting. Some of these effects are not necessarily obvious and therefore care must be taken in interpreting results.

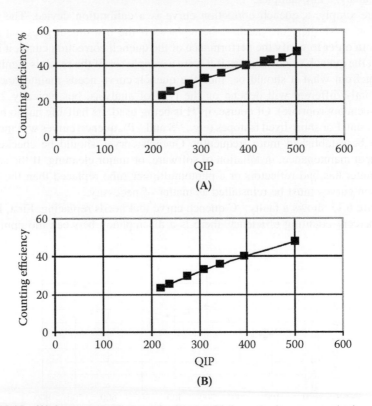

Figure 16.14 (A) A poor quench curve for ³H and (B) the quench curve repaired.

6.7.1   Luminescence

Luminescence can sometimes be a serious problem and can lead to spuriously high results. Luminescence is divided into two types; chemiluminescence and photoluminescence. There is also bioluminescence (i.e., luminescence arising from biological action) but this is rarely an issue in the current context. Irrespective of the type, luminescence is the production of photons, independent of radioactive events. While radioactive events lead to the production of multiple photons (around 10 photons per KeV of energy), luminescence produces single photons.

6.7.2   Chemiluminescence

Chemiluminescence is the production of photons due to a chemical reaction taking place in the scintillation cocktail and it can produce high numbers of photons, sometimes sufficient to overwhelm the photomultipliers. Alkaline solutions, hydrogen peroxide and solubilizers are the main causes of chemiluminescence. It can be a major problem and the effect can last for several hours. Leaving samples for a period before counting can alleviate the problem. Warming the sample (35°C), thereby speeding up the reaction and taking it to completion quicker, sometimes helps. Solid scintillators do not suffer from chemiluminescence.

6.7.3   Photoluminescence

Photoluminescence results if the scintillator (solid or liquid) is exposed to ultraviolet light. Samples should therefore not be prepared in direct sunlight. With liquid scintillants photoluminescence is short-lived and leaving vials in the dark for a short time prior to counting solves the problem (this is known as dark adapting). Solid scintillators suffer significantly from photoluminescence. Upon replacing a solid scintillation cell in a flow counter, the cell must be left for several hours to dark adapt before it can be used.

6.7.4   Correcting for Luminescence

Most luminescence occurs in the 0 to 6 KeV region of the spectrum. For certain isotopes, such as ^{14}C with an E_{max} of 156 KeV, the lower-energy region can be set to 6 KeV, but for ^{3}H this is not appropriate, as the E_{max} is only 18.6 KeV. In addition, with highly quenched samples, the energy spectrum is shifted toward the lower region and therefore, ignoring the 0 to 6 KeV region may not be appropriate.

To some extent, photons arising from chemiluminescence can be eliminated by coincidence counting. A delay time is added to one of the photomultipliers so that it counts both in coincidence with its partner and with a delay equal to the coincident time interval. The counts from the sample are collected with and without the delay. Single photon luminescence events will be detected by the delayed photomultiplier tube but they will not detect the multiphoton events of the radioactive decay. With the introduction of multichannel analyzers it is possible to subtract channel by channel one set of counts from the other and leave only those from the radioactive decay.

6.8 STATIC

Static occurs when there is an electrical imbalance due to the removal or addition of ions on the surface of the vial. Laboratory gloves may also contribute to static. The apparatus used to dispense liquid scintillator can introduce static into the vial itself. If the air is very dry, then there is a greater chance of static becoming a problem. In these situations increasing the humidity will usually reduce or remove the problem.

Static usually leads to increased background. Most modern scintillation counters will contain an electrostatic controller that generates a 360° electrical field, which neutralizes static on the surface of the vial. These are not always totally effective, and it is advisable to include other precautions. Plastic vials have a greater propensity to build up static on their surface compared to glass. There are also antistatic plastic vials commercially available, which have a thin coating of antistatic material on them. Some users routinely wipe the surface of the vial with either an antistatic wipe or a tissue dampened with methanol or ethanol.

Solid scintillation counters can suffer significantly from static. Highly nonpolar solvents such as hexane can induce significant levels of static in flow cells (Section 6.15).

6.9 WALL EFFECT

Organic solvents can penetrate the plastic wall of some scintillation vials. This has the effect of turning the plastic into a separate scintillator, which may contribute to the Compton spectrum, when the vial is irradiated with the external standard. In recent years, the organic solvents used in scintillation cocktails are less liable to cause this effect, and so it has been largely eliminated. The only precaution necessary is to count plastic vials without delay and then discard them. The wall effect may manifest itself in plastic vials that have been stored for prolonged periods.

6.10 CHERENKOV* COUNTING

Photons of light are produced when charged particles travel thorough transparent material with a speed that is greater than the speed of light in the same material. This phenomenon was named after the Russian scientist P.A. Cherenkov[3] in recognition of his research on the subject. The exchanged energy produces localized electronic polarizations along the path of the charged particle. As these polarized molecules return to their ground state, they release photons of light. In water, about 200 photons are produced corresponding to about 400 eV/cm. The upshot of the Cherenkov effect is that providing the nuclear decay is of sufficient energy, the radioactivity can be measured by liquid scintillation counting in the absence of the usual scintillation cocktail.

---

* There are two spellings, Cherenkov and Cerenkov.

As a general rule, it is better to use a larger volume of photon-producing solvent, as there is then a greater opportunity for the Cherenkov effect to occur. With water, at least 10 mL should be used.

The lowest energy (E_{min}) for Cherenkov counting is shown in Equation 6.4:

$$E_{min} = 0.511 \left(\sqrt{\left(1 - \frac{1}{n^2}\right)} - 1 \right) \tag{6.4}$$

where 0.511 is the rest mass of the electron in MeV and n is the refractive index of the medium.

If the medium is water, then the threshold is 263 KeV. In general terms, only isotopes with an E_{max} greater than 263 KeV are suitable for Cherenkov counting, which, in the present context, probably only leaves ^{32}P with an E_{max} of 1710 KeV (it has a Cherenkov counting efficiency in water of around 53%).

Cherenkov counting is little affected by chemical quench and may be ignored for the purposes of quench correction. Color quench, however, does affect counting and it may be necessary to produce a suitable quench curve, although external standards used in scintillation counting do not have sufficient penetrating power to produce a Cherenkov effect, unless ^{152}Eu is used (Section 8.6).

6.11 DUAL-LABEL COUNTING

It is possible to label a drug with two different isotopes (Section 3.6.2) and then measure the radioactivity from each isotope separately. This is known as dual labeling.[4] Each isotope has its own spectrum, which may be shifted by quench. Addition of the spectra forms a composite spectrum with overlapping energies that are difficult to deconvolute. For this reason, only radioisotopes with sufficiently different spectra can be analyzed by dual counting. ^{3}H and ^{14}C are the most commonly used dual isotopes, but $^{3}H/^{32}P$, $^{3}H/^{35}S$, and ^{14}C /^{32}P are all feasible. Figure 6.15 shows how a composite spectrum results from the individual spectra of ^{3}H and ^{14}C.

The composite spectrum has more counts in the lower region than a single ^{14}C spectrum would have. The spectra are deconvoluted by calculating what is known as the spill-up and spill-down values of the two isotopes. If a discriminator setting is placed at the 12 KeV value on the x-axis, counts below that energy value will contain ^{3}H and ^{14}C. The counts recorded above that value will also contain ^{3}H and ^{14}C, but there will be a lower proportion of ^{3}H. To differentiate the two isotopes, it is necessary to establish the different proportions of one isotope to the other in both counting regions. In the main, this is done by using two quench correction curves, one for each of the isotopes. The scintillation counter measures the lower-energy quench correction curve first (channel A). In the lower-energy region the efficiency of counting will be almost the same as counting a single radioisotope and the shape would not be much different from the normal quench curve. The quench curve in the upper energy region (channel B) will have a lower efficiency, as there will be

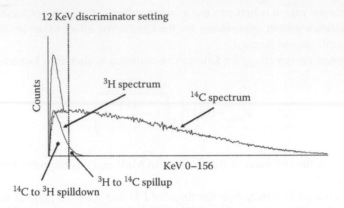

Figure 6.15   Composite spectra of ^{3}H and ^{14}C (not to scale).

fewer counts in that region. The separate dpm values for the isotopes can then be calculated using Equation 6.5A and B:

For calculating the dpm for ^{3}H:

$$dpm_A = (cpm_{H3A} \times E_{H3A}) - (cpm_{c14A} \times E_{C14A}) \qquad (6.5A)$$

For calculating the dpm for ^{14}C:

$$dpm_B = (cpm_{c14B} \times E_{c14B}) - (cpm_{H3B} \times E_{H3B}) \qquad (6.5B)$$

where cpm_A is the observed cpm in channel A, cpm_B is the observed cpm in channel B, E_{H3A} is the fraction efficiency of counting ^{3}H in channel A, E_{C14A} is the fraction efficiency of counting ^{14}C in channel A, E_{C14B} is the fraction efficiency of counting ^{14}C in channel B, dpm_A is the dpm of ^{3}H, and dpm_B is the dpm of ^{14}C.

The spill-down and spill-up effects are now taken into consideration. In practice, the spill-down from ^{14}C to ^{3}H can have an effect, but the spill-up from ^{3}H to ^{14}C is unlikely to be significant (illustrated in Figure 6.15). Corrections are made for spill-down of ^{14}C to ^{3}H using Equation 6.6:

$$dpm_{totalc14} = dpm_B + (cpm_{c14A} \times E_{c14A}) \qquad (6.6)$$

6.12 GAMMA COUNTING

Gamma counting is conducted with a solid scintillator. While in liquid scintillation counting photons are produced within the sample vial, with γ counting, the scintillation event takes place in the detector. The reason for this difference is that

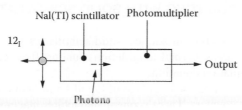

Figure 6.16 Gamma counter.

unlike β emission, γ has sufficient energy to reach and enter the detector from a distance.

The γ counter consists of a solid scintillator in front of a photomultiplier (Figure 6.16). The scintillator in most modern γ counters is thallium-activated sodium iodide crystal, NaI(Tl), discovered by Robert Hofstadter in 1948.[5-7] NaI(Tl) crystals have a relatively short decay time with a high light output and the short-lived pulse of light helps eliminate interference from other emissions. The decay time of NaI(Tl) is 250 nsec with a light output of 40,000 photons/MeV energy deposit. The main drawback of NaI(Tl) crystals is that they are hydroscopic and so they have to be kept dry and well sealed. Furthermore, they have a rather low density, which means it will not stop strong γ emissions. The detector crystal may lose resolution due to absorbed moisture or due to cracks arising from thermal or mechanical shock. This results in broad or malformed peaks in the spectrum. Good-quality NaI crystal will display sharp, narrow peaks. NaI(Tl) crystals are the principal scintillators for ^{125}I detection (and as an aside, are also used in positron emission tomography and γ scintigraphy; Chapters 11 and 12, respectively). The sample may be solid, liquid or gas.

With the detector itself generating photons, a dual photomultiplier tube assembly using coincident counting becomes redundant and so γ counters use a single tube. Even without coincidence counting, background must still be eliminated. Gamma counters usually contain a multichannel analyzer, which enables a spectrum to be constructed using a range of bins from 0 to 2000 KeV. A background spectrum is therefore taken and used for background subtraction. The ability to store a background spectrum also allows the instrument to monitor for contamination of the counter over time.

Most modern counters allow the use of the chi-square statistical calculation. This involves the repetitive counting of a single sample to enable good counting statistics. The chi-square value generated is used as an indication of the stability of the instrument, and on most modern counters, it can be stored and followed over a period.

If the γ counter consists of several detectors, they have to be normalized to each other so they will give the same response to the same amount of radiation. Some γ counters have as many as 20 detectors to increase throughput.

Quench curves are not used with γ counters, as the highly penetrating radiation is not subject to significant quench. Since the photons are produced in the counter itself, there is no color quench. Counters do have a counting efficiency, but this is constant, and so therefore the output of γ measurement is quoted as cpm.

6.13 β COUNTING WITH SOLID SCINTILLATORS

In terms of drug metabolism studies, solid scintillators for the detection of β⁻ are used in three main areas: normal scintillation counting, flow scintillation counting and microplate scintillation counting.

Solid scintillators can be used in place of liquid scintillators in conjunction with standard scintillation counters. There is one manufacturer that emphasizes the application of such a system; this is covered in Section 8.7. Solid scintillators can be used in multiwell plates where multiple samples are analyzed simultaneously (Section 6.14). Flow scintillation analysis applies to high-performance liquid chromatography (HPLC), where the eluate is passed through a flow cell containing a solid or liquid scintillator (Section 6.15).

Solid scintillators have a brighter output and produce larger numbers of photons per KeV of energy than liquid scintillators. For example NaI(Tl) will produce approximately 25 photons per KeV and CaF_2(Eu) will produce approximately 19 photons per KeV. The counting efficiency of solid scintillators is, however, lower. The counting efficiency of ^3H is in the region of 28 to 54% and that for ^{14}C is around 80 to 90%.

With solid scintillators, the β⁻ decay nuclide has to be in direct contact with the scintillator, and hence there is no energy loss due to chemical interaction; that is, there is no chemical quench. The photons, however, still have to travel from the scintillator to the photomultiplier and so there is still the potential for color quench. In practice, constructing quench curves with solid scintillators is challenging and on the whole data are expressed as cpm, rather than dpm. This is a potential drawback with solid scintillation counting, although instrument manufacturers have attempted to tackle the problem in various ways (Section 8.8).

6.14 MULTIWELL PLATE SCINTILLATION COUNTING

Traditionally, analysis of samples by scintillation counting has been carried out one sample at a time. Each sample is placed into its own vial, a batch of vials (which could be several hundred) is placed into a liquid scintillation counter, and each vial in turn is presented to the photomultipliers.

In the mid-1980s, scintillation counters were developed around multiwell plate technology, where wells are arranged in a plastic plate to allow for multiple-sample analysis. These plates were developed mainly for automation systems and typically come as a 8 × 12, 96-well array, although 384 and 1536 versions are available. These systems are also known as microplates, as the sample volume is usually quite small, although 24-deep-well plates are available, capable of handling several milliliters.

Plate scintillation counters are capable of scintillation counting in liquid, solid, and Cherenkov formats, as well as γ-emitters; it is in their application that they differ from standard scintillation counting. Multiwell plates can be used with liquid scintillation cocktail (essentially standard scintillation counting on a small scale), solid scintillator coated on the bottom of the well of the multiplate, and scintillator impregnated into the plastic of the multiplate. The simultaneous analyses, along with the potential for automation and robotics, have increased sample throughput considerably.

There are essentially two designs of instrument. One uses a standard coincidence counting circuit with the photomultipliers turned around (one above, one underneath) so that the microplate is read between the tubes. Because the microplate has to be transparent, there is the possibility that the coincidence circuit will detect photons originating from adjacent wells. This requires some compensation for the cross talk of signal. To combat this phenomenon, there are microplates available where the well of the multiplate is clear on the bottom and opaque on the side.

The other design uses one photomultiplier tube positioned above the microplate and exploits the properties of the photon pulse to discriminate real from background events. The different types of instrument are covered in more detail in Section 8.8.

Solid scintillator multiwell plates allow recovery of the sample for further analysis, such as mass spectrometry (Section 3.5.12) or nuclear magnetic resonance spectroscopy (NMR; Section 3.5.13), but it is not possible to recover samples once mixed with liquid scintillant.

6.14.1 Multiwell Plates and Fraction Collection

Multiwell plates can be used for routine analysis, but often they are used to collect multiple fractions of HPLC eluate. Flow scintillation counting (Section 6.15) is not very sensitive, and so if radioactivity in the HPLC peak is low, greater sensitivity can be achieved by collecting fractions (every 10 to 30 sec), analyzing each fraction separately, and then reconstructing the chromatogram. The disadvantage of fraction collection is that there is a loss of peak resolution. Continuous flow analysis will record the level of radioactivity at periods as short as 1 sec (the dwell time; see Section 6.15.1). In fraction collecting, physical restrictions do not allow fractions to be collected every second. Indeed, if conventional liquid scintillation vials are used to collect fractions, about one fraction every 30 sec is the norm. Multiwell plate technology has gone some way to alleviate this difficulty, as it is possible to collect fractions over much shorter times; the limitations are really in the design of the fraction collector. Nevertheless, 10 sec is not unrealistic, and 5 sec is possible with the right configuration of the fraction collector.

An application used in multiwell plates is to collect the eluate fraction in a plate that contains either the solid scintillator coated on the bottom of the multiplate well or the scintillator as part of the plastic construction of the well. The distance from the analyte to the scintillator in either case must be as short as possible, and consequently, the sample is dried down prior to analysis. It is, of course, important that the analyte itself is not volatile.

6.14.2 Sample Drying

There are considerations that must be taken into account when drying samples in microplates. If the liquid in the wells is dried too fast, then there is an opportunity for the radioactive material to be deposited on the wall of the well of the microplate and not on the scintillator, which is on the bottom of the well. Care must be taken in the drying process to ensure that the material is deposited where it can be detected. It is recommended that tests are carried out on the type of material to be collected so that the recoveries on the microplates may be established.

As with any solid scintillator, microplates suffer from photoluminescence and they have to be left in the counting instrument for some time prior to analysis, to allow them to dark adapt.

6.15 FLOW SCINTILLATION COUNTING

The principle of operation of flow scintillation counters is similar to a standard scintillation counter, with the exception that the vial is replaced by a coiled tube located in a cell that sits between the photomultiplier tubes. Instead of the sample vial being placed in the scintillation counter, the sample (eluate from an HPLC column) passes through the cell, which is sited permanently between the photomultiplier tubes. Radioisotopes such as ^{35}S, ^{32}P, and ^{33}P can all be readily analyzed using liquid or solid cells. Gamma emitters can also be analyzed using flow counting.

For the purposes of ADME, there are two types of flow cell, one based on the use of a solid scintillant and the other on a liquid scintillant, although the general design of the instrumentation is the same (Figure 6.17). Liquid flow cells use scintillation cocktail, and once mixed with the HPLC eluate, the drug and metabolites cannot be recovered for further analysis, such as mass spectroscopy (Section 3.5.12) or nuclear magnetic resonance spectroscopy (Section 3.5.13). Drug and metabolites can be recovered from solid cells and they are particularly useful where the eluate passes from the HPLC, through the flow cell, and then directly into a mass spectrometer.

In liquid flow cells the eluate stream is mixed with scintillation cocktail prior to entering the flow cell. In this case, the flow cell is just an empty coil of low-friction, nonadsorbent material tubing such as PTFE. Liquid flow cells are generally 500 μL in volume, although 1 mL cells are often used. The choice of flow cell is a compromise, as the bigger the cell, the better the sensitivity (Equation 6.7), but the poorer

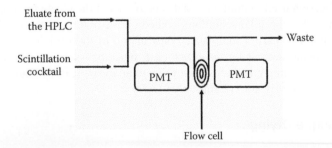

Figure 6.17   Diagram of flow scintillation counter. PMT, photomultiplier tube (shown arranged as part of a coincidence circuit). The flow cell can be of solid or liquid scintillant design. In solid cells, there is no scintillation cocktail introduced into the system.

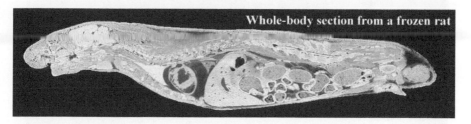

Figure 5.1 A 30-μm-thick section obtained from a male rat.

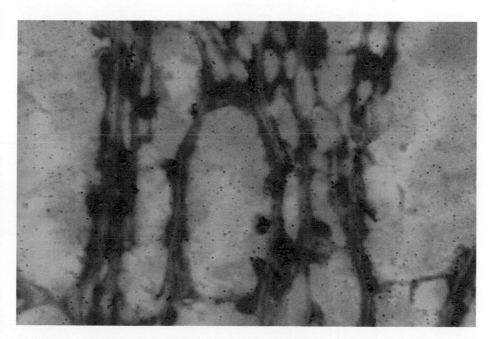

Figure 5.11 Microautoradiogram of the fundic stomach region in a rat.

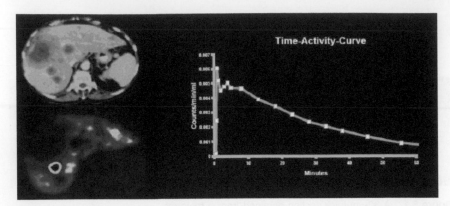

Figure 11.4 Schematic representation of isotope generation in a cyclotron. Injected H⁻ ions are accelerated to high speed by magnetic fields. Passage through carbon foil leaves accelerated protons, which are fired at the target material to produce the required isotope.

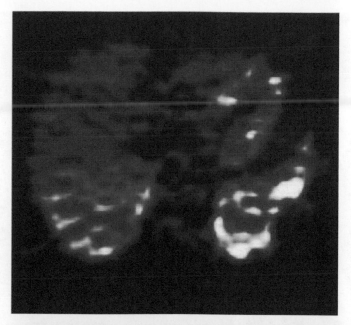

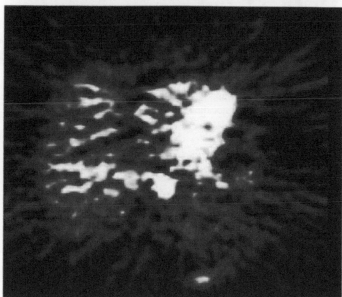

Figure 11.6 Transverse PET images of the chest after injection of (a) ^{15}O-labeled water and (b) ^{11}C-labeled DACA. (a) Increased signal intensity is seen in the blood pool of the heart and in the right lung. The tumor is poorly perfused and cannot be seen. (b) Increased uptake of ^{11}C-DACA is seen in the myocardium (upper-right-hand corner) and in the tumor (mesothelioma, lower-right-hand corner).

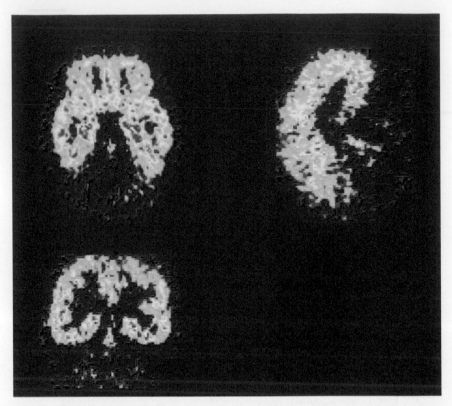

Figure 11.7 PET image of the serotonin 5-HT1A-receptor in the human brain with the radio-ligand [^{11}C]-WAY-100635. (Image courtesy of Prof. C. Halldin and Prof L. Farde, Karolinska Institute, Stockholm.)

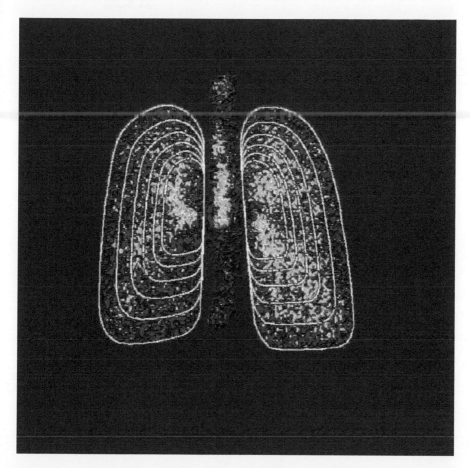

Figure 12.4 Regional lung analysis in gamma scintigraphy. The lung is divided into six concentric lung-shaped zones centered on the hilum. (From Newman, S.P. et al., *Adv. Drug Del. Rev.*, 55, 851, 2003. With permission.)

the chromatographic resolution. The sample–liquid scintillator mixture generates photons, which are recorded as cpm. Liquid flow cells require a flow scintillation cocktail, of which there are many types. They are all non-viscous and should, under no circumstances, be allowed to form a gel in the flow cell. The correct choice of flow cocktail cannot be overstated. The author has experience of cells becoming damaged by inappropriate flow cocktails, resulting in leaks from the cell and damaged electronics.

Solid scintillator materials are typically solid beads of yttrium silicate. Usually solid scintillator flow cells are much smaller in volume, around 200 µL. This ensures that chromatographic resolution is good, but they are not as sensitive. A drawback of the solid scintillator cell is that it can easily become contaminated. HPLC systems are used in ADME studies for a variety of different biological samples, and a lot of these may contain particulate material that will become attached to the solid scintillator material and thus reduce the cell's performance, or even render it inoperative. Solid scintillator cells have been developed with interchangeable scintillator cartridges to help overcome these problems. Solid scintillators are also prone to static and for this reason the cell is often fitted with a grounding wire.

For the detection of tritium, liquid flow cells are recommended. The path length of the tritium β^- particle is about 6×10^{-3} mm in water, and therefore there is little opportunity for it to interact with the solid scintillant. Solid cells for tritium analysis are available, but they have very low counting efficiencies — no greater than 10%.

It has been reported that liquid systems have higher counting efficiencies and lower backgrounds than solid scintillator systems. However, the costs of operating a liquid system are much higher, as they can use a significant quantity of scintillation cocktail in the course of an HPLC run (plus disposal costs). For this reason, some laboratories have explored the use of small-bore columns that have low flow rates (100 to 300 µL/min) but there should be a corresponding reduction in the choice of cell size.

Solid scintillator systems are more expensive to purchase, but they have much lower running costs.

6.15.1 Data Acquisition

Flow systems use a different method of recording cpm and converting into dpm than do standard counters. In a standard scintillation counter the sample does not move and the counts are accumulated over a given time. The total counts accrued over the analysis time are then divided by that time (in minutes) to yield cpm, which are then converted to dpm via a quench method. In a flow system the sample is constantly moving and is only in the detection area of the photomultiplier tube for a short period. If the flow cell is 500 µl and the flow rate is 1 mL/min of eluate and 3 mL/min of scintillation cocktail, then any one part of the sample is only exposed to the cell for 0.125 min or 7.5 sec. This time is called different names by different manufacturers. Some call it the residence time, some the time of flight or the transit time. For the purposes of this publication residence time will be used. Residence time is given by Equation 6.7:

$$RT = \frac{V}{F} \tag{6.7}$$

where RT is the residence time (min), V is the cell volume (mL), and F is the flow rate (mL/min).

The counts per minute in a flow system are calculated by Equation 6.8:

$$cpm = \frac{C}{RT} \tag{6.8}$$

where C is the total number of counts and RT is the residence time.

It is important to note that it is essential the volume of the flow cell is very accurately manufactured, as the calculations of residence time are dependent upon it.

For background subtracted results, Equation 6.9 is used:

$$CPM_{net} = \frac{C - C_b}{RT} \tag{6.9}$$

where cpm_{net} is the cpm value (C) minus the background (C_b).

As the eluate–cocktail mixture flows through the system there has to be a period of time to accumulate the radioactive events. These events are random, and so the longer the accumulation time, the better. The count time, however, is governed by the residence time. Therefore, the accumulation period, often called the update time or dwell time, cannot be longer than the residence time. The accumulation period is often kept at 1 sec but on some systems it is 6 sec. On all systems it is configurable. As the flow counter measures each time period it will accumulate a series of data points (at each update time) that, when graphed together, will draw a chromatogram in the same way as the HPLC.

On normal liquid scintillation counters, the limit of detection is simply defined as a multiple of the background. Calculation of the limit of detection in a flow cell is not as simple, as the chromatographic peak width has to be taken into account, and so Equation 6.10 is used:

$$MDA = \frac{B \times W}{RT \times E} \tag{6.10}$$

where MDA is the minimum detectable activity (dpm), B is the background cpm, W is the chromatographic peak width (min), RT is the residence time (min), and E is the efficiency percent divided by 100 (i.e., if the efficiency is 80%, then E = 0.8).

The question that immediately arises is, "How is efficiency calculated?" The answer is with great difficulty. It can be estimated by injecting a known amount of radioactivity, then recording the cpm value. The percentage difference between cpm and dpm is then an estimate of efficiency. The problem with this, however, is that it bears little relevance to the real situation, with chromatographic peaks. Given the variation in peak shape, solvent composition during a gradient separation, possible color of the analyte and performance of the cocktail, it is impossible to measure quench to convert cpm to dpm with an accuracy equivalent to a standard scintillation counter. For this reason, flow counter data are routinely recorded in cpm.

This also raises the possibility that if metabolites are quantified using radio-HPLC (Section 3.6.8) and the quench differs across the chromatogram, the values obtained from early peaks may not be comparable with those with later retention times. It is, however, common practice to ignore these potential issues. If there are concerns, then chromatographic peaks should be collected and analyzed offline with a liquid scintillation counter. The quantification of metabolites is routinely based on the relative amounts in the radio-HPLC peaks (Section 3.6.8). A simple check can be made by measuring the cpm in a late and early eluting peak, collecting these peaks in a fraction collector and measuring the dpm offline. If the ratio of the cpm values between the peaks is similar to that measured by dpm, then metabolites can be reliably quantified. If significant differences arise, then quench may be having an effect and offline quantification should be considered. The collected peaks from a liquid flow cell will already contain scintillant and this can be used in the offline liquid scintillation counter, providing an appropriate quench correction curve is used.

Flow scintillation analysis is not particularly sensitive and, as a rule of thumb, several hundred dpm are required in each HPLC peak to achieve an acceptable signal to noise.

REFERENCES

1. Thomson, J., Di-isopropylnapthelene: a new solvent for liquid scintillation counting, in *Liquid Scintillation Counting and Organic Scintillators*, Ross, J., Noakes, E., and Spaulding, J.D., Eds., Lewis Publishers, Chelsea, MI, pp. 19–34, 1991.
2. Te Wiel, J. and Hegge, T., Advances in scintillation cocktails, in *Liquid Scintillation Counting and Organic Scintillators*, Ross, J., Noakes, E., and Spaulding, J.D., Eds., Lewis Publishers, Chelsea, MI, pp. 51–67, 1991.
3. Cerenkov, P.A., *Dokl. Akad. Nauk. U.S.S.R.*, 2, 451, 1934.
4. Kobayashi, Y. and Maudsley, D.V., Practical aspects of double isotope counting, in *Current Status of Liquid Scintillation Counting*, Bransome, Jr., E.D., Ed., Grune and Stratton, New York, 1970, pp. 76–85.
5. Hofstadter, R., Alkali halide scintillation counters, *Phys. Rev.*, 74, 100–101, 1948.
6. Hofstadter, R., Properties of scintillation materials, *Nucleonics*, 6, 70–72, 1950.
7. Lempicki, A., The physics of inorganic scintillators, *J. Appl. Spectrosc.*, 62, 209–231, 1995.

CHAPTER 7

Statistics in Liquid Scintillation Counting

Simon Temple

CONTENTS

7.1 INTRODUCTION

Statistics are a tool to enable the user to report results to a level of confidence and are particularly important when the observed counts are close to the background.

The intention of this chapter is to provide a set of examples that may be used in everyday analysis and also to provide the basis for the statistical results printed on most commercial scintillation counters.

7.2 STANDARD DEVIATION

As mentioned in Section 2.7, radioactive decay is random. It therefore fits the model of normal distribution (Gaussian distribution). It is impossible to determine when any individual nuclear decay might occur and so statistical analysis is used to describe the average behavior of all the nuclear decays within a sample. Counting statistics are then applied to calculate the probability of obtaining a given count

Table 7.1   The Same Sample Counted 10 Times

Count No.	$CPM\chi$
1	86,287
2	86,301
3	85,910
4	86,084
5	86,498
6	86,277
7	86,346
8	86,039
9	86,212
10	86,227
Total	862,181
$\bar{\chi}$	86,218

Note: $CPM\chi$ = the counts for each analysis;
$\bar{\chi}$ = the mean of the counts.

within a defined confidence limit. Thus, when a count is reported, it should be qualified by the confidence level.

If, for example, a sample is counted and the result gives 65 cpm against a background count of 40 cpm, with a count time of 10 min, an investigator would not have much confidence in the result. Intuitively, there is just not enough information to form an opinion that would stand up to scrutiny. Statistics will mathematically tell you why it does not stand up.

Table 7.1 shows data from the same sample counted 10 times, for the same period of time.

As can be seen from the data, the counts are all different, even though it was the same sample counted under the same conditions. So what is the correct value? The mean value could be calculated, as shown in Table 7.1, but that alone does not give any measure as to the confidence that number carries with it. We could calculate the standard deviation of counting these 10 samples using Equation 7.1. (In reality, most people these days simply push the button on the calculator to calculate the standard deviation, but it is worth remembering how it is derived.)

$$\sigma = \sqrt{\frac{\Sigma\left(\chi - \bar{\chi}\right)^2}{i - 1}} \tag{7.1}$$

where σ is the standard deviation, Σ stands for the sum, $\chi = $ CPM , $\bar{\chi}$ is the mean CPM, and i is number of times the sample was counted.

Entering the data from Table 7.1,

$$\sigma = \sqrt{\frac{254893}{9}} = \sqrt{28321} = 168.289$$

Table 7.2   Data in Table 7.1 Arranged to Show the
             Number of Times Data Points Appear
             within a Defined cpm Range

Occurrence	cpm Range
1	85,900–86,000
2	86,000–86,100
0	86,100–86,200
4	86,200–86,300
2	86,300–86,400
1	86,400–86,500

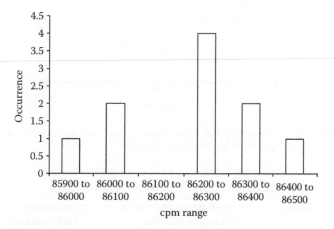

Figure 7.1   Distribution vs. time of the data shown in Table 7.2, demonstrating a normal distribution.

The standard deviation is 168.29.

The results of the 10 sample counts would be expressed as the mean, with the standard deviation recorded after it: 86,218 ± 168 cpm. Note the use of ±; we will come back to this in a moment.

Why is that a better representation of the results? To explain this, we will display the data as a normal distribution. First the data are grouped as shown in Table 7.2. These data are then plotted as shown in Figure 7.1.

There are only a few data points represented in Figure 7.2, but nevertheless, the shape of a normal distribution curve is evident. If many more analyses were conducted, then a classical normal distribution curve would be obtained, as shown in Figure 7.2. There is what is known as the central limit theorem, which states that the mean of any set of variants with any distribution having a finite mean and variance tends to the normal distribution. The upshot of this is that many common attributes, such as the height of people within a population, the temperature taken at noon each day for a year, or the number of letters per word in this book, all follow a normal distribution.

The middle value on the distribution curve is known as the median, and the most frequently observed occurrence is known as the mode. A normal distribution has the fortunate property that the median and mode are the same, and these are also

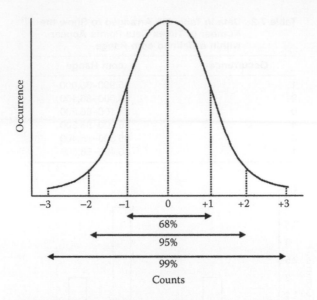

Figure 7.2   A normal distribution curve, showing the approximate confidence intervals for one, two, and three times the standard deviation.

Table 7.3   Standard Deviation (σ) and Corresponding Probability

Standard Deviation (σ)	% Probability of a Value Falling within the σ	% Probability of a Value Falling outside the σ
1σ	68.27	31.73
2σ	95.45	4.55
3σ	99.73	0.27

equal to the mean. This, in fact, simplifies the mathematics and is shown in Figure 7.2 as the line marked 0 on the x-axis. Values for one, two, and three times the standard deviation on either side of the mean have been added to the x-axis in Figure 7.2. Because we are dealing with a normal distribution, we can say that the probability of a value falling within ±1 standard deviation is 68%.* This value, 68%, is called the confidence limit. In other words, 68% of the time the observed count would be within ±1 standard deviation of the true count. In the example shown in Table 7.1, the mean value was 86,218 and the standard deviation was 168 cpm. So for 68% of the time the counts would be 86,218 ± 168, or between 86,050 and 86,386. This also means, of course, that 31.73% of the time the counts will fall outside 1 standard deviation of the true count. This level of confidence is not high enough to be used in nuclear counting, and so 2 standard deviations are used, which brings us to a 95.5% confidence level. If three standard deviations were chosen, the confidence level would rise to 99.73%. The percent probabilities for given standard deviations are shown in Table 7.3.

---

* The mathematic derivation of this value is not important here, so please take this on trust.

7.3 USE OF %2σ IN SCINTILLATION COUNTING

When measuring radioactivity in a sample, you are taking a sample of the total number of possible disintegration events over a finite period. The counts are therefore accumulated over this period. It is not possible to measure radioactivity in real time, as may be done with other detection methods, such as absorbance or fluorescence. At the end of the counting period, the number of counts is divided by the time, thus producing the cpm value. The longer the count time, the larger the number of counts, and therefore the higher the precision. The 95.5% confidence interval for any count can be calculated from Equation 7.2:

$$2\sigma = 2 \times \sqrt{\text{total counts}} \qquad (7.2)$$

(Note that for the 99.73% confidence level, the formula is $3\sigma = 3 \times \sqrt{\text{total counts}}$)

Take an example. A sample is counted and a total of 10,550 counts are accrued (this is the total counts over the counting period, not cpm). Using Equation 7.2,

$$2\sigma = 2 \times \sqrt{10,550} = 2 \times 102.7 = 205.4$$

Thus, we are 95.5% confident that the true count for our sample is between 10,344.5 and 10,755.4.

In practice, the sample being analyzed is of unknown activity and so if we just guessed at a count time of, say, 10 min and the sample contained 10 cpm, the total counts would be only 100. On the other hand, if the sample contained 100,000 cpm, the total count would be 1 million. Putting these values into Equation 7.2, we would be 95.5% confident that the true value for the 10 cpm sample fell between 8 and 12 cpm (two standard deviations = 2). We would be 95.5% confident that the true value for the 1,000,000 cpm sample fell between 998,000 and 1,200,000 cpm (two standard deviations = 2000). For the 10 cpm sample, the range is ±20% of the result. For the 1,000,000 cpm sample, the range is ±0.2% of the result. The conclusion would be that if the sample contained 10 cpm, it was not counted for long enough, and for the 1,000,000 cpm sample, it was counted for longer than necessary. What we need to do, therefore, is to count the sample for long enough so the percentage explained above is adequate but not overdone. Percentages commonly used are 2% for most counting, 5% where the value required is more approximate and 1% where greater precision is needed. This value is known as the %2σ (i.e., 2%2σ, 5%2σ, etc.). The notation is sometimes expressed simply as %2σ, without defining the actual percentage. Although strictly speaking this is not entirely correct, it is the convention for %2σ.

%2σ is calculated from Equation 7.3:

$$\%2\sigma = \frac{200}{\sqrt{\text{counts}}} \qquad (7.3)$$

(Note that %1σ would be calculated using $\dfrac{100}{\sqrt{\text{counts}}}$)

All manufacturers of liquid scintillation counters use computer assistance to gather the results, and this allows the results to be expressed in terms of the %2σ. This also allows the counter to be set so that it counts a sample until a certain value of %2σ is reached. The time required to achieve a desired %2σ value is given in Equation 7.4:

$$T = \frac{1}{\text{cpm}} \left(\frac{200}{\%2\sigma} \right)^2 \tag{7.4}$$

Let us go back to our examples of 10 and 100,000 cpm. Putting these values into Equation 7.4, we find that the instrument count times to achieve 2%2σ are:

$$T = \frac{1}{10} \left(\frac{200}{2} \right)^2 = 1000 \text{ min (16.6 h)}$$

$$T = \frac{1}{1,000,000} \left(\frac{200}{2} \right)^2 = 0.01 \text{ min (0.6 sec)}$$

Equation 7.4 is very useful practically. If you have a rough estimate of the amount of radioactivity in a sample, you can calculate approximately how long it will take to count. Modern counters can be set to count to %2σ or for a maximum amount of time, whichever is reached first. The sample containing 10 cpm in the example above is probably not significant in terms of the radiotracer study, and therefore counting to a lower level of precision to save counting time is acceptable.

Finally, note that cpm have been used throughout the above examples. Since it is cpm that the counter records, these are the values that should be used for the statistical calculations. The dpm values are derived from the cpm via quench correction. If an estimate of the dpm values is required, then the statistics should be calculated on the basis of cpm, and then an estimate for the counting efficiency can be factored in. Remember that the resulting dpm values are only estimates, as it will depend upon the actual level of quench in any given sample.

7.4 LOW ACTIVITY COUNTING

When counting high-activity samples, the issue of the background decay events caused by outside sources (instrument/environmental/cosmic) is unlikely to make a significant contribution to the overall result. If the cpm of a count that contains only scintillation cocktail and nonradioactive sample is, say, 25 cpm and an active sample is giving 98,000 cpm, then the background as a percentage of the total cpm is only 0.025%. If a different sample were counted giving 1000 cpm, then the background as a percentage of the sample count would be 2.5%. Again, this may be considered insignificant (depending upon the experiment). If a sample was counted and found to be 100 cpm, then the background count becomes a massive 25% of the total count.

A cpm value with the background subtracted is called the net cpm value. Net counts therefore have two separate components (background and sample) and each will have its own associated uncertainty. The uncertainty of the two parameters may be expressed using the rules for the propagation of the error (Equation 7.5):

$$\sigma Cn = \sqrt{\sigma(Cx)^2 + \sigma(Cb)^2} \qquad (7.5)$$

where Cx is the sample activity (which includes the background activity), Cb is the background activity, Cn is the net count, and σ is the standard deviation.

If the %2σ for the net cpm is required, this is calculated from Equation 7.6:

$$\%2\sigma = 200 \frac{\sqrt{\left(\frac{\sqrt{Nx}}{Tx}\right)^2 + \left(\frac{\sqrt{Nb}}{Tb}\right)^2}}{Cx - Cb} \qquad (7.6)$$

where Nχ is number of counts in the sample (total counts, not cpm), Tχ is the time the sample was counted, Nb is the number of counts in the background (total counts, not cpm), Tb is the time the background was counted, Cx is the cpm in the sample, and Cb is the cpm in the background.

Let us take the example we first started with (Section 7.2), where a sample was counted for 10 min and the result gives 65 cpm against a background count of 40 cpm:

$$\%2\sigma = 200 \frac{\sqrt{\left(\frac{\sqrt{650}}{10}\right)^2 + \left(\frac{\sqrt{400}}{10}\right)^2}}{65 - 40}$$

The answer is 25%2σ. It was said in Section 7.2 that intuitively this was not a good result — well, now we know why.

7.5 LIMITS OF DETECTION

Experience shows that every institute and even every department has historical methods of determining the limits of detection of any system of analysis. The same is true in the case of the counting of radioactive events. In 1968, a paper written by

Lloyd Currie established a high level of uniformity in the calculation of determining the limits of detection.[1] There are three limiting levels for qualitative and quantitative analysis, as follows:

- The critical level L_c — the level above which an observed instrument signal may be reliably recognized as being detected. This is a qualitative decision and is subject to two kinds of errors: concluding that a signal is true when it is not and failing to conclude that it is true when it is true.
- The detection level L_d — the true net signal level that will lead to detection.
- The determination level L_q — the signal level above which quantitative measurement can be performed with the relative uncertainty stated.

Each of these levels is calculated by the following criteria. The first is the standard deviation of a background or blank sample. Choosing a probability for an error of the first kind, for falsely deciding that the signal is present when it is not allows calculation of the critical level L_c. Choosing a probability for an error of the second kind, which decides that a signal is not present when it actually is, allows calculation of the detection level L_d. Finally, specifying the maximum tolerated error in the quantitative measurement allows the determination level L_q to be calculated.

For the purposes of scintillation counting, L_c and L_d are normally the ones calculated and then decisions are made as to the level of L_q. Formulae for calculation of these detection limits are shown in Equation 7.7 and Equation 7.8:

$$L_c = 2.33 \sqrt{\text{blank}} \qquad (7.7)$$

(the blank counted under the same conditions as the sample, but without the active element)

$$L_d = 4.65 \sqrt{\text{blank}} \quad (\text{blank as in } L_c) \qquad (7.8)$$

Let us take an example where a blank vial gives a count of 12 cpm. (We will assume that the vial was counted for a sufficiently long time. A count time of 2 h will give a value of $5.3\%2\sigma$; see Equation 7.3.) Thus, $L_c = 8.07$ cpm. This, according to the Currie equation, is the level above which an observed instrument signal may be reliably recognized as being detected. $L_d = 16.1$ cpm. This, according to the Currie equation, is the true net signal level that would lead to detection.

REFERENCES

1. Currie, L.A., Limits for qualitative detection and quantitative determination: application to radiochemistry, *Anal. Chem.*, 40, 586–593, 1968.

FURTHER READING

Kessler, M.J., Statistical computations in counting, in *Handbook of Radioactivity Analysis*, Annunziata, F.L., Ed., Academic Press, San Diego, 387–406, 1998.

CHAPTER 8

Instrumentation for Detection of Radioactivity

Simon Temple

CONTENTS

8.1 INTRODUCTION

The reader should be familiar with the theory and general principles of scintillation counting, which are described in Chapter 6.

Over the past 50 years or more, commercial manufacturers have produced a range of instrumentation for the measurement of radioactivity. Undoubtedly, strong competition among the manufacturers drove forward some fundamental developments, particularly with background reduction and quench correction. The upside of these competitive developments is the refined, sensitive, and user-friendly instruments we have today. The downside is that much of what goes on inside the instrument to convert simple flashes of light into usable data is hidden from the user. The fundamentals of the methodology have therefore become entwined with the instrumentation. Scintillation counting may not be unique in this respect, as computing has universally revolutionized instrument control and data acquisition. Nevertheless, unlike so many other analytical instruments, scintillation counters do have an unusual longevity. As a consequence, there are in existence many different instruments with a variety of background correction and quench correction routines, some of them fundamental to the way the data are gathered. It is therefore impossible to separate a discussion of background subtraction and quench correction from the instruments themselves.

In addition to scintillation counting other technological developments have been made in the field of radiodetection and this chapter provides a general review of the methods and instrumentation available.

8.2 HISTORY

The first instrument that could be called a scintillation counter was developed in 1903. William Crookes designed a system that he called the spinthariscope (from the Greek *spintharis* — "a spark"). The instrument consisted of a phosphorescent screen of zinc sulfide placed over a minute trace of a radium salt (which had been supplied to Crookes by Marie Curie). The α-particles emitted by the radium salt caused visible flashes of light (scintillations), which were observed and manually counted through a microscope, making the instrument cumbersome and time-consuming. While modern scintillation counters use photomultipliers for detection (Section 6.3), the detector in the very first scintillation counter was the human eye.

As discussed in Chapter 6, the design of scintillation counters made significant gains in the early 1950s. Scintillation counting offers excellent sensitivity and results that are little affected by the mass of the radioactive tracer. As always in scientific endeavor, the lowest detection levels are demanded from scintillation counting and instrument manufacturers have constantly strived to develop products with improved sensitivity. This has in general been achieved by increasing the efficiency of the counting process and at the same time reducing the background. There have also been many developments in the design of liquid scintillation cocktails. (It is nevertheless true that results from the best instrument in the world will only be as good as the sample. There is no substitute for good sample preparation — see Chapter 9.)

Although there is some debate about what constitutes low-level scintillation counting, for the purposes of this book, low-level counting is considered to be the quantification of less than 100 dpm of ^{14}C or less than 200 dpm of ^{3}H. As with any analytical instrumentation, the lower the background, the better the signal to noise and the better the sensitivity. In scintillation counting there are a variety of sources of background and so a combined approach has to be taken to reduce noise.

In addition to noise reduction, the manufacturers have developed numerous methods to handle quench correction. Although modern methods are all based on the use of an external standard (Section 8.6), some complex and sophisticated mathematical algorithms have been developed to handle the data. Different manufacturers developed their own systems and the principle methodologies are discussed in Section 8.4.

8.3 BACKGROUND REDUCTION

In the early days of scintillation counting the preferred method of ensuring a low background was to add lead shielding to block cosmic rays. This worked to some extent but there were other sources of noise where shielding had no effect, for example, where material in the construction of the scintillation counters unavoidably contained levels of natural radioactivity. In addition, the design of the instrument itself may produce effects that are incorrectly read as radioactive background. The material of the vial and the scintillation cocktail can also produce background.

Background is divided into two different types: unquenchable and quenchable. Approximately 32% of the total background spectrum is quenchable and 68% is unquenchable.[1]

Unquenchable background is that produced by events outside the scintillator material. Examples of unquenchable background are cosmic radiation interacting with the glass of the vial or the face of the photomultiplier tube, producing secondary Cherenkov events or γ rays. There may be naturally occurring radiation in the material of the vial (e.g., ^{40}K in the glass*). The use of high-density polyethylene vials is often recommended, as they have a lower background than glass vials. In addition to background originating from aberrant radioactivity, there will also be electronic cross talk between the photomultipliers and general instrument electronic noise. Static on the scintillation vial will also contribute to background (Section 6.8). It is impossible to quantify unquenchable background because of its nature. It is possible to some extent, however, to recognize unquenchable background and reject it from the counts.

Quenchable background is that produced by naturally occurring radioactivity in the scintillator material or cosmic radiation passing through it. It is possible to measure quenchable background and largely subtract it from the counts. As a consequence of having quenchable and unquenchable background, the value for background can only be quoted as cpm, not dpm — a fact rarely understood. If a background is quoted in dpm, it will contain a correction for quenchable background, but it will still contain a contribution from the unquenchable background, which by its nature cannot be quantified. Since the relative amounts of quenchable and unquenchable background vary, there is no way of defining the precise contribution of each. For this reason, background is measured in cpm, the background cpm are subtracted from the sample cpm, and then this value is used to derive dpm from the quench curve. All scintillation counters that have a background subtraction facility subtract background cpm from sample cpm, and then derive the dpm. If background subtraction is conducted manually (or by a proprietary program), the same algorithm should be used. It is incorrect to background subtract dpm from dpm. In practice, errors resulting in subtracting dpm from dpm are not significant unless the counts are low (below about 100 and 200 cpm).

8.3.1   Instrument Design

Scintillation counters measure the photons produced by the scintillator. These photons are produced in proportion to the intensity of the energy of the isotope being analyzed. The intensity and number of photons are registered by photomultipliers (Section 6.3). The signal from the photomultiplier ultimately ends up as a data readout. Between the photomultiplier and the readout are the electronics and it is here where there has been concentrated effort to reduce the signals from background noise. Without doubt, the use of coincidence counting (Section 6.3) contributed substantially to the reduction of background, and this was followed by improvements in photomultiplier tube design and low-activity lead shielding, often combined with other metals.

8.3.2   Active Guard Detectors

As lead shielding increased, so did the weight of the instruments (and some would say so did the construction of the laboratory floors to hold them). The guard detector was developed in response to this problem. A guard detector has a volume of scintillating material (liquid or solid) with an additional pair of photomultiplier tubes in anticoincidence to the sample photomultiplier tubes. Penetrating radiation,

---

* This is why glass for scintillation vials is especially selected to be low in ^{40}K.

external to the instrument, passes through the guard detector and then on to the detector, where it would normally be registered as an event. The scintillator in the guard detector, however, also registers an event. If the coincidence circuit on the guard detector registers an event within the same time window (approximately 20 nsec) as the sample detectors, the event is disregarded. In addition to rejecting events from cosmic and low-level environmental radiation, cross talk from Cherenkov events caused by cosmic activity on the face of the photomultiplier tubes and glass vials is also rejected.

An example of an instrument that makes good use of the guard detector is the 1220 Quantulus, introduced by Wallac. The guard detector in the scintillation counter comprises an anticoincidence guard of mineral oil scintillators with optically coupled photomultiplier tubes. The 1414 Guardian counter, also produced by Wallac, used a similar process, but the scintillator in the guard detector was constructed of plastic. In addition, the 1220 Quantulus employed extensive multichannel analyzers, allowing the background spectrum to be viewed as well as the sample spectrum.

8.3.3 Pulse Height Analysis

When the photons produced by a scintillation event reach the photomultiplier tubes, their intensity and number are recorded. The output of the photomultiplier is an analog signal; that is, it is continuous, like the volume control on a radio. On modern instruments, the analog signal is electronically converted to a digital signal, that is, one consisting of distinct packages of data. In early scintillation counters the conversion was done on a pulse height analysis (PHA) basis, which directly converted the analog signal into a digital number. The analog signal from the photomultiplier (summed by the summation circuit; see Section 6.3) was converted to a digital signal by an electronic circuit known as the analog-to-digital converter (ADC). The ADC converts the analog signal into a number that it allocates to that particular intensity.

In pulse height analysis, the operator selects an upper-level discriminator and a lower-level discriminator. If a count has an intensity above the lower-level discriminator and below the upper-level discriminator, it is recorded (Figure 8.1). It is not necessary to form a spectrum to achieve pulse height analysis. The system works by eliminating those counts that fall outside the required discriminator values, thus eliminating counts at the lower end of the spectrum where luminescence and static tend to appear. It also removes higher-energy background and cosmic radiation from the counts. Although at one time this was a standard method of background reduction, nowadays the electronics are a little more sophisticated.

8.3.4 Pulse Shape Analysis

When a packet of photons is released from the scintillator to the detector, this is called a pulse. A pulse can be described in two parts: (1) a prompt pulse or fast component and (2) a delayed pulse or slow component.[2]

Pulse shape analysis (PSA) works by looking at the shape of the pulse to determine if the pulse has the shorter component of an actual event or the longer

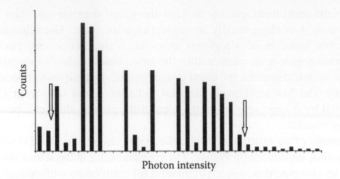

Figure 8.1   Pulse height analysis for background reduction. The arrows show the discriminator
settings. The signals below the lower arrow and above the upper arrow are
rejected.

component of background (Figure 8.2). The shape of the pulse and the length of the
tail of the pulse are scintillator and sample dependent; thus, the pulse shape depends,
at least in part, upon the analytical conditions. Overall, however, the prompt pulse
will be in the region of 2 to 5 nsec long and the delayed component will be in the
region of 900 nsec.[3]

The properties of pulse shape have been used to identify the difference between
β- and α-events because the delayed component of the α is much longer than the
delayed component of the β. The properties of pulse height can also be exploited in
determining the level of background originating from cosmic and other background
radiation interacting with glass vials, as this results in the emission of long pulses.

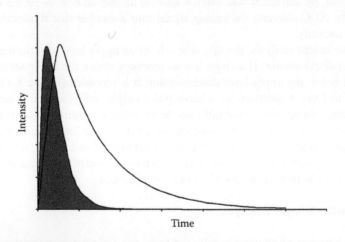

Figure 8.2   Pulse shape analysis. The pulse (represented by the black area) is an actual event
from the sample. The pulse (represented by the white area) originates from the
background. (Produced from original material by kind permission of Beckman
Instruments.)

Using pulse shape analysis may reduce the background by up to 50%, but it may also reduce the counting efficiency. Pulse shape analysis has been used by both Beckman and Wallac scintillation counters.

8.3.5 Pulse Amplitude Comparison

Pulse amplitude comparison (PAC) makes use of the fact that the amplitude of the pulses of light the photomultiplier tubes record are different if they are produced inside the scintillation vial or external to the scintillation vial. If an event takes place inside the scintillation vial, the photons detected by the two photomultipliers will be of approximately the same intensity and will be recorded as a real event. If the event takes place outside the vial, the pulses will not be of the same intensity and the signal will be rejected on the grounds of the different pulse heights. Some scintillation counters have programs that allow for the setting of the pulse amplitude comparator, which involves the use of a pure β^--emitter and a background sample.

8.3.6 Time-Resolved Liquid Scintillation Counting

This technique, introduced in 1986, is an extension of pulse shape analysis, but with a greater depth of analysis into the shape of the pulse. As stated in Section 8.3.4, the scintillation pulse originating from a scintillator is a burst of photons lasting about 2 to 8 nsec and is called the prompt or fast component. The pulse originates from direct fluorescence of the excited singlet states of the secondary scintillator (i.e., the state where all electrons in the molecule are spin paired). The slow or delayed component of a pulse is due to the delayed fluorescence emission from a process called triplet–triplet annihilation (The triplet state is where one set of electron spins is unpaired.) From studies of the way the pulses are formed it is possible to distinguish between the different types of pulse using time resolution. The prompt or fast component is usually much larger than the after-pulses since it contains a large number of photons emitted in a very short time. This is effectively a large group of photoelectrons emitted in a burst, and the electronics combine them as one large pulse (Figure 8.3A and B). The delayed or slow components (the after-pulses) are fewer in number and spread over a longer time period, and are distinguishable as single photoelectrons. The composition of the liquid cocktail or the solid scintillator has an effect on the characteristics of the pulse. For example, oxygen in a liquid scintillation cocktail will reduce the after-pulses as it scavenges triplets. The effect can be reduced or removed by purging the vial with inert gas. Solid scintillators behave differently. The triplet states in glass are not quenched, and hence any background events, caused by the glass, are exhibited with the delayed component in evidence. The electronics are able to recognize these delayed components and eliminate them. Furthermore, this enables time-resolved counting to be used to discriminate against unquenchable background such as cosmic activity and Cherenkov events in the glass of the vial or photomultiplier tubes. When the prompt pulse is identified by the electronics, the number of pulses are counted over a set period. The total number of bursts is known as the pulse index. Events that have a higher pulse index are treated as background.

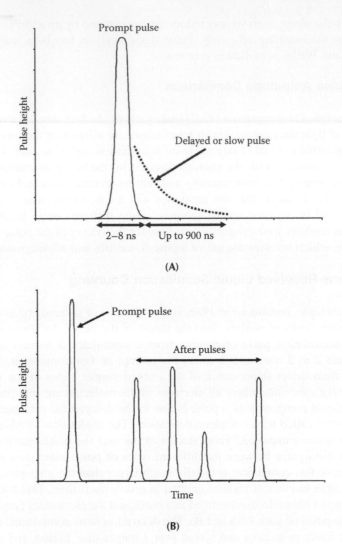

Figure 8.3 (A) A scintillator pulse consists of a prompt pulse and a delayed or slow pulse. (B) Following the prompt pulse, a series of after-pulses are observed. The prompt pulse and delayed or slow pulse in A is equivalent to the black area shown in Figure 8.2. The after-pulses in B represent greater detail of the area represented by the dotted line in A. (Produced from original material by kind permission of PerkinElmer Life and Analytical Science.)

Time-resolved counting also allows the user to optimize for the scintillator or isotope being analyzed. The pulse index is applied in different ways, depending upon the instrument. PerkinElmer states that there are four different count modes: normal, high sensitivity, ultra low level, and super low level. The normal count mode is used for normal everyday counting and is recommended for samples above 750 dpm. The low-activity/high-sensitivity count mode is recommended for samples to a level of 50 dpm. The ultra-low-level count mode is recommended for those samples that approach background levels and discriminates heavily against background counts. The super-low-level count mode employs a BGO guard detector (Section 8.3.7). In each case the criteria selected by the count mode use different limits to determine whether the observed pulse is accepted as a true count or rejected as a background. Each successive mode of counting uses a shorter time for pulse rejection. As more pulses are rejected as background, there will inevitably be a quantity of real events that are rejected, thus reducing the counting efficiency. This does not, of course, change the limit of detection, but it may demand longer count times (for the calculation of counting times, see Section 7.3).

The use of time-resolved liquid scintillation counting has enabled instruments to place less emphasis on shielding and to achieve higher levels of sensitivity.

8.3.7 TR-LSC Guard Detectors

The Packard Tri-Carb XL models combined the benefits of time-resolved counting with a guard detector. On these instruments, the detector assembly is surrounded with a slow scintillating plastic material optically coupled to the photomultiplier tubes. The decay time of the plastic scintillators is slow compared to the typical pulse speed of a sample event. Thus, cosmic and environmental radiation striking the guard detector produces a pulse with the slower resolution, which can be electronically recognized and eliminated. This removes the necessity to have a second set of photomultiplier tubes, specifically for the guard detector. One drawback of plastic scintillators, however, is that they are susceptible to the ingress of moisture, which reduces their efficiency and overall performance. Nevertheless, the models show excellent background reduction without recourse to additional photomultiplier assemblies and larger guards.

The Packard Instrument Company introduced a guard detector for time-resolved liquid scintillation counting (TR-LSC) using bismuth germanate ($Bi_4Ge_3O_{12}$, BGO).[4] BGO is a non-hygroscopic scintillator with low afterglow and high stopping power, which makes it especially useful as a guard for cosmic radiation. BGO has long been used in positron emission tomography (Chapter 11). Events that strike the BGO exhibit long-duration pulses that are therefore easily identified by the electronics. The duration of the pulse generated by a BGO is approximately 10 times the duration of an α- or β^--pulse. Backgrounds of 3 cpm in the region of 0 to 156 KeV have been observed while using a normal count mode. This performance allows the user to retain higher counting efficiencies as well as benefit from the reduction in background.

8.3.8 Other Background Issues

Although some sophisticated electronics are available for background reduction, there are also some simple everyday precautions that should be taken. Perhaps because of their simplicity they tend to be forgotten. Below is a reminder.

Attention should be paid to the location of the scintillation counter. The counter should be kept away from natural sunlight or strong fluorescent light. Ideally, the scintillation counter should be in a separate room with subdued lighting, temperature and humidity control.

The selection of vials is very important. It is difficult to be exact about the difference between background counts in glass compared to polyethylene. Different scintillation counters behave differently in different locations. However, the background counts in a 20-mL high-density linear polyethylene vial will be in the region of 15 cpm, when counting with 10 mL of scintillation cocktail in the 0 to 156 KeV region on a counter using normal count conditions. A glass vial would give in the region of 22 cpm under the same conditions. Small (7 mL) polyethylene vials give even lower backgrounds.

Not surprisingly, the choice of liquid cocktail is very important, as it is the cocktail that acts as the primary detector. There are many types of scintillation cocktails on the market and it is often difficult to make a choice. There is a saying that "you get what you pay for," and generally the more expensive the scintillation cocktail, the better its performance. It is nevertheless worth trying out different cocktails before committing to purchase. Some cocktails are sold especially for low-background work, but because so many different sample matrices are used, it is impossible, in practice, to be sure they will be suitable until they are tested in your own laboratory.

Perhaps it is stating the obvious but the counter should be kept clean and free from contamination. Vials should be wiped before being placed into the counter (also see static, Section 6.8). It is bad practice to use the racks holding the vials in the counter as test tube racks on the bench, as they can easily pick up contamination. In the most fastidious laboratories, counters used for the lowest-level work are kept in especially clean areas and are not used for higher-level analysis.

8.4 QUENCH CORRECTION: GENERAL CONSIDERATIONS

In practice, users may not have a choice as to which method of quench correction to use, as their laboratory may only have one model of counter. The intention here is to provide information on how various counters solve the problem of quench; it is not intended to imply that one method is superior to any other. I would promote a healthy skepticism for any result that is produced by a scintillation counter that does not have some standard against which to normalize the result. In general, using standards that can be traced to regulatory bodies such as the National Institute for Standards and Technology in the U.S. or the U.K. Accreditation Service provides the best means to substantiate experimental results. I would also promote regular and recorded calibration of instrumentation. This is often done automatically on modern instruments and in some cases the data are retained electronically so that they may be viewed at a later date. This facility, however, is often an optional extra and it is just as easy to retain the paper copies.

As explained in Chapter 6, the introduction of the multichannel analyzer made possible the graphical display of the spectrum of the isotope under analysis. This has been refined by many manufacturers and the use of the spectrum to assist in the optimization of the scintillation counter has become common. Quench correction based on spectral shift is now the norm and, as with background subtraction, the manufacturers have been busy developing their own specific systems, the principal ones of which are reviewed below.

8.5 QUENCH CORRECTION WITHOUT AN EXTERNAL STANDARD

8.5.1 Efficiency Tracing (Packard and PerkinElmer)

Efficiency tracing as a method of quench correction does not rely on spectrum analysis or a quench correction curve. It is applicable to all β^- and mixed β/γ emitting isotopes, so long as their E_{max} is greater than 40 KeV.[5]

Liquid scintillation counters in the Packard and PerkinElmer range of instruments use a ^{14}C unquenched standard for calibration and normalization. While doing this, they also measure the counts per minute in the following regions: 0 to 2000, 2 to 2000, 4 to 2000, 6 to 2000, 10 to 2000, and 20 to 2000 KeV. As the dpm in the unquenched standard is accurately known, the counting efficiency of the standard can be calculated in each of the regions. Efficiency is then plotted on the x-axis vs. sample cpm on the y-axis. The 100% counting efficiency point is established on the x-axis by the method of least squares.

Samples are then counted in the same six regions of interest. The counting efficiencies of each region, measured with the ^{14}C standard, are then applied to the unknown sample and the points plotted in the same way as above. Values in dpm are then plotted and extrapolated to the 100% value using the best squares fit of the points. This works very well and allows the user to measure any isotope, even with dual labeling. The precision of this system is well within 2%, and it is quick and easy to use. The system does rely on good statistics (sufficient counts) in the six regions of interest. It is therefore necessary to limit the use of this technique to samples with activity greater than 1,500 cpm.

If a situation arises where the quench standard set is generated by the user and only one counter is available that has a faulty quench curve, efficiency tracing can be used to verify the amount of radioactivity in the standard. Fitting of the curve at the lower-energy levels is error-prone, and so it is not advisable to use efficiency tracing for samples of less than 40 KeV, such as ^3H.

8.5.2 Auto-DPM (Beckman)

Auto-DPM is a method of quench correction that does not rely on quench correction curves. Auto-DPM extrapolates the dpm value for any pure α or β^- emitter from the characteristics of the shape of the energy spectrum. It provides an accurate dpm determination over a large quench range using a dpm extrapolation procedure. It should be noted that Beckman uses a multichannel analyzer on the 6500 series that has 32,768 channels, which is eight times the resolution of other scintillation counters.

This method is applicable to high and low-level samples, as the calculations are based on the accumulated cpm per channel of the sample. A patented Beckman curve fit is used to extrapolate to the y-axis and the actual dpm of the sample.

Beckman reports one limitation in that this method is not suitable for ^3H samples that have counting efficiencies below 30%.

8.5.3 Spectral Index of the Sample (PerkinElmer)

The spectral index of the sample (SIS) is a value derived from the average energy of the sample spectrum. It is not commonly used and therefore it is covered here only briefly.

In practicality, the spectrum of the sample is integrated and a balance point is established (one side of the integrated area of the spectrum equals the other). An algorithm is applied and a value is derived that approximates to the E_{max} of the bulk of the spectrum, which is then used as a measure of quench. This value is in fact the degree by which the spectrum of a sample has moved toward the zero-energy point.

There are advantages to using the actual spectrum of the sample to calculate the level of quenching:

1. There is no need for internal or external standardization, as it uses the spectrum of the sample itself.
2. It is count rate independent.
3. It is independent of sample volume.
4. It is independent of wall effect (Section 6.9), scintillation cocktail, or vial type.

However, because the sample itself provides the spectrum, it relies on there being enough data (counts) in the sample for statistical accuracy. This method should therefore not be used as a quench correction method if the activity is below 1000 cpm.

8.5.4 Spectral Quench Parameter of the Isotope (Wallac/PerkinElmer)

This quench parameter uses the logarithmic scale to derive what is known as the spectral quench parameter of the isotope (SQP(I)). This is not a widely used method and instruments using this method are no longer manufactured. The SQP(I) indicates the channel number on the scale on the QIP that corresponds to the center of gravity or balance point of the spectrum distribution. This channel number indicates the mean pulse height of the spectrum and allows the operator to view the position of the sample spectrum itself, and hence give the operator an indication of the level of quench. However, as with all measurements of quench that depend on the sample spectrum alone, it is dependent on there being sufficient counts to give any level of confidence in the result.

8.6 METHODS OF QUENCH CORRECTION USING EXTERNAL STANDARDS

Modern methods of quench correction use an external standard (Section 6.6.6). The type of external standard can vary from model to model, but it is always a γ

emitter, which has high energy but a short path length, so that it may be easily shielded. There are four external standards: ^{133}Ba, ^{137}Cs, ^{152}Eu, and ^{226}Ra. Those used most commonly are ^{133}Ba and ^{137}Cs. Both are good all-round external standards but neither has sufficient energy for Cherenkov counting (Section 6.10). ^{152}Eu is not commonly used, but it is suitable for Cherenkov counting. ^{226}Ra was in common use but it is no longer used in present-day counters. As an aside, disposal of the external standard can be a major issue when decommissioning counters, especially ^{226}Ra.

Before the sample is counted for activity, the external standard is brought into close proximity to the sample vial. The γ element of the external standard causes photons of light to be produced due to the Compton scattering effect in the scintil-lation cocktail solvent. The effect of this is to give the vial a huge number of counts that simulate those that arise from the sample itself. This is known as the Compton spectrum and shifts in the Compton spectrum allow the extent of quench to be measured (Section 6.6.6). The irradiation is only carried out for a short period, then the external source is removed and the cpm of the sample determined. The position of the Compton spectrum is compared with the calibration standard's unquenched Compton spectrum on a scale determined by each manufacturer. Some scintillation counters look at the sample spectrum first for a short period and remove this from the Compton spectrum so that only the external standard is used in the quench calculation. When the external standard has generated enough counts to satisfy the degree of confidence (usually 0.5%2σ; Section 7.3), the external standard is removed and takes no further part in the operation.

Having determined (1) the degree of quench and the (2) cpm in the sample, the efficiency is determined from the quench correction curve (Section 6.6.7) and the dpm in the sample is calculated.

Different manufacturers use different methods of measuring quench. There are many older counters still in use and so there are a variety of quench correction methods still in use today.

8.6.1 Linear vs. Logarithmic Representation

In the determination of the level of quench it is vital to establish the endpoint of the spectrum so that the spectral shift can be determined. It is in this area that the manufacturers have developed their own unique approaches. The spectrum may be in either linear or logarithmic format. Figure 8.4 shows the difference between the shapes of linear and logarithmic spectra.

If the logarithmic scale is used, it ensures that the spectrum has a clearly defined endpoint as the spectrum is forced to the center of the graph. The disadvantage with using the logarithmic scale is that the early part of the spectrum is distorted and the user is not able to view the scale in KeV. The logarithmic scale is used by Wallac and Beckman.

The linear scale shows the spectrum as it actually is. It does not suffer as much from lower-end energy distortion. Establishing the endpoint of the linear spectrum, however, is more difficult as it approaches the background.

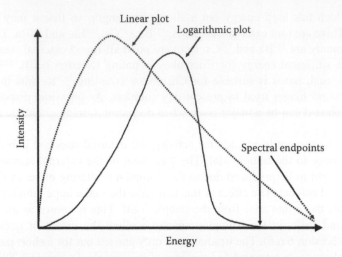

Figure 8.4   Comparison of the shape of energy spectra plotted as if the x-axis were either linear (----) or logarithmic (–).

8.6.2   External Standard Count–External Standard Ratio (Packard and LKB)

This is very similar to sample channels ratio (Section 6.6.5), but instead of using the sample itself to provide the information for the ratio calculation, it uses the information generated by an external standard. There are two preset regions, and the movement of the Compton spectrum is calculated by the scintillation counter instead of the postcount calculation of the sample channels ratio. It suffers from the same problems as the sample channels ratio in that it has a limited dynamic range, and as quench levels increase, the errors of calculation also increase. It is not often used and there are no commercial instruments available that supply the system.

8.6.3   H# or Compton Edge (Beckman)

In this method, the spectra are on a logarithmic scale, producing the characteristic hump shape seen in Figure 8.4 in the Compton spectrum. As the quench increases, the Compton spectrum will move toward the lower-energy region and the shape of the spectrum will alter. The H# (pronounced H-number) is calculated by using the inflection point at the edge of the Compton spectrum at the observed E_{max} point (Figure 8.5). A ^{137}Cs γ source is used as the external standard so that sufficient counts are available at the endpoint of the spectrum to enable determination of the inflection point with accuracy. Providing a reliable enough spectrum for the inflection point to be established becomes increasingly difficult as the volume of the sample decreases. To this end the technique is somewhat sample volume dependent and volumes of less than 200 μL are to be avoided. Severe

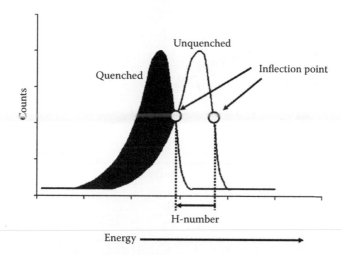

Figure 8.5 H# or Compton edge method of quench correction. (Produced from original material by kind permission of Beckman Instruments.)

color quench may also flatten the spectrum, making it difficult to establish the precise inflection point.

This method works very well, produces good results, and is the method used by most Beckman scintillation counters.[6]

8.6.4 Transformed Spectral Index of the External Standard (Packard and PerkinElmer)

The transformed spectral index of the external standard (tSIE) is another method using the Compton scattering spectrum generated by the solvent in the scintillation cocktail in the presence of the [133]Ba gamma source. There is, however, a fundamental difference between this and other methods. Instead of the raw spectrum being used, there is a prior transformation performed to correct for spectral distortions.

The Compton spectrum may be distorted by artifacts such as the wall effect, the sample volume, the cocktail type, and whether the vial is glass or plastic. Other external standard QIP parameters address these artifacts by choosing to ignore part of the Compton spectrum or by specifying the type of vial and cocktail type used to eliminate or compensate for the spectral shape. There is a further advantage of the [133]Ba source in that the Compton spectrum produced closely approximates the shape of a ^{14}C spectrum.

The reverse transformation technique operates by using channel-by-channel summation. In Figure 8.6A, the total counts of the highest-energy channel are stored in channel S1. The value of S1 is then added to the value of S2. The sum of S1 and S2 is added to S3, and so on. This continues until all channels have been transformed. The resulting transformed spectrum is shown in Figure 8.6B. Two points are located on the transformed spectrum (1 and 2 in Figure 8.6B), and a line is drawn between them to intersect the x-axis, which has the effect of removing spectral interferences

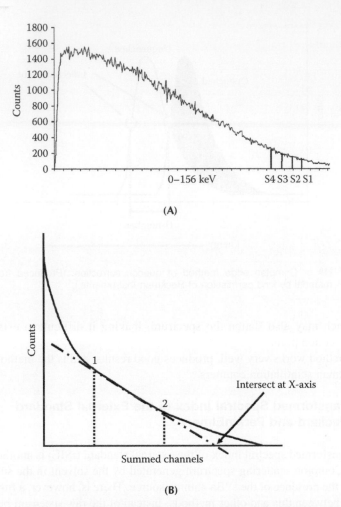

Figure 8.6   The transformed spectral index of the external standard (tSIE) method of quench
correction. (A) Reverse transformation. The total counts in channel S1 are added
to S2, and so on down the spectrum. The figure is not to scale (the spacing
between each channel is extremely small). The resulting transformed spectrum is
shown in B. The value at the far right of the x-axis is the value for S1; the next
point to the left on the x-axis is S1 + S2, then S1 + S2 + S3, and so on. Two
points are located on the transformed spectrum (labeled 1 and 2), and a line is
drawn down, intersecting the x-axis. The intersection is the measure of quench.
(Produced from original material by kind permission of PerkinElmer Life and
Analytical Science.)

by eliminating the top and bottom of the spectrum. The intersection with the x-axis
is used as the measure of quench. The scale of quench, called the transformed spectral
index of the external standard (tSIE), is determined by using the ^{14}C unquenched
calibration standard to set the 1000 tSIE value. All other tSIE values are then
measured against that value.[7]

8.6.5 Spectral Quench Parameter of the External Standard (Wallac and PerkinElmer)

The spectral quench parameter of the external standard (SQP(E)) is derived from the endpoint of the spectrum produced by the Compton scattering effect and is similar to the tSIE. The spectrum is stored in a logarithmic multichannel analyzer that has 1024 channels. The external standard used is ^{152}Eu, which is a high energy emitter with low activity. The area covered by the Compton spectrum is integrated, and 0.5% of the total area is removed from the total. The channel number where 99.5% of the total counts are accumulated becomes the SQP(E) number and the indication of quench. This method is influenced by the type of vial, due to wall effect, and also to the type of cocktail solvent. This is allowed for in the protocol conditions and compensated for in the calculation of the quench value.

SQP(E) is often used in later Wallac instruments in conjunction with a technique called digital overlay technique (see below). SQP(E) is an effective method of quench indication.

8.6.6 Digital Overlay Technique (Wallac)

The digital overlay technique is a factory set method of dual-label quench correction. The instrument software has a library of 60 to 80 standards of a given isotope at various quench levels. The SQP(E) and SQP(I) are established for each quench level. The spectra corresponding to this quench level is compared to the factory set information library and a best fit is made. The dpm values are then calculated using the library. The benefit of the system is that it conducts the quench correction without using quench curves. However, the user has little access to the quench library and is dependent on the information and data installed at the factory. In order to be able to gather good information for the curve fit, it is essential that there are sufficient counts in the sample to provide a spectrum that can be fitted.[8,9]

8.7 SOLID VS. LIQUID SCINTILLATION COUNTING

The majority of conventional scintillation counters use liquid scintillants. Beckman, however, has a system whereby samples of up to 200 µL are dispensed into caps containing a solid scintillant (yttrium silicate), which are then analyzed in a conventional counter. The sample is usually dried prior to counting.

Solid scintillators exhibit longer pulse delay times in comparison with liquid scintillators. The pulse lifetime of a liquid scintillator will be in the region of 20 nsec, whereas the pulse lifetime of a solid scintillator will be 100 to 200 nsec. Coupled to this, the higher photon production will lead to the spectrum being shifted toward a higher-energy region. Although it is usual to merely adjust the energy window to account for the higher-energy spectrum, Beckman has increased the coincidence time to 100 nsec to ensure that none of the solid scintillator pulses are eliminated. Solid and liquid scintillants are also used in microplate counters (Section 8.8) and in flow scintillation counting (Section 8.9 to Section 8.11).

8.8 MICROPLATE SCINTILLATION COUNTERS

The general principles on the use of microplate technology are covered in Section 6.14. Multiwell plates consist of an array of wells in a plastic plate in a 24, 96, 384, or 1536 well configuration. They can be used in conjunction with solid or liquid scintillators.

There are two configurations of microplate scintillation counter. One uses two photomultipliers in coincidence, the other uses a single photomultiplier. The principal instruments currently on the market are the MicroBeta Trilux range (Wallac/PerkinElmer), which uses coincidence counting, and the TopCount instrument (Packard/PerkinElmer), which uses a single photomultiplier. The configuration of the two systems is illustrated in Figure 8.7A and B. Both the TopCount and Micro-Beta range can be configured so that up to 12 wells may be counted simultaneously (i.e., up to 12 photomultipliers on the TopCount and 24 on the MicroBeta range). There is also an instrument on the market made by Hidex Oy, but this can also measure a range of other analytical endpoints, such as fluorescence, absorbance, etc.

For what seems a very straightforward situation, there is immense confusion surrounding plate counters. This probably stems from the fact that the dual and single-photomultiplier systems work on entirely different principles.

8.8.1 Background Reduction

Multiplate counters that operate with two photomultipliers use standard coincidence counting (Section 6.3) as the method of background reduction. They use the normal principles of scintillation counter and operate with standard liquid scintillants. Where solid scintillants are used, they are generally incorporated into the plastic of the plate but some users may operate with the yttrium silicate-based plates.

Where there is a single photomultiplier used, as stated in Section 6.3, it will exhibit significant background noise. Since there is only one photomultiplier, coincidence counting cannot be used for background noise reduction; instead, these instruments use a form of time resolution (Section 8.3.6). Under normal operation, time resolution uses the length of the scintillation pulse to discriminate against noise. In microplate counters, the opposite effect is used; there is a deliberate lengthening of the pulse by the use of a slow scintillator. Time resolution is used to discriminate against the short-duration pulse as background and accept the long-duration pulse as real. Solid scintillators already have the long pulse characteristics, but normal liquid scintillants do not. The liquid scintillators for single-photomultiplier instruments use dimethylanthracene as the secondary scintillator, which exhibits the appropriate long pulse shape.

8.8.2 Quench Correction Methods

Microplate scintillation counters using 96-well microplates are not able to use external standards in the same way as liquid scintillation counters, as they are largely incompatible with the instrument architecture. In the main, therefore, microplate scintillation counters use cpm results rather than dpm. If dpm is required, then a

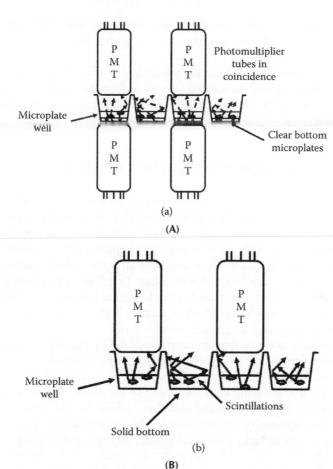

Figure 8.7 Microplate solid scintillation counter using (A) coincidence counting with dual photomultipliers (MicroBeta Trilux) and (B) single photomultipliers using time resolution to reject background (TopCount).

form of internal standard correction is necessary (Section 6.6.4). If many samples of the same type are being analyzed, then it is probably reasonable to assume the quench in each will be equivalent. The degree of quench can then be measured in representative samples and a generic correction then applied.

It is possible to use quench correction curves, but the method of construction is by using the spectrum of the sample rather than by using an external standard. The TopCount instrument (Packard/PerkinElmer) may be fitted with an external standard, but it can only be used on a 24-well plate and is not available for a 96-well plate (at the time of writing in 2005). The MicroBeta Trilux (Wallac/PerkinElmer) uses two photomultipliers in coincidence on either side of the microplate and so there is no room to install an external standard.

The TopCount uses a quench correction routine known as the transformed spectral index of the sample (tSIS). This is a modification of the SIS (Section 8.5.3), except the spectrum, is transformed in a way similar to that of the tSIE (Section 8.6.4). The MicroBeta Trilux uses the spectral quench parameter of the isotope (SQP(I)) (Section 8.5.4).

Generating a quench standard in the microplate is a very difficult process given the size of the plates. There are methods available from the manufacturers, but they are little used in ADME studies at present and consequently, they will not be considered here.

8.9 FLOW SCINTILLATION COUNTING

The general principles of flow detection are covered in Section 6.15. As with all scintillation counting, the reduction of background is an important consideration in the design of instrumentation and efforts have been made to reduce the background of flow counters to improve their sensitivity. Improvements in photomultiplier design, passive shielding and the flow cell have all helped reduce background.

Most flow counters can be fitted with either 1 or 2 inch photomultipliers. One inch photomultipliers have lower backgrounds but are less sensitive than the conventional 2 inch photomultipliers. With all matters in flow counting, however, there is a compromise between background and sensitivity.

The Radiomatic range of flow counters produced by Packard and subsequently by PerkinElmer, introduced time-resolved liquid scintillation counting technology (Section 8.3.6). The TR-LSC range of flow cells has a different type of flow cell window that has a scintillating material as part of the plastic. This has the effect of enhancing environmental background radiation striking the cell, which can then be recognized and eliminated by the electronics. This reduces background from around 30 to 40 cpm to 3 to 10 cpm, with a subsequent increase in sensitivity.

8.10 STATIONARY ELUATE ANALYSIS

The StopFlow™ system holds the eluate in the flow cell, effectively increasing the residence time and thereby increasing sensitivity. This is achieved by temporarily pausing the eluate flow and the flow of the scintillation cocktail. This gives much better statistics to the count and allows the user to achieve very good sensitivities. The action is similar to the counting of fractions with the exception that the fractions do not need to be collected and counted in a scintillation counter.

8.11 MULTICELL ELUATE ANALYSIS

A very recent development in flow counting is a novel system produced by raytest GmbH that uses the standard flow of a high-performance liquid chromatography (HPLC), but instead of one flow cell there are actually four flow cells in series, each with its own coincidence circuit (i.e., eight photomultipliers) The system is called the Mira Star. The eluate flows through each cell in turn and the data are combined for all four cells, accumulated in phase and added to one chromatographic peak profile. There is an increase in sensitivity, but the system can only be used with micro-HPLC columns, with flow rates of around 10 to 100 µL/min.

8.12 WIRE SCANNERS

Wire scanners are used to image a flat surface such as a thin-layer chromatography (TLC) plate. There are one-dimensional scanners (linear scanners) that quantify one lane on the TLC plate at a time. There are also two-dimensional scanners that are used to visualize and quantify radioactive regions on two-dimensional TLC plates. Wire scanners use a proportional wire that is housed in a gas-filled atmosphere. The ionizing radiation is detected by the proportional wire in the presence of the gas, which is usually an argon methane mixture. The scanners are very sensitive, but they suffer from being only able to view a small portion of the object. They have been largely superseded by phosphor imagers that are covered below. An exception to this is for the determination of radiopurity (Section 2.13), where the speed of wire proportional counting is an advantage, as sensitivity is rarely an issue.

8.13 RADIOLUMINOGRAPHY

Radioluminography is used in quantitative whole-body autoradiography (Section 5.3.7) and for the visualization and quantification of radio-TLC plates (Section 5.4.5).

Radiolabeled samples are exposed to phosphor screens, which store their energy in the photostimulable crystals ($BaFB_r:Eu^{2+}$). The energy of the radioisotope ionizes the Eu^{2+} to Eu^{3+}, which liberates the electrons to the conduction band of the phosphor crystals. The electrons are trapped in bromine vacancies, which are introduced in the manufacturing process. Exposure to stimulating laser light at 633 nm releases the photons at about 390 nm, which are detected by a photomultiplier. There are currently three instrument manufactures: Fuji, Molecular Dynamics, and PerkinElmer.

APPENDIX 1: LIST OF INSTRUMENT MANUFACTURERS AND SUPPLIERS

Hamamatsu Photonics KK
314-5, Shimokanzo, Toyooka-village, Iwata-gun, Sizuoka-ken, 438-0193, Japan
http://www.hamamatsu.com

PerkinElmer
549 Albany St., Boston, MA, 02118
http://www.perkinelmer.com
PerkinElmer acquired Wallac in the 1990s and acquired Packard Bioscience, Inc., in
November 2001.

Beckman Coulter, Inc.
2500N, Harbor Blvd., P.O. Box 3100, Fullerton, CA, 92834-3100
USA http://www.beckman.com

Raytest Isotopenmessgerate GmbH
Benzstrasse 4, 75334 Straubenhardt, Germany
http://www.raytest.de/

IN/US Systems, Inc.
5809 North 50th St., Tampa, FL 33610-4809
http://www.inus.com

National Diagnostics, Inc.
305 Patton Dr., Atlanta, GA 30336
http://www.nationaldiagnostics.com

Zinsser Analytic U.K., Ltd.
Howarth Road, Maidenhead, SL6 1AP, Berkshire, U.K.
http://www.zinsser-analytic.com/

Molecular Dynamics, Amersham Biosciences Corp.
800 Centennial Ave., P.O. Box 1327, Piscataway, NJ 08855-1327
http://www4.amershambiosciences.com

Berthold Technologies GmbH & Co. KG
Calmbacher Strasse, 22D-75323 Bad Wildbad, Germany
http://www.berthold.com

Hidex Oy
Mustionkatu 2 FIN-20750 Turku, Finland
http://www.hidex.com/

REFERENCES

1. L'Annunziata, M.F., Ed., *Handbook of Radioactivity Analysis*, Academic Press, London, 1998.
2. Roessler, N., Valenta, R.J., and Cauter, S.V., time resolved liquid scintillation counting, in *Proceedings of the International Conference on New Trends in Liquid Scintillation Counting and Organic Scintillators*, Ross, H., Noakes, J.E., and Spaulding, J.D., Eds., Chapter 44, Lewis Publishers Inc., Chelsea, MI, 1989.
3. Wright, G.T., Scintillation decay times of organic crystals, *Proc. Phys. Soc.*, 69B, 358, 1956.
4. Noakes, J.E. and Valenta, R.J., The Role of $Bi_4Ge_3O_{12}$ as an Auxiliary Scintillator for α, β⁻ and γ Liquid Scintillation Counting and Low Level Counting, paper presented at the International Conference on Advances in Liquid Scintillation Spectrometry (LSC '94), Glasgow, 1994.
5. Ishikawa, H., Takine, M., and Aburai, T., Radioassay by an efficiency tracing technique using a liquid scintillation counter, *Int. J. Appl. Radiat. Isot.*, 35, 463–466, 1984.
6. Horrocks, D.L., A new method of quench monitoring in liquid scintillation counting: the H number concept, *J. Radioanal. Chem.*, 43, 489–521, 1978.
7. Kessler, M.J., Application of quench monitoring using transformed external standard spectrum (tSIE), in *Liquid Scintillation Counting and Organic Scintillators*, Ross, J., Noakes, E., and Spaulding, J.D., Eds., Lewis Publishers, Chelsea, MI, pp. 51–67.
8. Caron, F., Sutton, J., Benz, M.L., and Haas, M.K., Determination of carbon-14 levels in heavy water and groundwaters, *Analyst*, 125, 59–64, 2000.
9. Kouru, H. and Rindt, K., Multilabel counting using digital overlay technique, in *Liquid Scintillation Counting and Organic Scintillators*, Ross, J., Noakes, E., and Spaulding, J.D., Eds., Lewis Publishers, Chelsea, MI, 1991, pp. 19–34.

CHAPTER 9

Sample Preparation for Liquid Scintillation Counting

Simon Temple

CONTENTS

9.1 INTRODUCTION

Absorption, distribution, metabolism and excretion (ADME) studies are a vital part of the comprehensive safety evaluation of a new chemical entity. The objective of these studies is to investigate the excretion rate and tissue distribution of the chemical entity and involves the collection and analysis of excreta from human studies and excreta and tissues from animal studies, following the administration of a radiolabeled test drug (Chapter 3).

The biological samples are quantitatively analyzed for radioactivity. The most widely used method for radioactivity analysis is liquid scintillation counting (Chapter 6). Some biological samples can be added directly to liquid scintillant, while others require a degree of preparation prior to analysis.

In general, all biological samples contain components not generally found in any other sample types. Nonbiological samples are comparatively simple and therefore their incorporation into a scintillation cocktail is much more straightforward. The components present in biological samples require either specialist cocktails or modified sample preparation techniques. Within the context of ADME studies, the samples generally encountered include urine, feces, blood, bile, serum, plasma, and tissues (liver, kidney, brain, muscle, etc.), and each will be considered in turn.

It is taken as read that results will be recorded in units of dpm (Section 2.5). Most biological sample preparations suffer from at least some degree of quench, and if purely machine counts (cpm) are used, then this is likely to lead to serious errors.

9.2 SOLUBILIZATION VS. OXIDATION

Samples of solid biological material such as tissues, feces, etc., will not dissolve directly in the liquid scintillation cocktail, and therefore, they have to be treated before analysis. There are two ways of doing this: (1) oxidation and (2) solubilization. In addition to rendering a sample suitable for analysis, oxidation can also be used on highly colored liquid samples, such as blood, which would otherwise cause unacceptable levels of colored quench (Section 6.6.2).

There has been a long-running discussion in the field of ADME comparing the benefits of solubilization over oxidation and vice versa. The process of oxidation is one that may only be used for ^3H and ^{14}C unless specialist equipment is employed. The principle of sample oxidation is that the sample is combusted in an oxygen-rich atmosphere and any hydrogen present is oxidized to water, while any carbon is oxidized to carbon dioxide. If tritium is present, then the combustion product will be ^3H_2O, and if ^{14}C is present, then the combustion product will be $^{14}CO_2$. In commercially available instruments, the water is condensed and then washed into a vial, where it is mixed with an appropriate liquid scintillation cocktail. The CO_2 is trapped by reaction with an amine, and the resulting product is again mixed with an appropriate cocktail. At the end of the combustion cycle two separate samples (a ^3H sample and a ^{14}C sample) are trapped at ambient temperature, thus minimizing cross-contamination.

Oxidizers are not particularly pleasant instruments to use. They may be considered tedious in operation, as the operator has the task of adding a sample, adding a vial, pressing a button, and then waiting for up to 2 min before any further action is needed (although robotized versions are available). The reagents used to trap the $^{14}CO_2$ have a distinctive smell that some find unpleasant and ventilation of the equipment is necessary. Oxidizers contain a lot of valves and pipework and may suffer failure due to cleanliness and operational problems.

Prior to use, and periodically while in use, standards have to be run through the instrument to ensure that the trapping efficiency is sufficient (usually around 90 to 100% is acceptable). A very annoying habit of oxidizers is that they start off giving efficiencies of over 90% at the start of the day, but then slowly (sometimes not so slowly) diminish as the day goes on. The periodic efficiency checks therefore need to be analyzed at the time of analysis, which necessitates a fast turnaround. In laboratories where there are limited scintillation counters with a high sample throughput, counter availability can be a problem in getting speedy results from the efficiency tests. For this reason, many laboratories use older counters for this, sometimes producing results only in cpm, which for this purpose is perfectly acceptable. Although oxidizers are very good at recovering radioactivity from biological samples, they have a reputation for being unreliable — one perhaps not entirely deserved with modern instruments. Nevertheless, probably for this reason, solubilization methods are becoming the norm.

Oxidizers are relatively straightforward to use and therefore they will not be covered in any further detail. Solubilization, however, is more sample dependent, and thus this area will be covered in some detail. Solubilization appears to be a more tedious process than sample oxidation, as each vial has to have more than one treatment during the process. However, if the samples are batched, throughput may be faster than with oxidation.

Many laboratories have undertaken their own validation projects with sample solubilization methods and there are probably as many methods as there are laboratories. The methods described below can be considered general and typical but by no means exclusive.

9.3 GENERAL CONSIDERATIONS

9.3.1 Sample Size and Scintillation Cocktail

Liquid scintillation cocktails have a finite capacity in that, depending upon the cocktail being used, there is a limit to the amount of sample that can be added.

Providing that the capacity is not exceeded, the amount of cocktail in the vial is not critical. The scintillation counter measures the total counts; the technique is independent of the concentration of the sample in the vial. The volume of the cocktail therefore is not important and does not require accurate dispensing. Indeed, if a sample is exhibiting color quench, one way of reducing the problem is simply to add more scintillation cocktail to the vial.

Accurate addition of the sample is, of course, critical. Many laboratories today conduct all sample analysis by weight, rather than volume. First, weights can be recorded to four (or even five or six) places of decimal. Second, if a pipette malfunctions and does not deliver the desired volume, there may be no way of knowing until a spurious result is obtained.

Laboratories conducting many thousands of assays can be equipped with data capture systems that record the weights and scintillation results directly into a database.

9.3.2 Sample Homogeneity

Cloudiness or color in a sample will lead to quench, and therefore, when developing any method for the first time, glass vials should be used, as opposed to plastic, as these allow visual inspection of the sample–cocktail mixture. In general, if a sample forms a homogeneous mixture with a cocktail and this mixture remains homogeneous for at least 15 min, then it will remain homogenous for an extended period provided it is not subjected to severe temperature change.

9.3.3 Safety

Since the purpose of sample preparation is to dissolve biological samples, some aggressive reagents have to be used. These should be treated with appropriate respect. In particular, with methods that require heating, samples should be well contained and consideration has to be given to the possibility of vials breaking in the oven or water bath. Also, reagents such as hydrogen peroxide produce oxygen gas, and if vials are tightly capped, as the oxygen pressure increases, they are liable to explode. When in doubt, leave the caps loose.

9.3.4 Chemiluminescence

If chemiluminescence (Section 6.7.2) is suspected, then resolution usually involves either selecting a specialist cocktail or allowing the chemiluminescence reaction to go to completion by allowing the sample–cocktail mixture to stand for a fixed time period before counting. To determine this period is straightforward using a nonradioactive sample:

1. Add cocktail to a glass scintillation vial.
2. Add the sample that does not contain radioactivity.
3. Place in the counter and arrange for repeat 2-min counts.

4. Continue repeat counting until the cpm stabilizes.
5. Calculate total time taken for cpm stabilization, and this becomes the fixed period the sample needs to stand before starting counting. The sample should be left in the dark so as not to promote photoluminescence (Section 6.7.3).

The above method can also be used in conjunction with samples and various scintillation cocktails in order to select the reagents with the lowest luminescence for the particular conditions of a laboratory.

Chemiluminescence is the result of a reaction between two chemicals. If allowing the sample to stand does not produce the desired effect, then the sample cocktail mixture may be cooled (e.g., 4°C) to reduce the rate of chemical reaction. If the scintillation counter has some form of cooling, then that will be so much the better but this is not a common feature on modern instruments. The last and final step if all the above fail is to add 200 µL of 20% (v/v) aqueous acetic acid, which will counteract the effects of the alkaline conditions that fuel chemiluminescence. This is a last resort, as there are already enough components in the scintillation cocktail sample matrix and addition of further material just adds to the general difficulty of counting.

9.3.5 The Radiolabel

Sample oxidation is limited to ^3H and ^{14}C. Solubilization can be used with most commonly encountered β^- isotopes, such as ^3H, ^{14}C, ^{25}S, and $^{32/33}P$. Weak γ-emitting isotopes such as ^{125}I will require sample preparation but stronger γ-emitters such as ^{131}I can, on the whole, be counted in γ-counters without sample preparation due to the penetrating nature of the radiation.

For solubilization methods, consideration has to be given as to the volatility of the drug or its metabolites in the sample. Clearly, heating vials with solubilizing agent will cause volatiles to evaporate and be lost. This tends to be less of a problem in drug development than it is in environmental work.

The methods described here refer to the analysis of total sample radioactivity. All the methods described are destructive, and if the drug or metabolite requires identification, then alternative extraction methods will be required.

9.4 URINE

9.4.1 Introduction

Normal urine consists of 95% water, with the remaining ingredients including waste products from the breakdown of protein, hormones, electrolytes, pigments, toxins and any abnormal components. The major waste product from cells in the body is ammonia, and the major waste product from blood is catabolized heme known as bilirubin. In the liver, ammonia is converted to urea and bilirubin is degraded to urobilins. Salt, water and urea are all colorless, but urobilins are yellow.

Freshly voided urine is generally clear and pale to deep yellow in color. The more concentrated the urine, the deeper the yellow color. An abnormal color may be due to certain foods or may be due to the presence of bile pigments or blood in the urine. Some drugs and vitamins may also alter the color of urine. Cloudy urine may indicate an infection in some part of the urinary tract.

The pH of urine varies, depending upon the species, but typically ranges from 4.5 to 8.0. The pH of normal human urine is around 7.4. Dog urine tends to be more acidic (5.5 to 7). A vegetarian diet, prolonged vomiting and bacterial infection of the urinary tract will all raise the pH of urine.

9.4.2   Sample Preparation

Urine can normally be added directly to liquid scintillation cocktail. From the point of view of sample incorporation into a cocktail, the components present that are likely to cause problems are color and divalent/trivalent ions. Individually these are relatively easy to manage but together they present an unusual problem. After the addition of urine to certain cocktails a wispy precipitate forms, usually just below the surface, which can be observed through a glass vial.

The precipitate can develop either rapidly (within 1 h) or slowly (over 1 day). This phenomenon is most probably due to the precipitation of dissolved urinary components as they mix with the relatively organic phase of the scintillant. This effect does not usually affect counting reproducibility, but if it is seen as a potential problem, it can usually be stopped by adding 10 to 15% isopropyl alcohol or ethanol. (Simply add 1.0 mL isopropyl alcohol to the 10.0-mL cocktail prior to adding the urine sample.) Since count times for urine samples in ADME studies are not usually excessive, this phenomenon can generally be dismissed unless very low levels are being measured (<100 dpm). For low levels of activity the count times are much longer and therefore stability is of major importance.

Divalent and trivalent ions (e.g., sulfate and phosphate) will adversely affect the microemulsion capability of many cocktails. However, the concentration of these ions in urine is usually so low that they should not cause a problem but in combination with the other ions present in urine (urea, sodium, potassium, magnesium, calcium, etc.) there can be difficulties, especially in concentrated urine samples. If the urine does not mix properly with the cocktail (forms a milky mixture), then such a problem has occurred. This can be resolved by either changing to a cocktail that is able to accept more concentrated solutes or diluting the urine sample with distilled or deionized water (1:1 urine:water). Urine from small animals (e.g., rat and mouse) is usually much more concentrated that that from humans. It is recommended, therefore, that the volume of sample from these animals is kept below 0.5 mL/10 mL cocktail. Specialist cocktail selection as well as dilution with water may be necessary to obtain a stable counting condition.

Chemiluminescence can occur with urine and this is characterized by the reduction of levels of cpm with time, as the luminescence dies away. Chemiluminescence is produced by an interaction between free peroxides and alkaline material. The free peroxides originate from the ethoxylate detergents present in the cocktail. Over time the ethoxylate polymer chain breaks down and the result is a free peroxide entity.

In general, freshly manufactured scintillation cocktail is peroxide-free but with prolonged storage the level of peroxide will increase and therefore attention should be given to the age of the cocktail being used in solubilization studies.

9.5 WHOLE BLOOD AND BILE

9.5.1   Introduction

Whole blood contains red blood cells, white blood cells, and platelets suspended in a watery fluid called plasma. A drop of blood the size of a pinhead contains approximately 5 million red blood cells, which get their color from the iron-containing protein hemoglobin.

Bile originates from the liver and contains bile acids as well as bilirubin. The principal bile acids are glycolic and taurocholic acids (sterols linked to amino acids).

9.5.2   Sample Preparation

Because of its complex nature and extreme color, blood should not be added directly to a cocktail. Such an attempt will result in a highly color quenched and non-homogeneous mixture that will not lend itself to accurate or reproducible counting. Bile is also highly colored, but it is a fluid without a cellular component. On occasions in ADME studies, bile can contain relatively high levels of radioactivity, and therefore only very small volumes are required for analysis, in which case bile can be added directly to the scintillant (10 µL of bile to 1 mL of scintillant).

Blood can be oxidized or it can be solubilized and decolorized. Bile does not require solubilization but is likely to require decolorization.

Solubilization is the action of chemical reagents on organic materials (such as animal tissue) that effects a structural breakdown (or digestion) into a liquid form that can then be directly dissolved in a liquid scintillation cocktail. The source of blood and the correct choice of solubilizer will significantly influence the results of digestion. In general, most of the sample preparation problems occur with blood samples from smaller animals such as rats and mice. In this case it may be necessary to consider smaller sample volumes and even then there can still be color quench problems.

The successful preparation of blood samples for liquid scintillation counting by solubilization can often be technically difficult and successful digestion can be largely dependent on the practical experience of the researcher. To process a sample, simply add the solubilizer and heat at 50 to 60°C until the sample is dissolved. After solubilization the sample may be colored and may require decolorization by treatment with hydrogen peroxide (as indeed may be the case with bile). The final step is to add the recommended liquid scintillation cocktail and the sample is ready for counting. Using this method, many samples can be processed simultaneously and then counted sequentially. Currently available on the market are two types of solubilizer: quaternary ammonium hydroxide in toluene/methanol and an inorganic alkali in water with added detergents. Examples of the former include Soluene®-350

(Perkin Elmer) and ScitiGest® (Fisher Scientific). The only version of an aqueous-based solubilizer is the Perkin Elmer product SOLVABLE®. The respective stepwise processes for solubilization with these different solubilizers are as follows:

Quaternary ammonium hydroxide method:
1. Add a maximum of 0.4 mL of blood to a glass scintillation vial.
2. Add, while swirling gently, 1.0 mL of a mixture of solubilizer and isopropyl alcohol (1:1 or 1:2 ratio). Ethanol may be substituted for the isopropyl alcohol if desired.
3. Incubate at 55 to 60°C for 2 h. The sample at this stage will be reddish brown.
4. Cool to room temperature.
5. Add 0.2 to 0.5 mL of 30% hydrogen peroxide in 100 μL aliquots. Foaming will occur after each addition; therefore, gentle agitation is necessary. Keep swirling the mixture until all foaming subsides and then repeat the process until all of the hydrogen peroxide has been added.
6. Allow to stand for 15 to 30 min at room temperature to complete the reaction.
7. Place in an oven or water bath at 55 to 60°C for 30 min. The samples at this stage should now have changed to slightly yellow. This is important, as heating destroys residual hydrogen peroxide, which if present can induce unwanted chemiluminescence.
8. Cool to room temperature and add 15 mL of recommended cocktail.
9. Temperature and light adapt for 1 h before counting.

Aqueous-based solubilizer:
1. Add a maximum of 0.4 mL of blood to a glass scintillation vial.
2. Add 1.0 mL of solubilizer.
3. Incubate the sample at 55 to 60°C for 1 h. Sample at this stage will be brown/green in appearance.
4. Add 0.1 ml of 0.1 M EDTA–disodium salt solution, which helps reduce foaming when the subsequent hydrogen peroxide is added. This reagent also complexes iron that has been released during digestion and produces a mixture that is less colored.
5. Add 0.3 to 0.5 mL of 30% hydrogen peroxide in 100 μL aliquots. Slight foaming will occur after each addition; therefore, gentle agitation is necessary. Keep swirling the mixture until all foaming subsides and then repeat the process until all of the hydrogen peroxide has been added.
6. Allow to stand for 15 to 30 min at room temperature to complete the reaction.
7. Place in an oven or water bath at 55 to 60°C for 1 h. The color will change from brown/green to pale yellow.
8. Cool to room temperature and add 15 mL of recommended scintillation cocktail.
9. Temperature and light adapt for 1 h before counting.

Both the above methods apply not only to blood, but also to any other biological tissue sample and the only modifications required concern the sample sizes. For bile, the procedure is picked up at the stage where hydrogen peroxide is added.

Since the products of such solubilization are in an alkaline mixture, there is a high degree of probability that chemiluminescence may be present. There are those who say that solubilization of blood when ^{3}H is involved is unsuitable due to unacceptably high chemiluminescence.

9.6 PLASMA AND SERUM

9.6.1 Introduction

Plasma constitutes about 55% of the blood volume. It serves as transport medium for glucose, lipids, hormones, products of metabolism, carbon dioxide and oxygen. Plasma contains about 10% protein consisting of albumins, globulins and fibrinogens. Around 60% of these proteins are albumins. Plasma is obtained by separating the liquid portion of blood from the cells by centrifugation. It is a straw-colored clear liquid, but a significant number of red and white blood cells, as well as platelets, are suspended in plasma.

Serum is the same as plasma except that clotting factors (such as fibrin) have been removed. Serum resembles plasma in composition but lacks the coagulation factors and is obtained by letting a blood specimen clot prior to centrifugation.

9.6.2 Sample Preparation

Plasma and serum samples can be added directly to liquid scintillation cocktails but consideration needs to be given to the presence of proteins, color, sample volume, cocktail compatibility and the biological origin of the sample.

The high concentration of proteins in plasma and serum produces a wispy precipitate just below the surface, similar to that seen with urine samples (although for different reasons). This can develop either rapidly (within 1 h) or slowly (over 1 day). This phenomenon is most probably due to protein unfolding in the presence of the detergents present in the cocktail. This effect does not usually affect counting reproducibility, but if it is seen as a potential problem, it can usually be stopped by adding 10 to 15% isopropyl alcohol or ethanol. (Simply add 1.0 or 1.5 mL of isopropyl alcohol to 10.0 mL of cocktail prior to adding the plasma or serum sample.)

Color is present to some degree in plasma and serum samples and the base effect of such color is quenching. The complex nature of plasma and serum means that these samples do not mix easily with most scintillation cocktails. Whatever cocktail is recommended for plasma, it should always be evaluated prior to commencing any work. The appearance of such samples will be somewhat different from others encountered in liquid scintillation counting in that they will appear opaque to a greater or lesser extent (sometimes described as a milky wispiness). Samples thus prepared should be allowed to stand at the counting temperature for at least 1 h for confirmation of stability. Providing there is no obvious two-phase separation, they will remain stable.

Whatever cocktail is selected the maximum sample volume will be low and most suitable cocktails will only accept 1.0 mL of plasma or serum in 10.0 mL of cocktail. Samples from small animals are even more problematic and although sample volume is usually 100 to 250 µL, compatibility with cocktail will be an issue. Two scintillation cocktails that are particularly good with plasma and serum samples are Pico-Fluor MI and Ultima-Flo M (both available from Perkin Elmer).

Alternative sample preparation methods include sample combustion and solubilization. If solubilization is being used, then either of the methods previously detailed under blood can be used and these are suitable for processing up to 1.0 mL of plasma or serum. Sample combustion is also suitable for processing plasma and serum samples but it should be remembered that this is only suitable for samples containing ^3H or ^{14}C.

9.7 BIOLOGICAL TISSUES

9.7.1 Introduction

There are four basic types of tissue: epithelium, connective tissue, muscle tissue, and nervous tissue. The epithelium is usually the layer of cells that resides closer to the outside world. The outermost layer of skin is composed of dead scaly or plate-like epithelial cells. Other examples are the mucous membranes lining the inside of mouths and body cavities. Internally, epithelial cells line the insides of the lungs, the gastrointestinal tract, the reproductive and urinary tracts, and make up the exocrine and endocrine glands. The primary functions of epithelial cells include secretion, absorption and protection. Loose connective tissue holds organs and epithelia in place and contains a variety of proteinaceous fibers, including collagen and elastin. Ligaments and tendons are a form of fibrous connective tissue. In most vertebrates, cartilage is found primarily in joints, where it provides cushioning. Muscle cells contain contractile filaments that move past each other, changing size as they do so. The most obvious examples of nervous tissue are the cells forming the brain, spinal cord and peripheral nervous system. The nervous system consists chiefly of two types of cells, neurons and Glia.

Organs are structures in the body that contain at least two different types of tissue functioning together. In ADME studies, organs such as the liver, kidneys, lung, heart, brain, spleen, GI tract, and gonads are commonly taken for analysis, along with samples of fat and muscle. Depending upon the study, other organs and glands may be taken from the pituitary through to Peyer's patches.

Most tissues and organs are homogenized to ensure any subsample is representative. The homogenates are then taken for scintillation analysis.

9.7.2 Sample Preparation

In order to be measured, radioactivity has to be accessible to the scintillation cocktail. Some form of destructive sample preparation is therefore necessary with tissues, in order to release or convert the radioactivity into a form that will mix with the scintillation cocktail. Samples can therefore be oxidized or solubilized. Solubilization usually involves alkaline hydrolysis. The recommended solubilization reagents are the same as mentioned previously under blood (Section 9.4), that is, a quaternary ammonium hydroxide in toluene/methanol and an inorganic alkali in water with added detergents.

For the purpose of sample preparation, some organs or biological samples can be grouped together; these are listed below:

- Muscle, skin, heart, stomach, brains, and stomach tissue
- Liver and kidney
- Fatty tissue

9.7.3 Muscle, Skin, Heart, Stomach, Brains, and Stomach Tissue

The method of solubilizing all of the above is relatively straightforward, and apart from possible color formation with certain tissue types, no major problems should be encountered during sample preparation and scintillation counting. The method is as follows:

1. Place selected sample (up to 200 mg) in a 20-mL glass scintillation vial.
2. Add an appropriate volume of solubilizer (1 to 2 mL, depending on sample size).
3. Heat in an oven or water bath at 50 to 60°C with occasional swirling until the sample is completely dissolved.
4. Cool to room temperature.
5. If color is present, add 100 μL of 30% (100 vol) hydrogen peroxide and allow to stand for 10 to 15 min or until any reaction has subsided. If no color is present, proceed to step 7.
6. Heat again at 50 to 60°C for 30 min to complete decolorization.
7. Add 10 mL of a recommended cocktail.
8. Temperature and light adapt for at least 1 h before counting.

There are two particular samples that cannot be solubilized with the aqueous-based solubilizer — vascular tissue (arteries and veins) and stomach. Both of these sample types are only very slowly or partially solubilized by an aqueous-based solubilizer and for complete solubilization the quaternary ammonium hydroxide type must be used.

9.7.4 Liver and Kidney

Both liver and kidney samples are brownish in color and, in addition, contain blood or blood decomposition products. As a consequence, sample preparation by solubilization will be similar to that used for whole blood, and as with blood, it is possible to use both solubilizers mentioned previously.

The methods for liver and kidney are as follows:

Quaternary ammonium hydroxide method:
1. Add a maximum of 100 mg of liver or kidney to a glass scintillation vial.
2. Add 1.0 mL of selected solubilizer.
3. Incubate at 55 to 60°C for 2 h.
4. Cool to room temperature.
5. Add 0.2 to 0.5 mL of 30% hydrogen peroxide in 100 μL aliquots. Foaming will occur after each addition; therefore, gentle agitation is necessary. Keep swirling the mixture until all foaming subsides, and then repeat the process until all of the hydrogen peroxide has been added.
6. Allow to stand for 15 to 30 min at room temperature to complete the reaction.

7. Place in an oven or water bath at 55 to 60°C for 30 min. The samples at this stage will now be slightly yellow. This is important, as heating destroys residual hydrogen peroxide, which if present can induce unwanted chemiluminescence.
8. Cool to room temperature and add 15 mL of recommended scintillation cocktail.
9. Temperature and light adapt for 1 h before counting.

Aqueous-based solubilizer:

1. Add a maximum of 100 mg of liver or kidney to a glass scintillation vial.
2. Add 1.0 mL of solubilizer.
3. Incubate the sample at 55 to 60°C for 1 h.
4. Add 0.1 mL of 0.1 M EDTA–disodium salt solution, which helps reduce foaming when the subsequent hydrogen peroxide is added. This reagent also complexes iron that has been released during digestion and produces a mixture that is less colored.
5. Add 0.3 to 0.5 mL of 30% hydrogen peroxide in 100 μL aliquots. Slight foaming will occur after each addition; therefore, gentle agitation is necessary. Keep swirling the mixture until all foaming subsides, and then repeat the process until all of the hydrogen peroxide has been added.
6. Allow to stand for 15 to 30 min at room temperature to complete the reaction.
7. Place in an oven or water bath at 55 to 60°C for 1 h.
8. Cool to room temperature and add 15 mL of recommended scintillation cocktail.
9. Temperature and light adapt for 1 h before counting.

Solubilization of liver and kidney always results in highly colored samples due to the presence of bilirubin, and in addition, such samples from small animals will produce even more color. It is strongly recommended that sample size should not exceed 75 mg for small animal samples. The aqueous-based solubilizer has proven to be better than the quaternary ammonium hydroxide solubilizer for these particular sample types, mainly due to significantly less color development at the end of the solubilization process. If excessive color still develops, then one way of reducing the interference is to increase the volume of scintillation cocktail from 15 to 20 mL. In effect, this is diluting the color but it is a solution to the problem.

9.7.5 Fatty Tissue

Fatty tissue contains adipose tissue and serves to cushion and insulate vital organs. Fat tissue is made up of fat cells, which are a unique type of cell. White fat cells are large cells that have very little cytoplasm, only 15% cell volume, a small nucleus and one large fat droplet that makes up 85% of cell volume. Due to the chemical nature of fats, they are difficult to solubilize and only the quaternary ammonium hydroxide type solubilizers are suitable. Even then the rate of solubilization is slow and may require up to 24 h until completion. Fat samples can be completely solubilized but it is a matter of time, temperature, and sample condition. Recommendations include:

- Cutting the fat samples into small pieces, which increases the surface area and hence the rate of reaction.
- Carrying out the solubilization at 60°C or even slightly higher.

- Adding a small amount of isopropyl alcohol.
- Other than the rate of solubilization, the only other problem that will occur is color formation. Solubilization of fatty tissue almost invariably results in yellow coloration of the final mixture.

The method is as follows:

1. Add a maximum of 100 mg of finely divided fat to a glass scintillation vial.
2. Add 1.0 mL of selected solubilizer and optionally 1.0 mL of isopropyl alcohol.
3. Incubate at 60°C until the entire fat sample is solubilized (may take 10 to 15 h).
4. Cool to room temperature.
5. Add 0.2 to 0.5 mL of 30% hydrogen peroxide in 100 μL aliquots. Foaming will occur after each addition; therefore, gentle agitation is necessary. Keep swirling the mixture until all foaming subsides, and then repeat the process until all of the hydrogen peroxide has been added.
6. Allow to stand for 15 to 30 min at room temperature to complete the reaction.
7. Place in an oven or water bath at 55 to 60°C for 30 min. The samples at this stage will now be slightly yellow. This is important, as heating destroys residual hydrogen peroxide, which if present can induce unwanted chemiluminescence.
8. Cool to room temperature and add 15 mL of recommended scintillation cocktail.
9. Temperature and light adapt for 1 h before counting.

9.8 FECES

9.8.1 Introduction

Feces are body waste formed of undigested food that has passed through the gastrointestinal system to the colon. A proportion of feces is inner gut lining. Normally, when blood cells become old, they are trapped and destroyed by the spleen. When this occurs, the hemoglobin is broken down in the liver to bilirubin, which is excreted in the bile and leaves the body in the feces. Its presence is the reason why feces are brown in color. Feces are made mostly of water (about 75%). The rest is made of dead bacteria, living bacteria, protein, undigested food residue (known as fiber), waste material from food, cellular linings, fats, salts, and substances released from the intestines (such as mucus).

9.8.2 Sample Preparation

Feces samples are thoroughly homogenized prior to analysis to ensure subsamples are representative. Feces can otherwise be a notoriously inhomogeneous sample. Homogenization is usually carried out with water, with the aid of a blender. Samples of the homogenate are then taken for scintillation analysis.

The digestion of feces strongly depends on the type of animal. It is possible to use both the quaternary ammonium hydroxide type and the aqueous-based solubilizers, but there can be problems with residual color and incomplete digestion due to the presence of cellulose type material present in feces from species such as the rabbit. The method is the same as shown previously for muscle, skin, heart, stomach, brains and stomach tissue.

An alternative method involves the use of a sodium hypochlorite solution. During this procedure the sodium hypochlorite solution decomposes and a small amount of free chlorine gas is produced. Care should be taken when opening the vials after solubilization, as chlorine gas will be present. It is recommended that this part of the procedure be carried out under an efficient fume hood. With this method, the choice of scintillation cocktail is critical. The addition of sodium hypochlorite to almost every cocktail produces an unusual form of chemiluminescence that manifests itself either immediately or gradually over a 24 h period. Until now the only scintillation cocktail that is unaffected by this phenomenon is the PerkinElmer cocktail Hionic-Fluor. When using this method isotope recoveries are greater than 98% for tritium.

The solubilization method used for processing is shown below:

1. Weigh 50 to 150 mg of feces into a 20-mL glass scintillation vial.
2. Add 0.5 mL of sodium hypochlorite solution and cap tightly.
3. Heat in an oven or water bath at 50 to 55°C for about 30 to 60 min with occasional swirling. All the brown color of the feces will disappear and a white fibrous material remains.
4. Cool to room temperature.
5. Remove the cap and blow out any remaining chlorine using a gentle stream of air or nitrogen.
6. Add 15 mL of Hionic-Fluor (PerkinElmer) and shake to form a clear mixture.
7. Temperature and light adapt for 1 h before counting.

After digestion, a small amount of white residual matter (most probably undigested cellulose) may remain; however, this should not affect the recovery.

Sodium hypochlorite is more commonly known as bleach and should have greater than 5% available chlorine if it is to be an effective solubilizer.

9.9 NON-COMMERCIAL SOLUBILIZERS

Many laboratories make their own solubilizers. This is usually done because of cost issues or previous practice, which may include standard operating procedures that have been in place for many years. Usually these formulations are easy to prepare but they often have the drawback of increased levels of chemiluminescence. Commercial preparations will carefully select their surfactants in this respect. A standard solubilization reagent may be 40% methanolic potassium hydroxide. Some laboratories prefer sodium hydroxide, as potassium tends to exhibit a high background. Other laboratories include small amounts of surfactant. Such homemade solubilizers are often used if large samples are being digested, such as residual rat carcass. This is often done under reflux. Homemade solubilizers tend to suffer from chemiluminescence, and therefore the precautions described above, in particular dark adaptation, should be taken.

ACKNOWLEDGMENT

The author acknowledges James (Jock) Thomson for his valuable assistance in the writing of this chapter.

CHAPTER 10

Biomedical Accelerator Mass Spectrometry

Graham Lappin

CONTENTS

10.1 THE BEGINNINGS OF ACCELERATOR MASS SPECTROMETRY

Accelerator mass spectrometry (AMS) is a nuclear physics technique, used for the measurement of rare isotopes. It was developed in the 1970s, principally as a method for carbon dating. In was not used in biomedical radiotracer studies, however, until the 1990s.

AMS is an extremely sensitive and precise technique for detecting and quantifying radiotracers. The reason it is so sensitive is that it detects individual atoms of the isotope, rather than relying on detecting radioactive decay events. Take ^{14}C as an example. The half-life of ^{14}C is 5730 years; thus, in 1 year about 0.0174% of the ^{14}C atoms in a sample decay to release detectable β^--particles.[1] Over a year, therefore, the other 99.983% of the ^{14}C atoms in a sample do not decay and are undetectable by radiodetection methods. AMS, however, acts like an atomic sieve, separating the ^{12}C, ^{13}C, and ^{14}C isotopes and measuring each isotope separately, making all the atoms in a sample detectable.

Willard Frank Libby won the Nobel Prize for Chemistry in 1960 for his method to use carbon-14 for age determination in archaeology, geology, geophysics, and other branches of science. Libby's technique, more commonly known as carbon dating, is based upon the fact that radioactive isotopes undergo radioactive decay at a very precise rate.

The Earth is some 4.5 billion years old, and ^{14}C has a half-life of 5730 years. Any ^{14}C that existed during the planet's formation has therefore long since decayed away. The atmosphere, however, is constantly replenished with small amounts of ^{14}C by bombardment of cosmic radiation on the upper atmosphere. This leads to the formation of ^{14}C from ^{14}N at a rate of approximately 2.5 ^{14}C atoms/cm^3 of air/sec.[1] Although ^{14}C is constantly being formed, it is still a rare isotope with a natural abundance of approximately $1.5 \times 10^{-10}\%$. Atmospheric ^{14}C readily forms $^{14}CO_2$, which is then fixed by plants during photosynthesis. Animals eat the plants, and thus all higher living organisms contain ^{14}C in equilibrium with the atmosphere. When the organism dies, respiration ceases and there is no further ^{14}C exchange with the atmosphere. Over time, the ^{14}C decays relative to the stable isotopes of carbon (^{12}C and ^{13}C). By determining the relative amount of ^{14}C remaining in the biological material, it is therefore possible to calculate the length of time since death.

Prior to the advent of AMS, carbon dating suffered from the fact that it was very difficult to determine with any degree of precision how much ^{14}C remained in an archaeological sample. In the early days of carbon dating, there were essentially two methods of measuring the amount of ^{14}C present in an archaeological sample: liquid scintillation counting or proportional counting.[2] Modern carbon, however, contains only about 0.01356 dpm/mg, due to the presence of ^{14}C, and of course, as the archaeological sample gets older, so the emission of radioactivity decreases. Thus, in order to obtain a sufficient number of decay counts, relatively large samples had to be used.

In 1977 two papers coincidently appeared in the journal *Science* reporting the development of accelerator mass spectrometry (AMS), a new technique for measuring isotope ratios.[3,4]

As stated above, the natural abundance of ^{14}C is around $1 \times 10^{-10}\%$, and AMS can measure this isotope ratio to a precision of less than 1% using a sample size of only a few milligrams. AMS opened up the field of carbon dating. The minute sample size allowed for the dating of artifacts such as the Turin Shroud,[5] and by comparison with uranium–thorium dating of lake sediments, carbon dating has been calibrated back 45,000 years.[6]

AMS was developed to measure levels of carbon much lower than those that exist as background (45,000 years is nearly eight half-lives). Biomedical AMS, however, is not concerned with samples with depleted ^{14}C; the samples are instead enriched with the isotope.

10.2 AMS INSTRUMENTATION

A degree of sample preparation is required prior to AMS analysis. For the measurement of carbon, for example, a biological sample must first be converted to carbon dioxide or more commonly graphite. This process is detailed in Section 10.4. AMS can be used to analyze a range of isotopes (Section 10.3), but for simplicity, we will stay with ^{14}C for the time being.

There are several types of AMS instrument, depending upon intended usage and age. Below is a description of the type of instrument most commonly used in the biomedical field currently. (Having said that, there are no more than a handful of biomedical AMS facilities at present.)

Figure 10.1 shows a schematic of a typical AMS tandem system. The cesium "sputter" ion source (A) contains the wheel (B) with the graphite samples (cathodes) and consists of a cesium oven, a heated ionizing surface, and an extractor, all under high-vacuum conditions. Vacuum pressures of approximately 10^{-6} Torr are maintained in the ion source and 10^{-9} Torr in the beam line (1 Torr = 13.595 Kg/m^2). Cesium vapor from the oven is ionized by the hot surface and the Cs$^+$ ions accelerate toward the cathode. Carbon atoms from within the sample preferentially sputter negative ions that are subsequently extracted by a series of plates held at several thousand volts more positive than the ion source. The resulting negative ions undergo energy analysis to

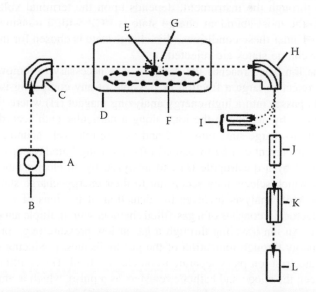

Figure 10.1 A schematic of an AMS. For A-L, see text.

select a narrow band of ion energies before entering an injection magnet (C). The injection magnet separates ions according to their mass (m) over charge (z). For carbon analysis, the injection magnet resolves to 1 m/z, allowing the ^{12}C, ^{13}C, and ^{14}C ions to pass through as a series of pulses in sequence by virtue of an electric field being bounced to modulate the speed of the ions. At this stage, molecular ions within the defined mass range, such as $^{13}CH^-$ and $^{12}CH_2^-$, may also be present. These also pass through the injection magnet since they are isobaric (i.e., essentially the same m/z) with ^{14}C. The pulsed negative ion beam enters into a tandem electrostatic Van de Graaff particle accelerator (D), where the negative ions drop through a very high potential difference toward a positive terminal, typically held at 1 to 5 million volts (E). The high voltage is generated by a rotating chain of alternate metal and plastic links, which transfers charge to the terminal (F). The accelerator is housed in a large steel tank containing insulating gas at high pressure (e.g., SF_6 at 3100 Torr). As the negative ions travel toward the positive high-voltage terminal their energy increases. The high-energy ion beam is focused to collide with argon gas molecules or a thin (0.02- to 0.05-μm) carbon foil in a collision cell (G) within the high-voltage terminal. This has the effect of stripping the outer valency electrons, and with the loss of electrons, the charge on the ions changes from negative to positive. This allows further acceleration of the ions as they leave the positive terminal. The positive ion beam is repelled by the high-voltage terminal and exits the tandem accelerator with an energy depending on the final charge state of the ions. The term *tandem accelerator* is derived from this two-stage pull–push effect.

Molecular charged ions such as the stable hydrides $^{13}CH^-$ and $^{12}CH_2^-$ do not survive the electron stripping process and are converted to atomic species. The electron stripping process leads to the formation of carbon ions with charge states from 1^+ to 4^+. The relative abundance of these particular charge states, and their transmission through the instrument, depends upon the terminal voltage. At 4.5 million volts, the most abundant charge state is $^{14}C_4^+$ with a transmission factor of 40 to 50%. Under these conditions, this charge state is chosen for measurement and the other charge states are rejected.

Before the ion beam reaches the detector, it is necessary to remove the stable isotopes and reject as large a fraction as possible of any competing isotopes. The ion beam thus passes into a high-energy analyzing magnet (H) where ^{12}C, ^{13}C, and ^{14}C are separated by deflecting the ions along a particular path according to their mass–momentum–charge state ratio. ^{12}C and ^{13}C are relatively abundant compared to ^{14}C, and their current can be measured off-axis using Faraday cups (I). The ^{14}C beam is focused by a quadrupole (J) and analyzed by an electrostatic cylindrical analyzer (K), which selects ions according to their energy–charge state ratio. The final stage in AMS analysis involves the detection of the ions of interest. A gas ionization detector (L) consists of a gas-filled chamber with multiple anode segments and a cathode. An ion traveling through a gas at low pressure (e.g., propane at 60 Torr) loses energy through ionization of the gas molecules, producing electron-ion pairs. These electron-ion pairs separate in an electric field. The resulting change in voltage between the anode and cathode registers as a pulse, which is amplified. The number of pulses is proportional to the number of ^{14}C ions entering the detector. The rate at which an ion loses energy in a material is proportional to the product of its mass and the square of its atomic charge, and inversely proportional to its energy. Measurement of the rate at which an ion loses energy (provided by the anode) and its total energy (provided by the cathode) therefore allows an isotope to be uniquely identified according to its mass and charge.

Along with carbon ions, other isobaric atomic species can also be formed in the AMS that can be potentially interfering. Whereas molecular species such as $^{13}CH^-$ and $^{12}CH_2^-$ are destroyed during ion stripping, some isobars are transmitted all the way through to the gas ionization detector. These ions with a mass–charge ratio equal to that of the radionuclide follow the same trajectory and reach the detector without any reduction in intensity. The principal isobar formed alongside $^{14}C_4^+$ is believed to be $^7Li_2^+$, although its origin is somewhat open to question. Although the lithium isobar enters the gas detector, at the very high energies involved in AMS (ca. 20 to 100 MeV) it can be separated from ^{14}C by virtue of its energy loss, and thus eliminated from the counting procedure. ^{14}N is not an interfering isobar of ^{14}C, as negative nitrogen ions decay in about 5×10^{-14} sec and hence do not reach the accelerator.

The instrument depicted in Figure 10.1 is approximately 25 m long and is capable of measuring a wide range of isotopes. Due to demands for biomedical use, more compact AMS instruments have recently been developed. These instruments are much smaller than those currently available, as they do not require a large insulating gas-filled tank to house the high-voltage terminal, nor do they operate on charged chains. In the compact design, the terminal is insulated using a vacuum and the high voltage is supplied by an external voltage supply. A gas stripper inside the terminal is used to break up molecular charged ions. Stable operation of these instruments can be achieved between 200 and 600 kV, and instead of gas ionization detectors, solid-state detectors are used.

10.3 ISOTOPES

Although AMS, in the drug development area, has been used mostly to quantify ^{14}C, the technique is by no means limited to this isotope. An element should conform to the following criteria if it is to be analyzed by AMS:

1. Since AMS is an isotope ratio technique, at least two isotopes for any given element are required, one of which should be rare. The natural abundance of the rare isotope determines the signal-to-noise ratio, and hence the sensitivity of the measurement. It is for this reason that ^{14}C is suitable for AMS and ^{13}C (natural abundance, 1.1%) is not. Some elements only have one stable isotope (Be, F, Na, Al, P, Sc, Mn, Co, As, Y, Nb, Rh, I, Cs, Pr, Pm, Tb, Ho, Tm, Au, and Bi), and therefore by definition their other (radio-)isotopes are rare or nonexistent in nature. This does not mean they are necessarily useful in AMS, as the radioisotope must have a usable half-life.
2. Elements with a low electron affinity (e.g., N, Mn, Pr, Pm, and Ho) do not readily form negative ions. These elements can still be measured by AMS, but analysis is more complicated and is based on molecular ion beams (e.g., MnH).
3. Since samples have to be prepared for AMS analysis, isotopes with short half-lives are impractical.

Isotopes of biological interest that have been studied by AMS include ^{3}H, ^{26}Al, ^{36}Cl, ^{41}Ca, ^{32}Si, and ^{129}I. Tritium (^{3}H), with a half-life of 12.3 years, is a useful tracer in the study of xenobiotic metabolism (Section 3.2.1) and has been analyzed by AMS. ^{26}Al is the only long-lived radioisotope of aluminum (with a half-life of 740,000 years). It has been suggested that aluminum could be involved in the development of anemia, Alzheimer's disease, and renal failures.[7] ^{41}Ca has a half-life of 103,000 years and can be used to investigate osteoporosis and other bone diseases.[8] ^{36}Cl and ^{129}I (with half-lives of 301,000 and 15.7 million years, respectively) are of interest in biomedicine, as they have importance in general metabolism. These isotopes can be measured down to a sensitivity of $>10^{-14}$ using AMS.[9,10] Elements such as Fe, Ni, and Se can be present in proteins and have vital metabolic functions in living organisms. The absorption and renal elimination of silicic acid in humans have been studied using ^{32}Si and AMS.[11] ^{32}S is a strongly interfering isobar of ^{32}Si, and a gas-filled magnet technique is required to separate them.

Routine measurement of the radioisotopes ^{55}Fe, ^{60}Fe, ^{59}Ni, and ^{79}Se may also become possible with AMS in the future.[10]

10.4 SAMPLE PREPARATION

Biological samples, such as blood, plasma, etc., cannot be placed directly into an AMS and a degree of sample preparation is required. Preparation procedures for a range of isotopes are given in Tuniz et al. (1998).[10] For example, ^{3}H is first converted to titanium hydride,[12] and organic carbon is converted to pure carbon (i.e., graphite).[13] The sample holder can be modified to allow CO_2 gas to be introduced directly into the ion source. This has several advantages: CO_2 gas from the sample eliminates the time-consuming process of graphite conversion and cross-contamination between successive samples is very low. Such gas sources are, however, less sensitive than graphite.

Figure 10.2 shows the process of the graphitization of carbon. The sample is aliquoted into a glass tube along with copper oxide (A). The size of the aliquot should be equivalent to approximately 2 mg of carbon. (Although in theory much smaller samples can be used, in practice, for samples enriched with ^{14}C, 2 mg is the most convenient.) The tube is sealed under vacuum (B) and placed in a furnace at ca. 900°C, where the carbon is oxidized to carbon dioxide (C). Once cooled, the tube containing the carbon dioxide is placed into one arm of a Y-piece. On the other arm there is a second tube containing titanium hydride and zinc powder as reductants and cobalt or iron (D). The tube containing the carbon dioxide is immersed in a mixture of solid carbon dioxide and organic solvent (E). The second tube is immersed in liquid nitrogen (F). The Y-piece is evacuated and the tip of the tube containing the carbon dioxide is snapped off. The carbon dioxide then cryogenically transfers into the second tube (F). This tube is also sealed and placed in a furnace at 500°C, where the carbon dioxide is reduced to graphite (G). Once cooled, the tube is snapped open (H) and the graphite is first gently placed into a cathode (I), then pressed into the cathode under high pressure.

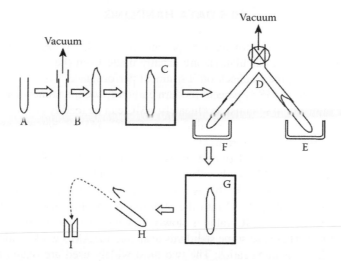

Figure 10.2 Graphitization of samples for AMS analysis. For A-I, see text.

Approximately 2 mg of carbon is required, to be pressed into cathodes, which are placed into the ion source of the AMS. The later stage of cryogenic transfer has been modified to include septa on the tubes, thus avoiding the glass-sealing stage.[14]

Although not absolutely critical, the amount of carbon in the biological sample is important. If the sample size is so small that less than about 0.5 mg of carbon is produced, then there is insufficient sample to press into the cathode. If the amount of carbon is too high, then the pressure in the sealed glass tubes can raise to a point that the tube bursts. The ideal amount of carbon is around 2 mg, but of course, different sample types contain different percentages of carbon, and so the aliquot volume has to be adjusted accordingly. It is therefore often necessary to determine the percentage of carbon in a sample before it is aliquoted into the first tube. This can be done using a standard carbon analyzer. Some sample types do not vary widely in their carbon content. For example, measurements made at Xceleron Ltd. have determined that plasma contains 4.14% carbon, and so a 50- to 60-μL aliquot contains about 2 mg of carbon. It should be noted at this point that AMS requires only very small sample sizes, as well as being extremely sensitive (just how sensitive we will see in moment).

There are situations where the sample contains too little carbon to enable a sample of sufficient size to be generated. Under these circumstances, carrier carbon is added. At first sight it may seem an odd thing to do; adding carbon to a sample will of course upset the isotope ratio. The answer is that carbon from immensely old petrochemical sources is used, which contain no ^{14}C. The isotope ratio is still diluted, but providing the amount of carrier carbon added is known, the effect on the isotope ratio can be corrected.

Because the biological samples are treated in such a way as to generate graphite, virtually any sample type can be used. No sample of biological origin will resist the harshness of the graphitization process.

10.5 DATA HANDLING

AMS provides a value for the isotope ratio of $^{14}C/^{13}C/^{12}C$. Because ^{12}C is the most abundant isotope, calculations are usually made from the $^{14}C/^{12}C$ ratio, with ^{13}C acting as a less precise check on instrument performance.

The raw unit for AMS is percent modern carbon (pMC), a somewhat confusing term for the biomedical scientist. Fortunately, pMC can be readily converted to units of radioactivity. First, however, an explanation of pMC, which is actually just another way of expressing an isotope ratio.

One hundred percent modern carbon (100 pMC) is defined as 98 amole* ^{14}C/mg carbon. The term 100 pMC is, however, a little misleading, as the pMC value for modern carbon is around 110. This is because the atomic bomb tests of the 1950s introduced some additional ^{14}C into the atmosphere. As the Earth's carbon cycle soaks up this ^{14}C, so the pMC value is slowly moving back toward 100 (Chernobyl notwithstanding). There are some standards available for AMS work, with precisely determined ^{14}C:^{12}C isotope ratios. The two most widely used are oxalic acid from the U.S. National Institute of Standards and Technology (NIST) and a crop of sugar harvested in Australia in the 1960s and certified by the Australian National University (ANU). The NIST oxalic acid standard has a pMC of 95, and ANU sugar has a pMC of 150.61. The higher pMC value of the latter standard reflects that it was harvested just after the height of the atomic bomb tests.

pMC is easily converted into a weight-by-weight isotope ratio (100 pMC = 98 amole ^{14}C/mg C), but how is this then converted to units of radioactivity?

For a detailed explanation on how to convert the quantity of isotope to units of radioactivity, see Section 2.9. Here, it is sufficient to know that 98 amole ^{14}C/mg C is equal to 0.01356 dpm. Take a moment to look at this value, however. It is saying that for a sample giving a value of 100 pMC by AMS analysis, this equates to 0.01356 dpm/mg of carbon. The significance of this statement is illustrated in Figure 10.3.

Assume both samples A and B give the same result on AMS analysis of 100 dpm/mg carbon. Assume both samples A and B weigh 100 mg. For sample A, 25% of this 100 mg is carbon. Thus sample A contains 25 mg of carbon. Since the AMS result tells us that every milligram of carbon in this sample equals 100 dpm, then the total radioactivity in the sample is 2500 dpm. Since the sample weighs 100 mg, then the concentration in the sample is 25 dpm/mg. Now do exactly the same calculation for sample B; the sample contains 5000 dpm, which equals a concentration of 50 dpm/mg sample. To convert an isotope ratio into a radioactive concentration, the amount of carbon in the sample has to be known.

The percent carbon in most samples can be measured using a carbon analyzer. Indeed, as stated above, if the amount of carbon is completely unknown, it is necessary to measure its content both so the radioactive concentration can be calculated and to ensure an appropriate amount of carbon is present for graphitization. If a sample contains so little carbon that it cannot be measured by a carbon analyzer, then carbon carrier is added. Under these circumstances, the amount of carbon in the carrier is usually used in the calculation of radioactive concentration.

---

* amole = attomole = 10^{-18} mol.

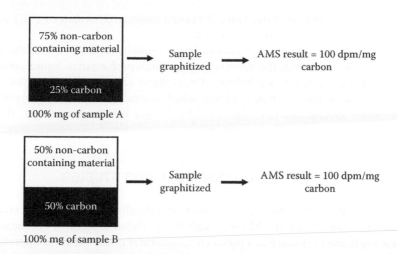

Figure 10.3 From AMS analysis, it is necessary to know the carbon content of the sample, in order to determine the dpm/g or mL value. See text for explanation.

If samples are taken from biological sources, for example, laboratory animals or clinical studies with humans, the samples will contain some background ^{14}C. For example, the background radioactivities for blood and plasma are approximately 1.5 and 0.6 dpm/g, respectively (the higher value for blood reflecting its higher carbon content). Interestingly, since the human body, on average, contains around 5.5 L of blood, then the blood alone contains about 8250 dpm of radioactivity due to ^{14}C. The total amount of radioactivity in a 70-kg human, due to ^{14}C, is about 3.7 KBq (100 nCi).

When calculating radioactive concentrations of biological samples from AMS data, it is important to subtract the background from the analytical sample. To do this, it is advisable to take samples from laboratory animals or humans prior to the administration of [^{14}C]-labeled xenobiotics, then use the results of these samples for background subtraction.

10.6 SENSITIVITY AND PRECISION OF AMS

The sensitivity of AMS is essentially one atom. In reality, the detector needs to count a minimum number in order to get a statistically significant value. As a rule of thumb, about 1000 atoms are required, putting the theoretical limit of detection of AMS in the zeptomole region. The practical limits of detection depend upon the sample workup and the level of background, or signal-to-noise ratio. The noise originates from background ^{14}C, and therefore the more carbon in a sample, the higher the noise level. For example, plasma has a background of around 0.6 dpm/g. AMS can measure an isotope ratio of modern carbon with a precision of less than 1%. For biomedical work, however, usually 5% is sufficient, as there is at least that level of variation in the biological systems being examined. Allowing for some variation, AMS can routinely measure ^{14}C from drug-related material that constitutes

10% of the sample radioactivity. Thus, if plasma contains 0.06 dpm of [^{14}C]-drug-related material, AMS can reliably detect it.

For some sample types, background carbon is virtually all removed and the only ^{14}C present originates from the xenobiotic (e.g., high-performance liquid chromatography (HPLC) samples; see below). Under these circumstances, radioactivity levels of 0.0001 dpm/mL can be detected, which is equivalent to 100 amole/mL at the maximum specific activity (Section 2.9). To put this in perspective, this is equivalent to around 60 million atoms/ml.

10.7 THE FIRST BIOMEDICAL AMS STUDIES

Before we move on to the use of AMS in drug development, it is worth considering the first applications of AMS in biochemistry. The measurement of macromolecular adducts after exposure to a potential genotoxin is of considerable importance in understanding the relationship between the level of exposure, the adduct level, and the biological effect. A variety of techniques have been used to measure adducts, including ^{32}P-postlabeling (Section 4.2.7), radioimmunoassay (Section 4.3), mass spectrometry (Section 3.5.12) and fluorescence. A commonly used experimental method is to label the potential toxin with ^{14}C, administer it to the test species, then isolate and analyze the DNA (Section 4.2). The difficulty with this is that the label is diluted in the body and the proportion that binds to DNA can be extremely small. The consequence of this is that conventional liquid scintillation counting techniques may not be sensitive enough to measure the level of radioactivity in the DNA sample. Enter AMS.

The heterocyclic amines, 2-amino-3,8-dimethylimidazo[4,5-f]quinoxaline (MeIQx) and 2-amino-1-methyl-6-phenylimidazo[4,5-b]pyridine (PhIP), are known food mutagens and are particularly prevalent in well-cooked beef and fish. They have been implicated in some cancers, such as cancer of the colon, prostate and breast. AMS has been used to study such DNA adducts at very low levels.[15-18] A dose–response relationship has been established with ^{14}C-MeIQx, with doses as low as 500 ng/Kg. The limit of detection was 1 adduct/10^{11} nucleotides or 1 adduct/approximately 100 cells (^{32}P-postlabeling is quoted as being able to detect about 1 adduct in 10^9 bases; see Section 4.2.7).[18]

As well as animal models, studies have been performed with [^{14}C]-PhIP, MeIQx, benzo[a]pyrene, and aflotoxin-B in humans.[19-21] It might be considered unusual to administer carcinogens to humans, but the amounts were below those already present in the diet, and therefore could be considered safe. For example, consenting human volunteers received just 20 μg, 182 KBq PhIP or 5 μg, 36 KBq of benzo[a]pyrene.[19] (Compare the radioactive doses used in these studies with those discussed in Chapter 3.)

The extreme sensitivity of AMS to ^{14}C made the above studies possible. Not only were very small amounts of compound administered, but the levels of radioactivity were also minimized.

10.8 AMS AND DRUG DEVELOPMENT

Although it is possible to administer radioactive tracers to humans, there are strict limits to the amounts that can be given. The limits are defined by national regulatory authorities, and although the regulations differ from country to country, the principles on which the limits are defined are the same. The regulatory limits are defined in units of equivalent dose, measured in Sieverts (Section 2.6 and Chapter 5, Appendix 1). Typically, a dose of 1 mSv is permitted — above this level and permission to conduct the experiment becomes increasing more difficult. Typically, for a drug with a plasma half-life of a few hours that does not accumulate in body tissues, around 3 to 4 MBq (around 100 μCi) can be administered without exceeding a 1-mSv ceiling. On the other end of the scale, however, for a drug with a plasma half-life of several days, it may only be possible to administer a fraction of this amount of radioactivity. The levels of radioactivity in the biological samples (e.g., blood, urine and feces) may therefore be too low to measure using liquid scintillation counting.

Perhaps not surprising, therefore, radiotracer studies on drugs with long plasma half-lives were the first to be conducted using AMS as the method of ^{14}C measurement.[22] In addition to determining rates and routes of excretion, AMS can be used to determine the metabolite profile. Unlike liquid chromatography–mass spectroscopy (LC-MS) (Section 3.5.12), there is no direct interface for AMS, although work is being conducted in the area.[23] Samples are analyzed by HPLC in the usual way (Section 3.5.9), and the eluate is collected as a series of fractions. Each fraction is then graphitized as described in Section 10.4 (or by using microplate technology as described in Section 6.14). The ^{14}C content of each fraction is converted to units of radioactivity (usually dpm) and plotted against retention time. Because background carbon is virtually eliminated during HPLC separation, the signal-to-noise ratio is also very low, and consequently, the limits of detection are particularly impressive. It is possible to generate a full metabolic profile consisting of a number of metabolites by injecting as little as 0.01 dpm into the HPLC column.

10.8.1 AMS as an Enabling Technology

AMS is now well established in drug development as a highly sensitive method of detecting radiotracers.[24-27] Although in its beginnings it was used merely to analyze samples where liquid scintillation counting had run out of sensitivity, it soon became apparent that the technology enabled whole new areas of research to be conducted that were previously impossible. Some of these areas are reviewed below.

10.8.2 Experimental Populations

Because of the restrictions on administering radioactivity to humans, it is only possible to conduct radiotracer studies in limited populations. For this reason, the majority of radiotracer studies are performed in healthy male volunteers (Section 3.5.4). The typical radioactive dose in a conventional radiotracer study of around 3 to 4 MBq per volunteer can be reduced a thousand-fold to 3 to 4 KBq if the study is designed around AMS. This reduction almost certainly puts the levels of radio-activity below the regulatory limits. In other words, although the drug contains a radiotracer, it is classified as a nonradioactive study. As stated in Section 10.5, the average human contains about 3.7 KBq of naturally occurring ^{14}C. The level of radioactivity administered is therefore about the same as that which is already present in the body. Moreover, the author has experience of doses as low as approximately 200 Bq being used.

Whereas conventional radiotracer studies are limited to certain populations of human volunteers, studies designed around AMS have no such limitations. This opens up the potential experimental population to include patients, pediatrics[28] and women of childbearing age. Patient studies can be performed in regular hospital wards, as opposed to specially designated radioactive areas. In one case, tables containing low levels of [^{14}C]-drug were prepared using conventional tabletting machinery.[29]

10.8.3 Phase I Studies

Given that normal patient populations can be used in radiotracer studies, there is no reason why low-level [^{14}C]-drug cannot be used in the phase I clinical studies. Information on the metabolism of the drug can therefore be obtained at the point it is first administered to man. Up until that point, the likelihood is that the only data on the drug's metabolism comes from *in vitro* experiments and the analysis of samples using nonradioactive methods from clinical trials. Going down the tradi-tional path, it is possible that human-specific metabolism only becomes apparent once the drug is in phase II (Section 1.5.3 and Section 1.7.1).

The first-in-man study involves a rising dose of drug and the monitoring of symptomatic endpoints as well as pharmacokinetics. If a small amount of ^{14}C is included in one of these doses, samples can be profiled (Section 3.5.9) and then the profiles compared to those obtained from the toxicology species from *in vivo* and *in vitro* studies. If human-specific metabolites are present, then the earlier in the development program they are identified, the better, and it may be possible to amend the design of the toxicology studies if necessary.

10.8.4 Absolute Bioavailability

The concept and experimental design of absolute bioavailability studies are explained in Section 3.6.7 and in Appendix 3 to Chapter 3. In short, human volunteers are administered an intravenous dose on one dosing occasion and an extravascular dose on another dosing occasion. Plasma samples are analyzed for parent drug concentration, and the areas under the curve (AUCs) for both doses are calculated. The intravenous dose represents 100% absorption (since it was administered directly into the bloodstream), and so comparison of the AUCs (relative to the doses admin-istered) gives the absolute bioavailability (see Equation 3.2).

The technique is open to criticism when the plasma concentrations of the intra-venous and extravascular doses are significantly different. The problem arises from the fact that the maximum dose that can be administered intravenously is limited by issues such as toxicity and solubility. If clearance is concentration dependent, then it is not correct to compare the AUCs resulting from widely different plasma concentrations.

In the 1970s, a method of determining absolute bioavailability using a stable isotope was developed.[30] An intravenous dose of N-acetylprocainamide, labeled with ^{13}C, was administered simultaneously with an unlabeled oral dose. There was therefore a single-dose occasion and a single set of plasma samples taken. By analyzing the plasma samples, it was possible to deconvolute the concentrations of the intravenous dose from the oral dose. Essentially, the method relies on isotopic dilution (Section 4.5). The intravenous and oral doses mix as they enter the bloodstream. The proportion of the oral dose that reaches the bloodstream is thus proportional to the degree of isotopic dilution of the intravenous dose. The plasma concentrations for the two doses were separated by virtue of the different molecular weights, using mass spectroscopy. Since it was possible to determine the concentrations of both the intravenous dose and the oral dose from the same plasma samples, any issues of dose dependency were eliminated, irrespective of the initial doses administered.

The use of ^{13}C suffered from poor sensitivity, because of its natural abundance of 1.1%. Other stable isotopes have lower natural abundances; for example, ^{15}N has a natural abundance of 0.36% and has been used for absolute bioavailability determinations,[31] but this is still well above the natural abundance of radioisotopes such as ^{14}C. Traditionally, there are restrictions on administering radioactivity to humans, and therefore the use of ^{14}C in bioavailability experiments was not routine.

With the advent of AMS, ^{14}C-labeled drugs can be administered to human volunteers using levels of radioactivity below those that demand regulatory acceptance. Volunteers are administered a $[^{14}C]$-drug intravenously, using typically 3 to 4 KBq. The physical amount of drug is also kept very low, typically below 100 µg. Such small doses are termed a microdose (this is expanded upon in Section 10.8.5). The extravascular drug is administered as the nonlabeled form at the therapeutic dose level. Plasma samples are collected over time, and the concentration of parent drug in each plasma sample is measured by LC-MS and HPLC, followed by AMS (Figure 10.4).

The above technique has an additional advantage in that toxicology data from the intravenous dose may not be required. Under normal circumstances, toxicological data using the intravenous route of administration would be required to enable an intravenous dose to be given to human volunteers. This is both costly and time-consuming and, for many orally administered drugs, would only be required for the absolute bioavailability study. Providing there were plasma concentration data from the oral dose that covered the concentrations that would be achieved from the intravenous microdose, then specific toxicity testing for the intravenous administration would be an unlikely requirement.

10.8.5 Microdosing and Human Phase 0

The three phases of clinical development (phase I to phase III) were explained in Section 1.1. Recently an additional phase has been introduced, prior to phase I, the so-called human phase 0 study. The purpose of such a study is to assist in the

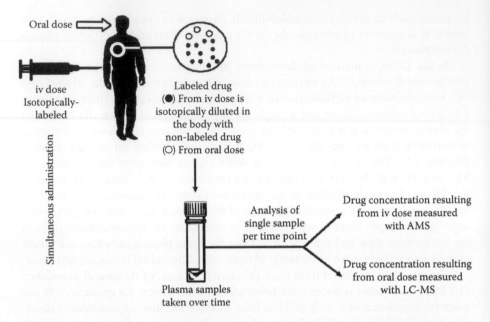

Figure 10.4 Schematic showing the experimental procedure for determining absolute bio-availability from the simultaneous administration of a labeled intravenous (iv) dose and an non-labeled oral dose.

drug selection process; it is not intended for regulatory submission. Selection of candidate drugs for clinical development is carried out largely on the basis of *in vitro* data and minimal amounts of animal data. Where metabolism or pharmacokinetics is important in the selection decision, then the human phase 0 study provides data from the target species, namely, humans, to assist in the process.

A microdose is defined as one 100th of the therapeutic dose (or predicted therapeutic dose), up to a maximum of 100 μg.[32] This very small dose is administered to human volunteers and plasma, urine and feces are collected in the usual way (as described in Chapter 3). Although in theory it is possible to administer nonlabeled microdoses and conduct the analysis with LC-MS, no metabolite profile can be generated and often LC-MS lacks the necessary sensitivity. Most microdosing is therefore conducted using radiolabeled drug.

Because such a small amount of drug is administered, the toxicology package required to enable a microdose to be administered to humans is much reduced. Some minimal animal data is all that is required. Human phase 0 studies can therefore be performed at a much lower cost than the full first-in-man study.

There has been much debate about pharmacokinetic linearity of microdosing.[33] Much of this debate, however, rather misses the point. In Chapter 1, it was explained that *in vitro* data are an aid to decision making, and that *in vitro* data are useful rather than precise. The same premise applies to human phase 0 studies. Precise linearity between the microdose and the therapeutic dose is not really required. It is true that if the microdose gave a wildly different set of pharmacokinetic parameters than the therapeutic dose, then the human phase 0 study might be misleading.

However, this situation already exists with reliance on *in vitro* and animal models. The intention of the human phase 0 study is to provide the extra data that are required, when they are required, to aid in the decision-making process. If microdosing reduces the drug attrition rate in clinical trials by only a few percent, then this represents many millions of dollars (see Figure 1.1 in Chapter 1). Microdosing and human phase 0 studies have to be applied intelligently, and in this respect, they are no different than any other experiment that may be conducted in the drug development program.

Microdosing has also been conducted using positron emission tomography (PET; Chapter 11).

10.8.6 The Future of AMS

There has been an inextricable drive toward risk reduction in society as a whole and in clinical research in particular. Providing the design of AMS instrumentation continues to be simplified and costs reduced, it seems inevitable that in the future all radiotracer studies with humans will be conducted using AMS as the analytical endpoint. Some would say this is an overstatement, but why would we continue administering a thousand-fold higher levels of radioactivity to humans than we really need to?

ACKNOWLEDGMENTS

My thanks to Darren Groombridge for the description of AMS instrumentation.

REFERENCES

1. Turteltaub, K.W., Felton, J.S., Gledhill, B.L., Vogel, J.S., Southon, J.R., Caffee, M.W., Finkel, R.C., Nelson, D.E., Proctor, I.D., and Davis, J.C., Accelerator mass spectrometry in biomedical dosimetry: relationship between low-level exposure and covalent binding of heterocyclic amine carcinogens to DNA, *Proc. Natl. Acad. Sci. U.S.A.*, 87, 5288–5292, 1990.
2. Theodorsson, P., *Measurement of Weak Radioactivity*, World Scientific, Singapore, 1996.
3. Bennett, C.L., Beukens, R.P., Clover, M.R., Gove, H.E., Liebert, R.B., Litherland, A.E., Purser, K.H., and Sondheim, W.E., Radiocarbon dating with electrostatic accelerators: negative ions provide the key, *Science*, 198, 508–510, 1977.
4. Nelson, D.E., Korteling, R.G., and Stott, W.R., Carbon-14 direct detection at natural concentrations, *Science*, 198, 507–508, 1977.
5. Wilson, I., *The Blood and the Shroud: The Passionate Controversy Still Enflaming the World's Most Famous Carbon-Dating Test*, Weidenfeld & Nicolson, London, 1998.
6. Kitagawa, H. and van der Plicht, J., Atmospheric radiocarbon calibration to 45,000 yr B.P.: late glacial fluctuations and cosmogenic isotope production, *Science*, 279, 1187–1190, 1998.

7. Moore, P.B., Day, J.P., Taylor, G.A., Ferrier, I.N., Fifield, L.K., and Edwardson, J.A., Absorption of aluminium-26 in Alzheimer's disease, measured using accelerator mass spectrometry, *Dement Geriatr. Cogn. Disord.*, 11, 66–69, 2000.
8. Barker, J. and Garner, R.C., Biomedical applications of accelerator mass spectrometry: isotope measurements at the level of the atom, *Rapid Commun. Mass. Spectrom.*, 13, 285–293, 1999.
9. Schmidt, A., Schnabel, C., Handl, J., Jakob, D., Michel, R., Synal, H.A., Lopez, J.M., and Suter, M., On the analysis of iodine-129 and iodine-127 in environmental materials by accelerator mass spectrometry and ion chromatography, *Sci. Total Environ.*, 223, 131–156, 1998.
10. Tuniz, C., Bird, J.R., Fink, D., and Herzog, G.F., *Accelerator Mass Spectrometry, Ultrasensitive Analysis for Global Science,* CRC Press, Boca Raton, FL, 1998.
11. Popplewell, J.F., King, S.J., Day, J.P., Ackrill, P., Fifield, L.K., Cresswell, R.G., di Tada, M.L., and Liu, K., Kinetics of uptake and elimination of silicic acid by a human subject: a novel application of 32Si and accelerator mass spectrometry, *J. Inorg. Biochem.*, 69, 177–180, 1998.
12. Chiarappa-Zucca, M.L., Dingley, K.H., Roberts, M.L., Velsko, C.A., and Love, A.H., Sample preparation for quantitation of tritium by accelerator mass spectrometry, *Anal. Chem.*, 74, 6285–6290, 2002.
13. Vogel, J.S., Production of carbon for accelerator mass spectrometry without contamination, *Radioacarbon*, 34, 344–350, 1992.
14. Ognibene, T.J., Bench, G., Vogel, J.S., Peaslee, G.F., and Murov, S., A high-throughput method for the conversion of CO_2 obtained from biochemical samples to graphite in septa-sealed vials for quantification of ^{14}C via accelerator mass spectrometry, *Anal. Chem.*, 75, 2192–2196, 2003.
15. Turteltaub, K.W., Vogel, J.S., Frantz, C., Felton, J.S., and McManus, M., Assessment of the DNA adduction and pharmacokinetics of PhIP and MeIQx in rodents at doses approximating human exposure using the technique of accelerator mass spectrometry (AMS) and ^{32}P-postlabeling, *Princess Takamatsu Symp.*, 23, 93–102, 1995.
16. Mauthe, R.J., Dingley, K.H., Leveson, S.H., Freeman, S.P., Turesky, R.J., Garner, R.C., and Turteltaub, K.W., Comparison of DNA-adduct and tissue-available dose levels of MeIQx in human and rodent colon following administration of a very low dose, *Int. J. Cancer*, 80, 539–545, 1999.
17. Turteltaub, K.W., Mauthe, R.J., Dingley, K.H., Vogel, J.S., Frantz, C.E., Garner, R.C., and Shen, N., MeIQx-DNA adduct formation in rodent and human tissues at low doses, *Mutat. Res.*, 376, 243–252, 1997.
18. Frantz, C.E., Bangerter, C., Fultz, E., Mayer, K.M., Vogel, J.S., and Turteltaub, K.W., Dose-response studies of MeIQx in rat liver and liver DNA at low doses, *Carcinogenesis*, 16, 367–373, 1995.
19. Lightfoot, T.J., Coxhead, J.M., Cupid, B.C., Nicholson, S., and Garner, R.C., Analysis of DNA adducts by accelerator mass spectrometry in human breast tissue after administration of 2-amino-1-methyl-6-phenylimidazo[4,5-b]pyridine and benzo[a]pyrene, *Mutat. Res.*, 472, 119–127, 2000.
20. Cupid, B.C., Lightfoot, T.J., Russell, D., Gant, S.J., Turner, P.C., Dingley, K.H., Curtis, K.D., Leveson, S.H., Turteltaub, K.W., and Garner, R.C., The formation of AFB(1)-macromolecular adducts in rats and humans at dietary levels of exposure, *Food Chem. Toxicol.*, 42, 559–569, 2004.

21. Turteltaub, K.W., Dingley, K.H., Curtis, K.D., Malfatti, M.A., Turesky, R.J., Garner, R.C., Felton, J.S., and Lang, N.P., Macromolecular adduct formation and metabolism of heterocyclic amines in humans and rodents at low doses, *Cancer Lett.*, 143, 149–55, 1999.

22. Young, G., Ellis, W., Ayrton, J., Hussey, E., and Adamkiewicz, B., Accelerator mass spectrometry (AMS): recent experience of its use in a clinical study and the potential future of the technique, *Xenobiotica*, 31, 619–632, 2001.

23. Liberman, R.G., Tannenbaum, S.R., Hughey, B.J., Shefer, R.E., Klinkowstein, R.E., Prakash, C., Harriman, S.P., and Skipper, P.L., An interface for direct analysis of (14)c in nonvolatile samples by accelerator mass spectrometry, *Anal. Chem.*, 76, 328–334, 2004.

24. Lappin, G. and Garner, R.C., Current perspectives of ^{14}C-isotope measurement in biomedical accelerator mass spectrometry, *Anal. Bioanal. Chem.*, 378, 356–364, 2004.

25. White, I.N. and Brown, K., Techniques: the application of accelerator mass spectrometry to pharmacology and toxicology, *Trends Pharmacol. Sci.*, 25, 442–447, 2004.

26. Garner, R.C., Goris, I., Laenen, A.A., Vanhoutte, E., Meuldermans, W., Gregory, S., Garner, J.V., Leong, D., Whattam, M., Calam, A., and Snel, C.A., Evaluation of accelerator mass spectrometry in a human mass balance and pharmacokinetic study-experience with ^{14}C-labeled (R)-6-[amino(4-chlorophenyl)(1-methyl-1H-imidazol-5-yl)methyl]-4-(3-chlorophenyl)-1-methyl-2(1H)-quinolinone (R115777), a farnesyl transferase inhibitor, *Drug Metab. Dispos.*, 30, 823–830, 2002.

27. Kaye, B., Garner, R.C., Mauthe, R.J., Freeman, S.P., and Turteltaub, K.W., A preliminary evaluation of accelerator mass spectrometry in the biomedical field, *J. Pharm. Biomed. Anal.*, 16, 541–543, 1997.

28. Leide-Svegborn, S., Stenstrom, K., Olofsson, M., Mattsson, S., Nilsson, L.-E., Nosslin, B., Pau, K., Johansson, L., Erlandsson, B., Hellborg, R., and Skog, G., Biokinetics and radiation doses for carbon-14 urea in adults and children undergoing the *Helicobacter pylori* breath test, *Eur. J. Nuclear Med.*, 26, 573–580, 1999.

29. Garner, R.C., Garner, J.V., Gregory, S., Whattam, M., Calam, A., and Leong, D., Comparison of the absorption of micronized (Daflon 500 mg) and nonmicronized ^{14}C-diosmin tablets after oral administration to healthy volunteers by accelerator mass spectrometry and liquid scintillation counting, *J. Pharm. Sci.*, 91, 32–40, 2002.

30. Strong, J.M., Dutcher, J.S., Lee, W.K., and Atkinson, A.J., Jr., Absolute bioavailability in man of N-acetylprocainamide determined by a novel stable isotope method, *Clin. Pharmacol. Ther.*, 18, 613–622, 1975.

31. Wilding, I.R., Davis, S.S., Hardy, J.G., Robertson, C.S., John, V.A., Powell, M.L., Leal, M., Lloyd, P., and Walker, S.M., Relationship between systemic drug absorption and gastrointestinal transit after the simultaneous oral administration of carbamazepine as a controlled-release system and as a suspension of ^{15}N-labelled drug to healthy volunteers, *Br. J. Clin. Pharmacol.*, 32, 573–579, 1991.

32. European Medicines Evaluation Agency (EMEA), Position Paper on Non-clinical Safety Studies to Support Clinical Trials with a Single Microdose, position paper CPMP/SWP/2599, June 23, 2004.

33. Lappin, G. and Garner, R.C., Big physics, small doses: the use of AMS and PET in human microdosing of development drugs, *Nat. Rev. Drug Discov.*, 2, 233–240, 2003.

CHAPTER 11

Positron Emission Tomography

Barbara S. Koetz and Patricia M. Price

CONTENTS

11.1 INTRODUCTION

Although the potential value of imaging with positron-emitting radionuclides was envisaged more than half a century ago, only more recent advances in radiochemistry, scintillation detection, electronics, and computer capacities for image reconstruction allowed further development of this functional imaging modality to become a valuable tool in research and drug development. Positron emission tomography (PET) now has the potential for *in vivo* imaging of drug pharmacokinetics, pharmacodynamic endpoints, molecular pathways, and gene expression. Human

studies with minute amounts of the labeled pharmacological compound, known as
PET microdosing, can be performed, which can avoid some uncertainties that arise
with respect to tissue pharmacokinetics from animal models and is hoped to reduce
the need for studies on animals in the future.

11.2 GENERAL PRINCIPLES OF PET

Multiple steps are involved in the PET process, which starts with the selection
of a suitable biological tracer, which is then labeled with a positron-emitting radioisotope, administered to an organism, and imaged *in vivo* in a quantitative way to
reveal its distribution. The biological tracer can theoretically be any molecule or
chemical compound that can be marked with a radionuclide. PET employs radionu-
clides of biologically important elements, such as ^{11}C, ^{13}N, ^{15}O and ^{18}F, which decay
by pure positron emission (Section 2.3.3) and are building stones in nearly every
molecule in living organisms.

Positron emitters are artificially produced, unstable, proton-rich or neutron-
deficient isotopes that achieve stability through emission of a positive electron. After
emission the positron collides with orbital electrons in the surrounding tissue and
thereby loses energy until it annihilates with an electron that is within 1 to 2 mm
of the labeled atom. The annihilation of a positron with an electron produces two
γ-rays, also called annihilation photons. These photons, each 511 KeV of energy,
leave in opposite directions with a relative angle of 180° and are simultaneously
detected by the PET camera, as shown in Figure 11.1.

PET scanners consist of a large number of scintillation detectors comprised of
inorganic crystals such as bismuth germanate (BGO; Section 8.3.7) placed on a ring
that encircles the patient. Four of these rings can be added to get an axial field of
view of approximately 15 cm.

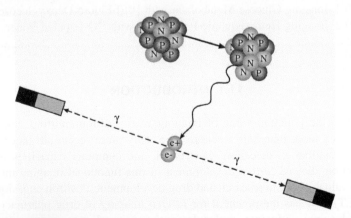

Figure 11.1   Schematic representation of positron emission and annihilation. The unstable
proton-rich nucleus emits a positron, which loses energy and eventually annihilates with an electron. Two back-to-back 511-KeV photons are produced that are
detected by the PET scanner.

The γ-ray photons arrive at the ring-shaped array of photoelectric crystals, where they are registered in coincidence, which is defined by two photons that are detected within a narrow time window of usually about 4 nsec (see Section 6.3). Coincidence lines — also referred to as lines of response (LORs) — provide a unique detection scheme for forming tomographic images with PET. Photon energy absorbed by the scintillation detector is reemitted as visible light and detected by photomultiplier tubes (PMTs; see Section 6.3). With the help of tomographic reconstruction algo rithms, the site of annihilation in the body can be determined (Figure 11.2)

11.3 SPATIAL RESOLUTION AND DETECTORS

Three main factors dictate the spatial resolution that can be achieved with positron emission tomography: the positron range, annihilation noncollinearity and detector size and efficiency.[1] Since the aim is to map the distribution of the positron-emitting radiotracer and not the distribution of the annihilation, the distance the positron travels prior to annihilation imposes a fundamental physical limitation of about 2 mm. A further limiting factor is called noncollinearity, which means that some positrons will not have lost all their energy during their journey through tissue and annihilate while in motion. To conserve this energy, the annihilation photons are emitted in less than a 180° angle. The scanner, though, will assume that these two photons were collinear and calculate a straight line to find the point of emission. The further the scintillation detectors are apart, the greater will be the contribution of noncollinearity to the limitation in spatial resolution, which is typically about 1.5 to 2.0 mm for whole-body scanners and only about 0.2 to 0.6 mm in small animal PET scanners.

Bismuth germanate (BGO) scintillation detectors for PET were first introduced in the late 1970s, because of their greater stopping power for 511-KeV photons compared to the thallium-activated sodium iodine crystals used in standard nuclear medicine gamma cameras.[2] For a PET scanner it is desirable to maximize the number of photons that deposit their energy in the detector, which depends on the stopping power of the crystal and will increase the sensitivity of the scanner.[3] Another important factor is the decay time of the deposited energy: a short decay time is desirable, as it reduces the recovery time of the crystal, which allows shortening of

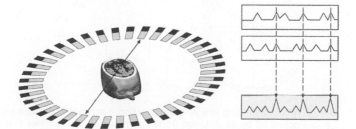

Figure 11.2   Schematic representation of coincidence detection. Opposing photoelectric crystals detect back-to-back γ-ray photons. Signals outside a narrow time window and defined energy level are rejected.

the coincidence time window while maintaining high count rates, leading to a better resolution. The recent introduction of new, faster scintillators with more light output, like lutetium oxyorthosilicate (LSO) and gadolinium oxyorthosilicate (GSO), have greatly improved the performance of PET scanners for clinical imaging and research.

11.4 DATA GATHERING AND INTERPRETATION

As the data acquisition in PET is based on coincidence event detection, it is substantially different from other nuclear medicine imaging modalities and single-photon emission computed tomography (SPECT) (Chapter 12).[4] Each coincidence detection is characterized by a line of response (LOR) that connects the two detectors involved in the detection. Each LOR can be characterized by the shortest distance between the LOR and the center of the gantry and by its angle of orientation, as shown in Figure 11.3. This information is plotted into a graph, also referred to as a sinogram.

PET data are acquired directly into sinograms, each detector pair corresponding to a particular point, or pixel. The value in each pixel represents the number of coincidence detections along the corresponding line of response, which consequently represents the amount of annihilations and hence radioactivity in that area. A separate sinogram is acquired for each slice at different angles and generated into images of tracer activity distribution. This map of activity is commonly related to corresponding anatomical areas with the help of magnetic resonance imaging (MRI) or computerized tomography (CT) imaging, as PET provides very limited anatomical information.

Image analysis refers to the process of extracting useful information on tissue function, like regional glucose metabolism or blood flow from PET images of radioactivity distribution. On the computer display, each pixel is assigned a display color according to the radioactivity, expressed as units of counts/time/pixel or volume of tissue. For a detailed analysis of a certain organ or tissue area, the corresponding region is outlined on the computer. The computer then calculates the mean value of the pixels in this region of interest (ROI). For biochemical and functional processes,

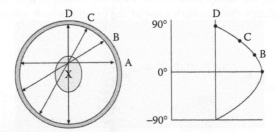

Figure 11.3 Sinogram formation and image reconstruction. Each line of response (LOR) can be characterized by its distance from the gantry of the scanner and its angle. This information is plotted into sinograms, which build the basis of image reconstruction.

the tracer uptake over time is of fundamental interest. In this so-called kinetic imaging analysis, the mean radioactivity value in a region of interest at several time points after the tracer administration is evaluated with a sequence of PET images. From these measurements time–activity curves are generated (Figure 11.4) and physiological and mathematical models are applied to quantify, for example, receptor density or blood flow.

11.5 ISOTOPE GENERATION USING A CYCLOTRON

Many chemical elements have several isotopes, which have the same number of protons in their atoms, but different numbers of neutrons (Section 2.1). In a neutral or stable state, the number of external electrons equals the sum of the protons and neutrons in the center. Radioisotopes are naturally occurring or artificially produced unstable elements with an imbalanced amount of neutrons and protons in their nucleus and surrounding electrons.

Because of their long half-lives, none of the naturally occurring radioisotopes are suitable for nuclear medicine. Short-lived proton-rich isotopes for PET research facilities are manufactured on-site with a cyclotron, a machine used for accelerating charged particles to high speeds. All cyclotrons are essentially made of the following components: an ion source and injection system, a vacuum chamber, an electromagnetic field, and the target material (Figure 11.5).

The ions used for acceleration are obtained from hydrogen gas, which is saturated with electrons producing a large number of H⁻ ions. These are injected into the vacuum chamber, forming an ion beam. Accelerated by a powerful electromagnetic field, the ions spiral along a circular orbit, thus gaining very high levels of energy. The electrons are finally stripped of the ions by passing the beam through a carbon foil, which leaves protons (H⁺). These protons are bombarded at the target material containing, for example, oxygen or nitrogen, depending on the isotope that is required. During the production of radioisotopes, which takes approximately 90 min, the cyclotron produces heat and radiation. The radiation is contained in the cyclotron

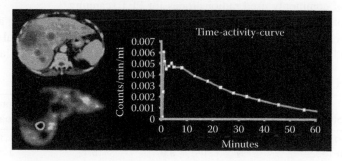

Figure 11.4 **(See color insert following page 178.)** A liver metastasis is outlined as the region of interest (ROI) on the computer-reconstructed image of tracer distribution. The average activity in the area at several time points after injection of the tracer is plotted in a time–activity curve.

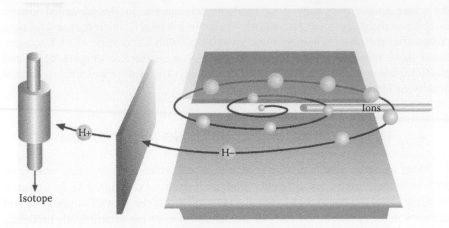

Figure 11.5 Schematic representation of isotope generation in a cyclotron. Injected H– ions are accelerated to high speed by magnetic fields. Passage through carbon foil leaves accelerated protons, which are fired at the target material to produce the required isotope.

enclosure, made of up to 2-m-thick concrete. A combination of cooling gases and chilled water is used to cool the target assembly.

11.6 CHOICE OF RADIOISOTOPES

The choice of isotopes requires careful thought, and several factors need to be considered when selecting an isotope for a particular investigation or study, including the radiation exposure, the half-life of the isotope, the chemical structure of the molecule to be labeled, the average distance a positron travels before annihilation (positron range), and, last but not least, the research question to be answered. Due to their short half-lives, most positron-emitting isotopes have to be produced on-site with a dedicated cyclotron, apart from [^{18}F]-fluorine, which can be manufactured off-site and delivered to the scanning facility. Table 11.1 gives an overview of the half-lives of commonly used radioisotopes for PET scanning.

Some of the factors that need to be taken into account when choosing an isotope can be demonstrated on the example of myocardial perfusion studies. Several radiotracers can and have been used, namely, [^{82}Rb]-rubidium, [^{13}N]-ammonia, and [^{15}O]-

Table 11.1 Properties of Some Positron-Emitting Isotopes

Isotope	Symbol	$t_{1/2}$ (min)	Range in Water (mm)	
			Max.	Mean
Carbon-11	^{11}C	20.4	4.1	1.1
Nitrogen-13	^{13}N	9.9	5.1	1.5
Oxygen-15	^{15}O	2.0	7.3	2.5
Fluorine-18	^{18}F	109.8	2.4	0.6
Rubidium-82	^{82}Rb	1.25	14.1	5.9

labeled water. Tracers such as ^{82}Rb or ^{13}N are retained in myocardium in proportion to the myocardial blood flow. The short half-life of [^{82}Rb]-rubidium of only 75 sec makes it generally suitable for repeated perfusion studies of the myocardium at rest and under pharmacologically induced stress conditions; however, in order to achieve adequate count statistics, relatively high doses need to be administered, in the region of 1480 MBq. Another disadvantage is the rather long positron range, which leads to degradation of the image quality. [^{13}N]-nitrogen has a positron range of only 1.5 mm, which leads to a comparatively better image resolution. The half-life of 9.9 min allows for a longer image acquisition time, which leads to higher count density, and hence a lower dose of radioactivity can be administered (about 550 MBq). However, the longer half-life also means that a longer time period of about 40 min is required to allow for the decay of radioactivity between resting and stress-induced flow studies. [^{13}N]-labeled ammonia as a tracer also has the disadvantage that it is partially metabolically trapped in tissue, so that its uptake may be influenced by factors other than myocardial blood flow.[5] [^{15}O]-labeled water was first used for cerebral blood flow studies, but has also been used and compared to [^{13}N]-ammonia as a tracer for myocardial blood flow. The shorter half-life of about 2 min and the relatively short positron range make [^{15}O]-oxygen almost an ideal isotope for repeated flow studies; however, the labeled water also distributes throughout the blood pool and adjacent anatomical structures. In the case of myocardial perfusion studies, the contamination from the blood pool needs to be corrected for, requiring additional scanning with inhaled [^{15}O]-carbon monoxide, which labels the red blood cells.

For pharmacokinetic studies the radionuclide must be an isotope of an element that is already present in the compound; otherwise, the radiolabeled derivate may behave very different from the parent compound, and no useful information can be derived from its biodistribution. Almost every compound contains carbon, and ^{11}C has the most potential in drug development with positron emission tomography.[6,7] The relatively short half-life of [^{11}C]-carbon of about 20 min limits its use to intravenously administered or inhaled drugs. Another disadvantage may occur if the drug to be studied has a long half-life compared to the short physical half-life of [^{11}C]-carbon,[8] in which case PET studies would reveal only a snapshot of the initial distribution rather than the full tissue kinetics. [^{18}F]-fluorine can be used if the substance has a fluoride atom and its longer half-life makes it the isotope of choice for investigating orally administered drugs, although the dose of radiation to the stomach wall needs to be considered. ^{18}F has, for example, been used in the pharmacokinetic evaluation of orally administered fluoroquinolone antibiotics.[9]

11.7 LABELED LIGAND AND DRUG SYNTHESIS

Labeling drugs or ligands to be researched with positron-emitting isotopes generally involves replacement of a carbon, nitrogen, oxygen, or fluoride atom of the native compound with ^{11}C, ^{13}N, ^{15}O, or ^{18}F, which means that the radiolabeled compound is chemically, biochemically, and pharmacologically identical. The ability to use these biologically common elements with their variety of half-lives is an important advantage of pharmacokinetic and pharmacodynamic studies with PET, but also imposes high demands on the synthesis of the labeled drug, and great expertise in radiochemistry is required. To maintain a high radioactive yield, expressed in units of radioactivity per chemical quantity, only about two to three half-lives are available to prepare the radiopharmaceutical for administration, which involves several complex production procedures and a number of quality control tests to ensure that injection into a patient is safe.

Steps generally involved are generation of the radionuclide in the cyclotron, followed by a series of chemical reactions that lead to the incorporation of the isotope into the biological compound, purification, and composition into a suitable formula for administration to the patient. Introducing the radionuclide as late as possible in the synthetic sequence and minimizing the synthesis time will increase the yield and the specific radioactivity.[10] Consideration needs to be given to the positioning of the labeled atom in the molecule, as this will be affected by the metabolism of the compound, and hence the information that can be derived from the PET imaging study. To minimize radioactivity exposure to the radiochemist, these steps need to be automated and performed in robotically controlled hot cells as far as possible.

11.8 PET APPLICATION: PHARMACOKINETIC STUDIES

11.8.1 Bioavailability and Kinetics

The aim of pharmacokinetic studies is to evaluate the time-dependent biodistribution of a pharmacological compound and to determine the optimum dose for further studies in humans accordingly. Presently this requires animal experiments, although due to the complexity of biological systems, the extrapolation of the results to the human body can be problematic. Owing to the high sensitivity of PET, which is about 10-fold greater than that of conventional SPECT, pharmacokinetic studies with very low doses of the labeled agents in the order of 1/1000 of the suggested phase I dose can be used. At these dose levels new compounds are unlikely to be toxic, and hence early evaluation of the biodistribution in humans can be performed.[11] After administration of the labeled compound the distribution of the radioactivity in different organs and tissues can be measured quantitatively. To determine the concentration of the drug in the vascular space, arterial blood sampling with measurement of the radioactivity in the probes is normally required, although occasionally these data have been derived from measurements of large vessels or the blood pool in the heart. Time–activity curves from regions of interest over various organs and tissues are then derived from the dynamic data acquisition and corrected for the regional blood flow. Through kinetic models, information on the distribution, metabolism and the blood–brain barrier penetration can be obtained. Pharmacokinetic studies of various classes of drugs, such as antibiotics, antineoplastics, and psychotropic drugs, have been performed over the last decade using PET technology. These include well-established drugs like the chemotherapeutic agent 5-fluorouracil,[12] various fluoroqinolone antibiotics and erythromycin,[13] as well as pharmacological compounds under development in animals or prephase I clinical trials in humans (Section 1.1).[11,14] Present limitations of pharmacokinetic evaluation with PET are the inability to distinguish the radiolabeled parent compound from its metabolites, which may be overcome by varying the labeling position in the molecule.

An example is the pharmacokinetic evaluation of a new compound with promising antitumor activity in a prephase I study in humans.[11] Carbon-11 radiolabeled DACA (N-[2-(dimethylamino)ethyl]acridine-4-carboxamide) was injected at a tracer amount of 1/1000 of the phase I starting dose in 24 patients with advanced cancer. Dynamic PET scanning of radioactivity in arterial blood and tissue was performed over 60 min. Biodistribution data for [11C]-DACA were acquired in discrete time frames ranging from 30 sec to 10 min and reconstructed into tomographic images, as shown in Figure 11.6. Regions of interest on tumor, liver, kidney, spleen, lung, myocardium,

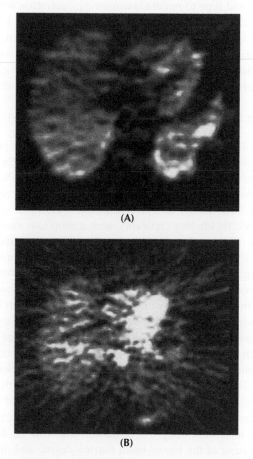

(A)

(B)

Figure 11.6 **(See color insert following page 178.)** Transverse PET images of the chest after injection of (A) 15O-labeled water and (B) 11C-labeled DACA. (A) Increased signal intensity is seen in the blood pool of the heart and in the right lung. The tumor is poorly perfused and cannot be seen. (B) Increased uptake of 11C-DACA is seen in the myocardium (upper-right-hand corner) and in the tumor (mesothelioma, lower-right-hand corner).

brain, and vertebral body were defined manually, and the radioactivity per unit volume over time for each region of interest was registered as time–activity curves (TACS).

From the TACs, C_{max} and t_{max} (see Chapter 3, Appendix 3) were calculated. The retention of radiotracer, which could be attached to either the parent drug or a metabolite, was also evaluated at 60 min. To obtain information of the plasma metabolites, discrete blood samples were taken at certain time points after the injection and analyzed by high-performance liquid chromatography (HPLC). The study could demonstrate that [^{11}C]-DACA underwent rapid and extensive metabolism with seven radioactive metabolites. The time to reach maximal tissue concentrations was short in lung, kidney, brain, spleen, and myocardium and longer in the liver. Tumor uptake and time to reach maximum concentration were highly variable in contrast to normal tissue. The maximum concentration was lowest in brain and vertebral body and highest in the liver, spleen and myocardium. From this data it was thought that neurotoxicity and bone marrow suppression were unlikely to be dose-limiting toxicities, but the high concentration in the myocardium alerted to possible cardiotoxicity, which subsequently occurred in the following phase I study.[15]

11.8.2 Receptor Ligand Imaging

The advantage of a nuclear imaging modality like PET is the potential for *in vivo* visualization and quantification of receptors at various sites in the body. The ligand is defined as a molecule that, due to its structure, is specific for the target of interest, e.g., a certain receptor on the cell surface. The ideal ligand for receptor imaging with radiotracers should have access across endothelial barriers, a high affinity to the receptor, low nonspecific binding capability, and appropriate metabolism and clearance characteristics. Known or newly developed receptor agonists or antagonists or, more recently, specific molecular antibody fragments can be employed.

The dopaminergic system of the brain has been most extensively studied, and the dopamine D_2-receptor was the first evaluated by PET in humans.[16,17] Dopamine is a key neurotransmitter, and involvement of its receptor system in numerous brain disorders like schizophrenia, Parkinson's disease, and other movement disorders has prompted intense research in this field. A classical example of quantitative receptor ligand imaging with positron emission tomography is the measurement of cerebral D_2-receptor occupancy with [^{11}C]-raclopride,[16] which was developed more than 20 years ago. Raclopride is a ligand with moderate affinity and high selectivity for the D_2 receptor. Imaging with [^{11}C]-raclopride for the assessment of new antipsychotic drugs uses an indirect approach, measuring receptor occupancy before and after treatment with the unlabeled drug.[18] Information that can be derived from these studies includes passage of the blood–brain barrier, degree and duration of receptor occupancy for a given dose, or the effect of other drugs on the receptor. PET studies also have established that there is a threshhold occupancy of the dopamine receptor at which extrapyramidal side effects occur. Another important neurotransmitter implicated in a number of psychiatric disorders, like anxiety and depression, is the serotonergic system, and several PET ligands for various serotonin receptors have been developed.[19,20] Figure 11.7 shows the distribution of the serotonin 5-HT1A-receptor in the human brain. Suitable radiotracer ligands for other important neu-

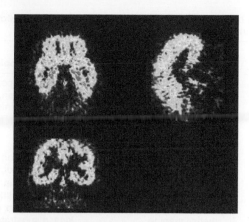

Figure 11.7 **(See color insert following page 178.)** PET image of the serotonin 5-HT1A-receptor in the human brain with the radioligand [^{11}C]-WAY-100635. (Image courtesy of Prof. C. Halldin and Prof L. Farde, Karolinska Institute, Stockholm.)

rotransmission systems, like the glutamate receptors, have yet to be found, and research in the area is ongoing.

Outside the central nervous system receptor expression on malignant tissue has been of major interest. Quantitative *in vivo* imaging of tumor receptors appears to be a very attractive tool for prediction of the response to receptor-targeted therapy. More than 15 years ago several steroid receptor ligands were developed for quantification of estrogen and progesterone receptor expression in breast cancer, and excellent correlation between uptake of the labeled estrogen on the PET images and tumor estrogen receptor concentration measured *in vitro* after excision of the tumors could be demonstrated.[21,22] A later study with [^{18}F]-labeled tamoxifen — an estrogen receptor antagonist used in the treatment of breast cancer — confirmed that PET receptor studies are also feasible to monitor treatment response.[23]

Increasing understanding of molecular biology led to the discovery of many more receptors involved in the development and sustained growth of tumor cells, and some targeted therapies, mainly in the form of monoclonal antibodies, have already entered mainstream medicine. Although a receptor-specific radiolabeled monoclonal antibody appears to be an ideal ligand, the use of intact antibodies has been hampered by their large molecular size, which causes a slow diffusion from vasculature into the tumor and prolonged clearance.[24,25] The slow kinetics of radiolabeled antibodies thus results in low radiolocalization and high systemic background levels of tracer activity. Enzymatically digested or genetically engineered low-molecular-weight antigen binding fragments, so-called diabodies or minibodies, are now developed to improve pharmacokinetic properties while maintaining high binding specificity. Evidence that engineered antibody fragments can serve as excellent PET imaging tools has been provided by a study by Sundaresan et al.[26] Carcino-embryonic antigen (CEA) is commonly expressed on colon carcinoma cells, and imaging with an ^{124}I-labeled anti-CEA minibody has been evaluated in tumor xenograft-bearing mice. The results demonstrated much improved image contrast due to better target-to-background radioactivity with excellent visualization of the tumor at 18 h after

Table 11.2 Examples of Pharmacodynamic Endpoints Studied, Radiotracers Used, and Applications in Drug Development

Pharmacodynamic Process	Radiotracer	Applications
Glucose metabolism	[^{18}F]fluorodeoxyglucose	Glucose transport and hexokinase activity in brain, myocardium, tumors, and infection
Protein synthesis	[^{11}C]methionine [^{11}C]leucine [^{18}F]fluoroethyl-L-tyrosine	Rate of protein synthesis in tumors; tumor viability
Cell proliferation	[^{11}C]thymidine [^{18}F]fluorothymidine	Cell proliferation rate in response to treatment in oncology
Oxygen consumption	[^{18}F]fluoromisonidazole	Tumor hypoxia for assessment of radiation sensitizers in oncology
Gene expression	[^{18}F]fluoro-3-hydroxy-methylguanine [^{18}F]gancyclovir	Herpes simplex virus 1–thymidine kinase substrates for imaging gene expression
Blood flow	[^{15}O]H$_2$O [^{13}N]ammonia	Regional cerebral blood flow; perfusion of myocardium, tumors, and normal tissues
Blood volume	[^{15}O]carbon monoxide	Blood pool in myocardial perfusion studies; cerebral blood volume in cerebrovascular disease
Apoptosis	[^{124}I]Annexin-V	Cell death in response to treatment in oncology
Enzyme activity	[^{11}C]choline [^{18}F]fluoro-thymidine	Choline kinase activity; thymidine kinase 1 activity
Multidrug resistance	[^{11}C]daunorubicin [^{11}C]verapamil	P-glycoprotein substrated to assess multidrug resistance phenotype in brain and tumors

administration. Research exploring the properties of radiolabeled engineered receptor–antibody fragments for PET imaging is now advancing fast, particularly in the field of oncology.[27,28]

11.9 PHARMACODYNAMIC STUDIES

Positron emission tomography has the potential to evaluate the effect of a drug *in vivo* in animal studies or the human body by measuring metabolic or hemodynamic responses in the tissue in question. Physiological functions like the glycolysis rate, protein synthesis, enzyme activity, tissue perfusion, oxygen consumption, or even gene expression can be quantified and used to construct dose–response evaluation, which may considerably reduce the cost of drug development in the future. Table 11.2 gives an overview of pharmacodynamic endpoints evaluated by PET and the radiotracers used.

11.9.1 Imaging Glucose Metabolism with [^{18}F]-Fluoro-Deoxyglucose

The most commonly used and first clinically approved radiotracer is [^{18}F]-fluoro-deoxyglucose. [^{18}F]-labeled 2-fluoro-deoxyglucose (FDG) is used in neurology, cardiology, and oncology to study glucose metabolism. FDG follows the same route as glucose into cells, where it is phosphorylated by hexokinase to FDG-6-phosphate. Unlike glucose, though, little further metabolism is possible and FDG-6-phosphate is trapped within cells, accumulating proportional to the rate of glucose utilization.[29] In neurology and psychiatry [^{18}F]-FDG is employed to image altered energy demands in the brain, and in cardiology to determine myocardial glucose metabolism, but has found its main application in oncology, where it has entered mainstream medicine and clinical trials. Increased glycolysis is among the key metabolic alterations marking the transformation from normal to malignant cells in most tumor types, and [^{18}F]-FDG-PET is now widely used to determine the grade and extent of tumors, as a prognostic indicator, and as a measure of tumor response to treatment.

[^{18}F]-FDG-PET's ability to assess response to anticancer therapy has been evaluated in pilot or phase I/II studies with both conventional chemotherapy agents and novel molecular targeted drugs.[7] Evidence of early tumor response may be particularly beneficial in the development of novel agents not amenable to traditional endpoint assessments, like maximum tolerated dose or structural tumor changes on anatomical imaging, because of their at least initially cytostatic, rather than cytotoxic, effect.

An example is the pharmacodynamic evaluation of the novel c-kit* signal transduction inhibitor imatinib with [^{18}F]-FDG-PET imaging in patients with gastrointestinal stromal tumors in several phase I/II studies.[30] PET revealed treatment responses as early as 24 h after initiation of therapy. Decrease of [^{18}F]-FDG uptake of 50% or more at day 8 of treatment, compared to a baseline scan, correctly predicted response in 89% of patients. On anatomic scans like CT and MRI these responses were not evident until weeks 4 to 16 of treatment.

To enable much needed comparison of smaller clinical studies and large multi-center trials, the European Organization for Research and Treatment of Cancer (EORTC) PET group has published guidelines for response assessment using [^{18}F]-FDG-PET imaging.[31]

Imaging of metabolic processes using [^{18}F]-FDG unfortunately has several imitations, including a high background uptake in normal brain tissue and increased uptake in inflammatory tissues.[7] Immune reactions induced by tumor tissue death may elevate the overall posttreatment [^{18}F]-FDG signal due to invasion by inflammatory cells. Furthermore, stressed tumor cells show an enhanced glucose transport prior to cell death, and this effect may vary according to tumor type and treatment from several days to even months, necessitating the development of alternative radiotracers. Progress has been made with [^{11}C]-labeled amino acids like leucine, tyrosine, and methionine, which have been evaluated as markers for protein synthesis in various tissues. Increased activity has been shown in proliferating tumors and abscesses. Changes in the rate of protein synthesis can hence serve as surrogate endpoints for the effectiveness of antibiotics or cytotoxic treatments.

---

* Stem cell factor and its receptor c-kit constitute an important signal transduction system regulating cell growth and differentiation in hematopoiesis, gametogenesis, and melanogenesis.

11.9.2   Imaging Hemodynamic Parameters with ^{15}O-Labeled Water

PET techniques for the quantitative evaluation of vascular parameters using intravenous [^{15}O]-labeled water were originally developed *for in vivo* studies of the brain.[32] Changes in neuronal brain activity are accompanied by an increase in glucose and oxygen demand, reflected by focal changes in regional cerebral blood flow (rCBF) and blood volume. The most common research applications for rCBF imaging have been functional brain mapping studies.[33]

The low dose of radiation exposure and the short half-life of ^{15}O allow repeated scanning of the same subject before and after performing different neuropsychological tasks, which gives vascular studies with [^{15}O]-labeled water preference over the metabolic evaluation of neural activity with [^{18}F]-fluoro-deoxyglucose. Pharmacodynamic studies have, for example, investigated changes in blood flow in the human brain during anesthesia and in response to opioid analgesia. Brain regions closely linked to pain-related responses demonstrated changes in blood flow during analgesia with fentanyl, a morphine derivative.[34] A strong correlation between the level of consciousness and reduced blood flow, indicating a decrease in neuronal activity in certain areas of the brain like the thalamus, basal forebrain, and occipitoparietal region, was found in response to the anesthetic drugs midazolam[35] and propofol,[36] and a dose-dependent impairment of the processing of tactile stimuli could be demonstrated.

In the field of cardiology, quantitative blood flow measurements with PET have been used for the evaluation of myocardial perfusion at rest and under pharmacologically induced stress conditions. The effects of cardiac drugs like α- and β-adrenoceptor blockers,[37,38] calcium channel blockers,[39] and inotropic sympathomimetics[40] on myocardial blood flow and flow reserve in healthy individuals and patients with heart disease have been assessed. Quantitative measurements of myocardial perfusion can also be used to examine possible side effects of drugs on the human coronary circulation, as in the example of a new selective 5-hydroxytriptamine receptor agonist for the treatment of migraine headaches. This study was particularly important, as serotonin analogs like ergotamine have been shown to constrict coronary blood vessels. The effect on myocardial blood flow of subcutaneous naratriptan was assessed under resting and hyperemic conditions with [^{15}O]-labeled water PET studies in a randomized, double-blind, placebo-controlled crossover trial in 34 known migraine sufferers with no evidence of ischemic heart disease.[41] The study demonstrated no difference between drug and placebo on resting myocardial flow, but a significant fall in blood flow and increase in coronary resistance with naratriptan under pharmacological stress conditions.

More recently, applications for hemodynamic studies with PET are evolving in oncology drug development. It has long been recognized that the growth of tumors beyond 2 mm depends on new blood vessel formation supplying the tumor with oxygen and nutrients.[42] Several drugs inhibiting angiogenic factors or receptors and targeting the tumor vasculature are in preclinical development and clinical trials.[43,44] Changes in tumor and normal tissue perfusion *in vivo* can be evaluated with PET methodology demonstrating biological activity in humans,[45] although the pharmacodynamic effects have not yet been validated to predict antitumor activity.

REFERENCES

1. Townsend, D., Physical principles and technology of clinical PET imaging, *Ann. Acad. Med.*, 33, 133, 2004.
2. Cho, Z. and Farukhi, M., Bismuth germanate as a potential scintillation detector in positron cameras, *J. Nucl. Med.*, 18, 840, 1977.
3. Bailey, D., Karp, S., and Surti, S., Physics and instrumentation in PET, pp 41–67, in *Positron Emission Tomography: Basic Science and Clinical Practice*, Valk, P., Bailey, D., Townsend, D., and Maisey, M., Eds., Springer-Verlag, London, 2003.
4. Fahey, F., Data acquisition in PET imaging, *J. Nucl. Med. Technol.*, 30, 39, 2002.
5. Huang, S., Schwaiger, M., Carson, R., et al., Quantitative measurement of myocardial blood flow with oxygen-15-water and positron computed tomography: an assessment of potential and problems, *J. Nucl. Med.*, 26, 616, 1985.
6. Fowler, J., Volkow, N., Wang, G., et al., PET and drug research and development, *J. Nucl. Med.*, 40, 1154, 1999.
7. Hammond, L., Denis, L., Salman, U., et al., Positron emission tomography (PET): expanding the horizons of oncology drug development, *Invest. New Drugs*, 21, 309, 2003.
8. Gupta, N., Price, P., and Aboague, E., PET for *in vivo* pharmacokinetic and pharmacodynamic measurements, *Eur. J. Cancer*, 38, 2094, 2002.
9. Tewson, T., Yang, D., Wong, G., et al., The synthesis of fluorine-18-levomefloxacin and its preliminary use in human studies, *Nucl. Med. Biol.*, 23, 767, 1996.
10. Antoni, G. and Långström, B., Progress in ^{11}C radiochemistry, pp 237–250, in *Positron Emission Tomography: Basic Science and Clinical Practice*, Valk, P., Bailey, D., Townsend, D., and Maisey, M., Eds., Springer-Verlag, London, 2003, chap.10.
11. Saleem, A., Harte, R., Matthews, J., et al., Pharmacokinetic evaluation of N-[2-(dimethylamino)ethyl]acridine-4-carboxamide in patients by positron emission tomography, *J. Clin. Oncol.*, 19, 1421, 2001.
12. Kissel, J., Brix, G., Bellemann, M., et al., Pharmacokinetic analysis of 5-[^{18}F]fluorouracil tissue concentrations measured with positron emission tomography in patients with liver metastases from colorectal adenocarcinoma, *Cancer Res.*, 57, 3415, 1997.
13. Tewson, T., Labeled antibiotics: positron tomography as a tool for measuring tissue distribution, *Drug Dev. Res.*, 59, 261, 2003.
14. Christian, B., Livni, E., Babich, J., et al., Evaluation of cerebral pharmacokinetics of the novel antidepressant drug, BMS-181101, by positron emission tomography, *J. Pharmacol. Exp. Ther.*, 279, 325, 1996.
15. Twelves, C., Campae, M., Coudert, B., et al., Phase II study of XR5000 (DACA) administered as a 120-h infusion in patients with recurrent glioblastoma, *Ann. Oncol.*, 13, 777, 2002.
16. Farde, L., Hall, H., Ehrin, E., et al., Quantitative analysis of D2-dopamine receptor binding in the living human brain by positron emission tomography, *Science*, 231, 258, 1986.
17. Wagner, H., Burns, H., Dannals, R., et al., Imaging DA receptors in the human brain by PET, *Science*, 221, 1264, 1983.
18. Farde, L., The advantage of using positron emission tomography in drug research, *Trends Neurosci.*, 19, 211, 1996.
19. Lemaire, C., Cantineau, R., Guillaume, M., et al., Fluorine-18-altanserin: a radioligand for the study of serotonin receptors with PET: radiolabeling and *in vivo* behaviour in rats, *J. Nucl. Med.*, 32, 2266, 1991.

20. Shine, C., Shine, G., Mozley, P., et al., ^{18}F-MPPF: a potential radioligand for PET studies of 5-HT$_{1A}$ receptors in humans, *Synapse*, 25, 147, 1997.

21. Dehdashti, F., McGuire, A., van Brocklin, H., et al., Assessment of 21-[^{18}F]Fluoro-16-alpha-ethyl-19-norprogesterone as a positron-emitting radiopharmaceutical for the detection of progestin receptors in human breast carcinoma, *J. Nucl. Med.*, 32, 1532, 1991.

22. Mintun, M., Welch, M., Siegel, B., et al., Breast cancer: PET imaging of oestrogen receptors, *Radiology*, 169, 45, 1988.

23. Inoue, T., Kim, E., Wallace, S., et al., Positron emission tomography using [^{18}F]fluorotamoxifen to evaluate therapeutic response in patients with breast cancer; preliminary study, *Cancer Biother. Radiopharm.*, 11, 235, 1996.

24. Jain, M. and Batra, S., Genetically engineered antibody fragments and PET imaging: a new era of radioimmunotherapy, *J. Nucl. Med.*, 44, 1970, 2003.

25. Jayson, G., Zweit, J., Jackson, A., et al., Molecular imaging and biological evaluation of HuMV833 anti-VEGF antibody: implications for trial design of antiangiogenic antibodies, *J. Natl. Cancer Inst.*, 94, 1484, 2002.

26. Sundaresan, G., Yazaki, P., Shively, J., et al., [124]I-labeled engineered anti-CEA minibodies and diabodies allow high-contrast, antigen-specific small-animal PET imaging of xenografts in athymic mice, *J. Nucl. Med.*, 44, 1962, 2003.

27. Kenanova, V., Olafsen, T., Crow, D., et al., Tailoring the pharmacokinetics and positron emission tomography imaging properties of anti-carcinoembryonic antigen single-chain Fv-Fc antibody fragments, *Cancer Res.*, 65, 622, 2005.

28. Robinson, M., Doss, M., Shaller, C., et al., Quantitiative immuno-positron emission tomography imaging of HER2-positive tumor xenografts with an iodine-124 labeled anti-HER2 diabody, *Cancer Res.*, 65, 1471, 2005.

29. Price, P., Saleem, A., and Aboague, E., PET in development and use of anticancer drugs, 829–841, in *Positron Emission Tomography: Basic Science and Clinical Practice*, Valk, P., Bailey, D., Townsend, D., and Maisey, M., Eds., Springer-Verlag Limited, London, 2003.

30. Van den Abbeele, A. and Badawi, R., Use of positron emission tomography in oncology and its potential role to assess response to imatinib mesylate therapy in gastrointestinal stromal tumors (GISTs), *Eur. J. Cancer*, 38 (Suppl. 5), S60, 2002.

31. Young, H., Baum, R., Cremerius, U., et al., Measurement of clinical and subclinical tumour response using [^{18}F]-fluorodeoxyglucose and positron emission tomography: review and 1999 EORTC recommendations, *Eur. J. Cancer*, 35, 1773, 1999.

32. Herscovitch, P., Markham, J., and Reichle, M., Brain blood flow measured with intavenous H$_2$[15]O. I. Theory and error analysis, *J. Nucl. Med.*, 24, 782, 1983.

33. Herscovitch, P., Cerebral physiologic measurements with PET, 283–307, in *Positron Emission Tomography: Basic Science and Clinical Practice*, Valk, P., Bailey, D., Townsend, D., and Maisey, M., Eds. Springer-Verlag, London, 2003.

34. Firestone, L., Gyulai, F., Mintun, M., et al., Human brain activity response to fentanyl imaged by positron emission tomography, *Anesthesiol. Analgesia*, 82, 1247, 1996.

35. Veselis, R., Reinsel, R., Feshenko, V., et al., Midazolam changes cerebral blood flow in discrete brain regions, *Anesthesiology*, 87, 1106, 1997.

36. Bonhomme, V., Fiset, P., Meuret, P., et al., Propofol anesthesia and cerebral blood flow changes elicited by vibrotactile stimulation: a positron emission tomography study, *J. Neurophysiol.*, 85, 1299, 2001.

37. Rimoldi, O., Spyron, N., Foale, R., et al., Limitations of coronary reserve after successful angioplasty is prevented by oral pretreatment with an alpha-1-adrenergic agonist, *J. Cardiovasc. Pharmacol.*, 36, 310, 2000.

38. Böttcher, M., Czernin, J., Sun, K., et al., Effect of beta-1-receptor blockade on myocardial blood flow and vasodilatory capacity, *J. Nucl. Med.*, 38, 442, 1997.

39. Neglia, D., Sambuceti, G., Giorgetti, A., et al., Effects of long-term treatment with verapamil on left ventricular function and myocardial blood flow in patients with dilated cardiomyopathy without overt heart failure, *J. Cardiovasc. Pharmacol.*, 36, 744, 2000.

40. Krivokapich, J., Czernin, J., and Schelbert, H., Dobutamine positron emission tomography: absolute quantitation of rest and dobutamine myocardial blood flow and correlation with cardiac work and percent diameter stenosis in patients with and without coronary artery disease, *J. Am. Coll. Cardiol.*, 28, 565, 1996.

41. Gnecchi-Ruscone, T., Bernard, X., Pierre, P., et al., Effect of naratriptan on myocardial blood flow and coronary vasodilator reserve in migraineurs, *Neurology*, 55, 95, 2000.

42. Folkman, J., Tumour angiogenesis: therapeutic implications, *N. Engl. J. Med.*, 285, 1182, 1971.

43. Eskens, F., Angiogenesis inhibitors in clinical development: where are we now and where are we going?, *Br. J. Cancer*, 90, 1, 2004.

44. Tozer, G., Measuring tumour vascular response to antivascular and antiangiogenic drugs, *Br. J. Radiol.*, 76 (special issue), S23, 2003.

45. Anderson, H., Yap, J., Miller, M., et al., Assessment of pharmacodynamic vascular response on a phase I trial of combretastatin-A4-phosphate, *J. Clin. Oncol.*, 21, 2823, 2003.

CHAPTER 12

Gamma Scintigraphy and SPECT

Stephen P. Newman and Gary R. Pitcairn

CONTENTS

12.1 THE DEVELOPMENT OF SCINTIGRAPHIC IMAGING

This chapter concerns the radionuclide imaging techniques of gamma scintigraphy (γ-scintigraphy) and single-photon emission computed tomography (SPECT), which are used widely to assess drug delivery by various routes. The drug formulation is radiolabeled with a γ-emitting radionuclide, which is usually ^{99m}Tc. Since the radiolabel is not generally incorporated into the structure of the drug molecule, γ-scintigraphy and SPECT do not usually enable drug absorption to be assessed, but they do allow quantification of parameters such as deposition of inhaled drug products in the lungs and the time after dosing at which orally administered products leave the stomach or begin to disintegrate.

12.1.1 Nuclear Medicine

The discovery of radioactivity took place at the end of the 19th century and has had profound effects on society, some of which have been good and some bad. One beneficial use of radioactive materials has been to provide information on the function of different organs and systems in the body — often information that could not be obtained any other way. Once nuclear reactor products became readily available after 1945, a range of diagnostic radiotracer tests was developed, and the discipline of nuclear medicine was born.[1] The majority of these tests involved γ-emitting radionuclides, the presence of which could be detected in the body by scintillation probes containing one or more photomultiplier tubes. Simple scintillation detectors only provide a γ-ray count rate, which is useful for comparing radiotracer uptake in different organs or for quantifying organ retention over time.[2] However, there was much interest in developing a scintillation device that could actually be used to image the radionuclide distribution in the body, thereby providing information not only on organ function, but also on structure. Initially, this was done using rectilinear scanners, in which a scintillation probe was moved in a series of parallel lines over the organ containing the radionuclide,[3] but in due course the γ-camera became the instrument of choice.

12.1.2 Gamma Camera Design

The γ-camera is a large radiation detector consisting of a disc-shaped crystal, usually composed of thallium-activated sodium iodide, and was invented by the American scientist Hal Anger.[4] In the earliest γ-cameras, used primarily for thyroid imaging, the disc was only 4 inches in diameter, and the light photons generated by interactions with γ-rays were viewed by an array of only seven photomultiplier tubes. The device used a pinhole collimator, and the image was displayed on an oscilloscope screen.[5] The first commercial γ-camera was introduced 40 years ago.[6]

Predictably, the sophistication of γ-cameras increased greatly during the second half of the 20th century. A modern γ-camera (Figure 12.1) has a crystal, typically around 10 mm thick and 500 mm in diameter, so that it can be used to image the larger organs of the body, such as the liver and lungs, and can cover the entire width of the patient. These instruments contain dozens of photomultiplier tubes, and there

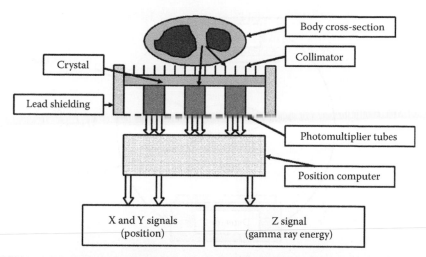

Figure 12.1 Schematic representation of a single-headed gamma camera used for gamma scintigraphy. The parallel-hole collimator only allows gamma rays moving approximately at right angles to the crystal to be detected.

is a lead collimator placed between the crystal and the organ of interest. The collimator is also disc shaped and has thousands of small circular or hexagonal holes drilled in it, usually all parallel and at right angles to the crystal surface. Gamma rays pass unrestricted through the holes in the collimator, but only pass to a very limited extent through the lead septa between the holes. This arrangement means that a signal will only be produced in the area of the crystal adjacent to the source of the γ-ray. X and Y coordinates can be assigned to the original location of the γ-ray event in the body, and hence an image can be built up of the distribution of radionuclide. The image is stored by a data processing system as counts in an array of picture elements (pixels), typically a 128 by 128 matrix. Computer-generated regions of interest may be drawn on the images, allowing the γ-counts from different organs, or parts of an organ, to be determined.

12.1.3 Gamma Cameras for SPECT

When used as described above, a γ-camera provides a two-dimensional representation of the radionuclide distribution. This is known as planar imaging. This imaging modality has proved to have great practical utility, but the data it provides are limited because the radionuclide is often distributed in a complex three-dimensional anatomical structure. Single-photon emission computed tomography (SPECT) can overcome this fundamental limitation. In SPECT imaging a γ-camera system, consisting usually of two or three detector heads, is rotated about the supine subject (Figure 12.2). The detector heads take images of the radionuclide distribution in the organ of interest from a series of different angles.[3,7] These images are stored and are then used to reconstruct the original distribution pattern by an algorithm such as filtered back-projection. Data are presented as counts in a three-dimensional array of volume picture elements (voxels).

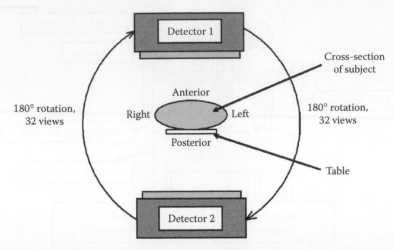

Figure 12.2 Schematic representation of a twin-headed gamma camera used for SPECT imaging. The detector-heads take a series of images from different angles during a 180° rotation, and these images are used to reconstruct the three-dimensional distribution of radionuclide in the organ being imaged. (From Pitcairn, G.R. et al., *Drug Delivery Syst. Sci.*, 3, 5, 2003. With permission.)

A typical SPECT protocol involves taking 32 pairs of images from different angles during a 180° rotation of the heads. In a double-headed camera, the heads may be placed either at an angle of 90° apart, or may be diametrically opposed. Some cameras have integral line sources of ^{153}Gd, and the γ-ray transmissions from these sources are used to make tissue attenuation corrections. SPECT requires the use of a larger quantity of radionuclide than in planar imaging, and this could place limits on the data that can be obtained, for instance, restricting the number of replicate administrations an individual subject may receive.

12.1.4 Extrapolation to Pharmaceutical Development

In the late 1970s and early 1980s, it was realized by pharmaceutical scientists that the imaging methods used in nuclear medicine could be extrapolated to provide key information about the drug delivery process by a variety of routes.[8–11] The majority of studies have involved gastrointestinal,[12] pulmonary[13] and nasal[14] drug delivery, but studies involving the ophthalmic,[15] buccal,[16] rectal,[17] vaginal[18] and parenteral[19] routes have also been undertaken. Initially, this involved two-dimensional imaging with a single-headed or double-headed camera, a procedure that has come to be known as γ-scintigraphy. More recently, nuclear medicine has embraced the three-dimensional imaging techniques of SPECT and positron emission tomography (PET; Chapter 11). PET now has a well-established role in the pharmaceutical industry for assessing receptor binding and *in vivo* pharmacokinetics.[20] This chapter will concentrate on the role of the single-photon imaging techniques of γ-scintigraphy and SPECT.

12.1.5 Choice of Radionuclide for Gamma Scintigraphy and SPECT

Not every γ-emitting radionuclide is suitable for use in drug delivery studies using γ- scintigraphy or SPECT. First and foremost, the radiation dose arising from γ-rays and any other particles emitted by the radionuclide must be acceptably low. This requirement favors radionuclides that emit relatively few beta particles during their decay process, have short physical half-lives, and do not accumulate extensively in any organ of the body. For instance, the radionuclide ^{131}I was used widely as a diagnostic agent in the 1950s and 1960s, but is now considered unsuitable, since it confers a high beta ray dose, has a half-life of 8 days, and localizes in the thyroid when in an unbound form. The shorter-lived radionuclide ^{123}I is now preferred.

Radionuclides commonly used in γ-camera studies are listed in Table 12.1. The radionuclide ^{99m}Tc is in many ways ideal as a γ-camera imaging agent, since it emits few beta rays and has a half-life of only 6 h, which reduces the exposure time, and hence the radiation dose, compared to longer-lived radionuclides. [99m]Tc has a flexible chemistry, which allows it to be labeled to a variety of compounds, thereby creating a useful range of radiopharmaceuticals. [111]In is often preferred to ^{99m}Tc for studies of gastrointestinal transit,[21] owing to its longer half-life (2.8 days). Dual-imaging studies are possible using two radionuclides with different γ-ray energies, such as ^{99m}Tc and [111]In. This makes it possible to radiolabel different components of the same formulation, e.g., the core and coating of a tablet preparation. The development of radionuclide generator systems permits the use of some radionuclides with physical half-lives of less than 1 min, such as the inert gas [81m]Kr for lung ventilation scanning. Of course, not all radionuclides can be imaged. The radionuclides ^{3}H and ^{14}C are widely used in drug metabolism studies, but are unsuitable for imaging since they do not emit any γ-rays.

The γ-ray energy of [99m]Tc (140 KeV) is very suitable for use with a γ-camera, because it allows the use of a collimator with a relatively small septal thickness, and hence can be detected efficiently. γ-Rays with energies between about 100 and 300 KeV are considered ideal for γ-camera imaging. Higher γ-ray energies require thicker septa in order to maintain image sharpness (resolution), but at the expense of reduced sensitivity. The design of the collimator varies according to the radionuclide to be used, but a general-purpose collimator would be typically 25 mm thick and would have around 20,000 parallel circular or hexagonal holes, each 2.5 mm in diameter.

Table 12.1 Radionuclides Commonly Used in Gamma Scintigraphic and SPECT Investigations of Drug Delivery

Radionuclide	Symbol	Gamma Ray Energy (KeV)	Physical Half-Life
Erbium-171	[171]Er	296,308	7.5 h
Indium-111	[111]In	173,247	2.8 d
Iodine-123	[123]I	160	13 h
Krypton-81m	[81m]Kr	191	13 sec
Samarium-153	[153]Sm	103	46.7 h
Technetium-99m	[99m]Tc	140	6 h

A radiolabeling approach that has proved very useful in studies of gastrointestinal drug delivery has involved the method of neutron activation.[22] At the time of manufacture a small amount of a rare earth oxide, usually samarium oxide in the isotopically enriched form of [152]Sm, is added to the formulation. Brief irradiation in a nuclear reactor converts [152]Sm to the γ-emitting radionuclide [153]Sm (γ-ray energy, 103 KeV; physical half-life, 47 h). The same strategy may be used to create [171]Er from erbium oxide. The advantage of this method is that the formulation can be prepared before irradiation, under normal conditions, and as a normal batch size, in the laboratories of the sponsor company.

Since SPECT involves the acquisition of multiple images, the entire SPECT procedure typically takes longer than planar imaging, and it is important that the radionuclide distribution should remain essentially static during the imaging process. This may render SPECT unsuitable for use in situations where the distribution in the body changes rapidly with time. Lung imaging with SPECT may be undertaken using radiotracers that remain in the lungs long enough to be considered essentially static during the course of the imaging process, such as ^{99m}Tc–diethyelenetriamine pentaacetic acid (DTPA) or ^{99m}Tc–technegas.[23,24] Rapid SPECT may be undertaken using short imaging times for radiotracers that are quickly absorbed via the lungs,[25] and corrections may be made to the data to allow for the effect of radiotracer absorption. It is very rare in either γ-scintigraphic or SPECT studies of drug delivery to incorporate a radiolabel into the structure of the drug molecule itself.[26] Positron-emitting radionuclides such as ^{11}C and ^{18}F have been used to directly radiolabel drug molecules, and a number of interesting studies have been carried out, notably involving pulmonary drug delivery.[27,28]

12.2 DATA GATHERING AND INTERPRETATION

12.2.1 Radiolabeling Strategies and Validation

The use of indirect radiolabeling strategies using radionuclides such as ^{99m}Tc,[111]In and [153]Sm requires that some kind of validation testing should be undertaken prior to the scintigraphic study. Often the validation program is very simple in nature. For instance, in studies of gastrointestinal drug delivery, demonstration that the *in vitro* dissolution rate of a capsule or tablet is the same for labeled and unlabeled products is generally sufficient.[29] In studies of pulmonary drug delivery involving solution formulations, it may generally be assumed that drug and radiolabel are homogeneously mixed within the formulation, so that every droplet in a spray produced from the formulation will contain drug and label in direct proportion to droplet volume.[30] Again, the amount of validation data required is minimal.

However, for pulmonary studies involving pressurized metered dose inhalers (pMDIs) and dry powder inhalers (DPIs), a much fuller program of work is needed. This normally involves particle sizing measurements undertaken to show the similarity of the size distributions of drug and radiolabel in the inhaled aerosol. It is accepted practice to quantify the size distributions of three quantities: (1) drug before labeling (in other words, the off-the-shelf product), (2) drug after labeling and (3) the radiolabel.[31,32] These data are generally obtained with either an Andersen cascade impactor or multistage liquid impinger.[33] Impaction devices are used because it is possible to wash out the stages of these instruments with a suitable solvent and to quantify the amount of drug and radiolabel associated with each size band. A series of replicate measurements are made, and the results plotted in such a way as to demonstrate the similarities or differences between the size distributions. A typical set of data is shown in Figure 12.3.

Comparison of before-labeling and after-labeling data shows that the size distribution has not been perturbed significantly by the labeling process, and comparison of drug and radiolabel data show that the radiolabel may be considered a valid marker for the drug across the full range of particle size bands. It is also helpful to quantify the mass of drug present in before-labeling and after-labeling samples, in order to ensure that the labeling process has not changed the delivered dose. In addition to validation data obtained prestudy, the actual study day inhalers should also be tested, for instance, to show that the distribution of radiolabel within different size bands lies within the range of values seen in the prestudy validation tests.[34]

12.2.2 Influence of Radiolabeling Strategy on Data Obtained

The strategy of radiolabeling the formulation rather than the drug molecule affects the type of data that it is possible to obtain from γ-camera and SPECT studies. In pulmonary studies, the validation data are used to show that the γ-camera data effectively quantify drug deposition, but once the formulation has been deposited on the airways, it is likely that drug and radiolabel will rapidly dissociate. It is therefore unlikely that sequential images will provide useful information about drug clearance or absorption. On the other hand, nonabsorbable radiotracers such as ^{153}Sm-oxide or ^{99m}Tc-DTPA in gastrointestinal studies are

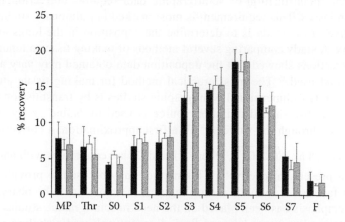

Figure 12.3 Typical radiolabeling validation data for a pulmonary product. The size distributions within an Andersen cascade impactor have been obtained for drug before labeling, drug after labeling, and radiolabel. MP, device mouthpiece; Thr, inlet "throat" to impactor; S0 to S7, impactor stages 0 to 7; F, final filter. ■, drug before labeling; □, drug after labeling; ▨, radiolabel.

suitable for tracing the passage of the formulation through the gastrointestinal tract, for determining the location of the formulation at any time, and for ascertaining when and where the formulation disintegrates.[12,35] Should information about drug absorption be required, then γ-scintigraphic or SPECT imaging can be combined with conventional pharmacokinetic assessment. This is a powerful combination, sometimes called pharmacoscintigraphy, which gives important insights into the drug delivery process.

12.2.3 Converting Gamma Camera Counts into Drug Delivery Data

Gamma scintigraphy provides powerful images that show how dosage forms behave in the body. However, γ-scintigraphy and SPECT are quantitative methods in which the radioactive count or count rate from an organ is converted into a form that enables the magnitude of drug delivery to be determined. In simple terms, the three corrections made to the data are the subtraction of background radiation, calculation of a geometric mean of anterior and posterior count rates (or right lateral and left lateral count rates), and adjustment to the count rate to allow for the effects of γ-ray attenuation and scatter that occur when γ-rays pass through overlying tissues on their way to the γ-camera.[36] Background subtraction is essential, unless the count rate from the body is so high that background is negligible in comparison. Whether the geometric mean and tissue attenuation corrections are required depends to some extent on the nature of the study and the data to be obtained. For instance, some studies involve images of an organ taken from one direction only, and a geometric mean count rate cannot be obtained. Many gastrointestinal studies involve sequential images, intended to show when the key events, such as tablet disintegration, gastric emptying, and colon arrival, occur. Correction of the data for γ-ray attenuation and scatter is not needed in order to obtain this information.

Accurate quantification of scintigraphic data requires correction for tissue attenuation losses. This requirement is most marked in pulmonary studies, where the objective of the study is to determine the deposition in the lungs and in the oropharynx. A study comparing several methods of making tissue attenuation and scatter corrections showed that the deposition data obtained may vary according to the method used.[37] The most practical method for making tissue attenuation corrections in two-dimensional scintigraphic studies is by transmission scans, in which a large disc-shaped radiation source is used to "shine" γ-rays of either ^{99m}Tc or ^{57}Co through the subject.[38] To a first approximation, a correction factor may be obtained as $\sqrt{(C2/C1)}$, where C1 and C2 are count rates with and without the subject present, respectively. This method may be used to provide separate correction factors for individual lung regions, the mouth and the pharynx.[39]

Great emphasis has been placed on the need in scintigraphic studies to attend carefully to quality control issues, including not only radiolabeling validation and attenuation corrections, but also factors such as γ-camera uniformity and the need to obtain counts from all possible sites in order to ensure a radiolabel mass balance.[40–42]

12.2.4 Gamma Scintigraphy vs. SPECT

Gamma scintigraphy and SPECT are both methods that provide quantitative information about the behavior of pharmaceutical dosage forms. In some situations, the additional three-dimensional information provided by SPECT is probably of little value. For instance, a study to quantify where and when a tablet preparation disintegrates in the gastrointestinal tract has been undertaken by SPECT,[43] but γ scintigraphy would probably have provided equally useful data. In studies of nasal drug delivery, SPECT could be useful to provide information on the regional distribution of drug formulations in the nasal cavity, but there have been no published studies to date. A significant factor that may explain this lack of data is the rapid movement of formulations in the nasal cavity by mucociliary clearance. The clearance half-times of formulations from the nasal cavity are often only a matter of minutes, and may be comparable to the time taken to acquire a sequence of SPECT images as the γ-camera heads rotate. PET imaging seems to offer more promise for the assessment of nasal drug delivery in three dimensions.[44]

For studies of pulmonary drug delivery, γ-scintigraphy can quantify accurately the total amount of drug deposited in the target organ (the lungs), but the information that can be provided about deposition in specific lung regions is more limited.[45,46] Gamma scintigraphic analysis of regional lung deposition data involves dividing the lung fields into a series of regions, following the definition of the lung edges either from a ventilation scan with a radioactive inert gas or from a transmission scan. Since the γ-camera views the complex three-dimensional structure of the lungs in only two dimensions, it is difficult to relate the distribution pattern to lung anatomy in any precise way. A recently described method used in the authors' laboratory involves dividing the lungs into six concentric lung-shaped zones that are centered on the hilum (Figure 12.4). The data may be quantified as the mass of drug or percentage of the dose in each zone, or as airway penetration factors, which are corrected for the area of each zone and then normalized according to the activity concentration of the lungs as a whole.[47,48] The innermost regions will comprise mainly large conducting airways, and the outermost regions mainly small conducting airways and alveoli, but there will be significant overlap of airways in the different zones, with many small airways and alveoli also being represented in the innermost lung regions.

SPECT overcomes this fundamental limitation of γ-scintigraphy by viewing the lungs in three dimensions. The regional deposition data may be expressed either as sections through the lungs in transverse, coronal, and sagittal planes, or as a series of concentric shells (Figure 12.5) that are the three-dimensional equivalent of the two-dimensional concentric zones in γ-scintigraphy.[49]

The lung outline in three dimensions may be determined either by x-ray computed tomography or by magnetic resonance imaging, the latter being preferable since it does not result in an additional radiation dose. Case study 2 below will give an example of the way in which SPECT was able to detect a difference in regional lung deposition between two products that had not been detected by γ-scintigraphy. An exciting further development of SPECT imaging is that starting with the distribution data in a series of concentric shells, it is now possible to estimate the amount

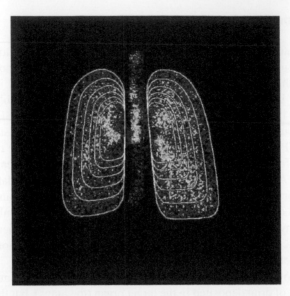

Figure 12.4   (See color insert following page 178.) Regional lung analysis in gamma scintigraphy. The lung is divided into six concentric lung-shaped zones centered on
the hilum. (From Newman, S.P. et al., *Adv. Drug Del. Rev.*, 55, 851, 2003. With
permission.)

of deposition taking place in different airway generations, thereby providing deposition data for specific anatomical regions of the lungs in a much more precise way
than was previously possible.[50] This approach has been validated using simulated
data,[51] with a good agreement shown between actual and estimated regional deposition patterns. In order for the data to be fully quantitative, it is necessary to make
corrections for the decrease in γ-ray counts in a region caused by tissue attenuation,
the increase in counts caused by γ-rays scattered into the region, and the partial
volume effect, which causes γ-rays to be wrongly assigned to a particular region
because of poor resolution.[52,53]

12.2.5 *In Vivo / In Vitro* Correlations

Scintigraphic studies of drug delivery by the pulmonary, nasal, and gastrointestinal routes can provide more useful and more clinically relevant data than more
traditional *in vitro* tests. The regulatory authorities place great importance on *in vitro*
particle size data for new pulmonary devices or formulations, but while these data
are vital for quality control purposes, they do not always reflect *in vivo* drug delivery
accurately. For instance, Figure 12.6 compares the fine-particle fraction (fraction of
particles contained in aerosol smaller than about 5 µm in diameter) measured by
cascade impaction and whole-lung deposition measured by γ-scintigraphy. Data are
shown for three inhaler devices: a liquid spray device (Respimat® soft mist inhaler,
Boehringer Ingelheim GmbH, Ingelheim, Germany), a DPI (Turbuhaler®, AstraZen-
eca PLC, London, U.K.) and a pMDI, all used to deliver inhaled corticosteroids.
For all three inhalers, the fine-particle fraction overestimated whole-lung deposition.

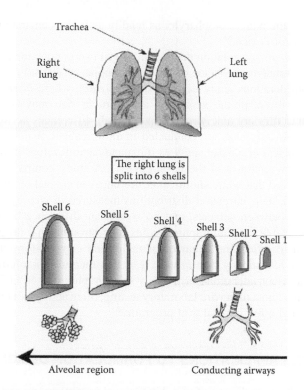

Figure 12.5 Regional lung analysis in SPECT. The lungs are divided into a series of concentric shells.

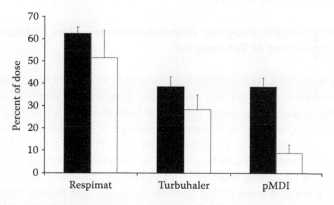

Figure 12.6 Comparison of fine-particle fraction (FPF) data as a predictor of lung deposition, and measured whole-lung deposition data by gamma scintigraphy, for three inhaler devices. ■, FPF; □, lung deposition. (Data from Pitcairn, G.R. et al., *J. Aerosol Med.*, 18, 264.)

For the pMDI, the differences between the fine-particle fraction and whole-lung deposition were very marked, probably because the rapidly moving pMDI spray cannot penetrate the human oropharynx as readily as it can penetrate the induction port of an impactor device.[54]

The *in vivo/in vitro* correlation may be improved using induction ports to impactor devices that simulate the shape of the human upper airways.[55]

Similar considerations apply to nasal drug delivery, where *in vitro* parameters such as spray pattern, plume geometry, and particle size may be measured so reproducibly that they are able to detect very small differences between products. Arguably, these *in vitro* tests are conducted in an unrealistic manner because they assess the parameters of a nasal spray as it expands and develops in free air, rather than in the narrow confines of the nasal cavity.[56] A study comparing two similar nasal sprays showed that while significant differences in several *in vitro* parameters could be detected, their intranasal distributions measured *in vivo* by γ-scintigraphy varied markedly between subjects, and no significant difference between the two sprays was detectable.[57] Scintigraphic studies of gastrointestinal drug delivery are also considered to reflect the behavior of tablet and capsule formulations in the human gut more realistically than *in vitro* tests that measure dissolution rates.[12,35]

Bearing these considerations in mind, γ-scintigraphic and SPECT studies can provide a useful adjunct to *in vitro* laboratory testing, often acting as a bridge between the laboratory and a full clinical trial program.[58]

12.3 APPLICATIONS TO FORMULATION DESIGN

In order to illustrate the use of two-dimensional γ-scintigraphy and three-dimensional SPECT, a series of case studies will be presented involving pulmonary, nasal, and gastrointestinal drug delivery.

12.3.1 Scintigraphic Imaging: Development of a New Pulmonary Formulation of Tobramycin

Patients with cystic fibrosis (CF) are susceptible to severe chest infections with pathogens including *Pseudomonas aeruginosa*. The lung secretions of CF patients are very viscous and cannot easily be cleared from the lung. Thus, infections have a chance to develop and lead to further lung damage. A formulation of the antibiotic tobramycin is marketed for pulmonary delivery (TOBI®, Chiron Corporation, Emeryville, CA), but this has to be given by jet nebulizer in a 5-mL volume over a treatment period of several minutes.[59] Jet nebulizers are bulky and inconvenient, deliver only a small fraction of the dose to the lungs, and require long treatment times. An alternative method of delivering tobramycin could therefore be advantageous. A formulation of porous dry powder particles[60] made by a proprietary spray-drying process (PulmoSphere® particles, Nektar Therapeutics, San Carlos, CA) has been developed for pulmonary delivery, and a proof-of-concept scintigraphic study was undertaken to compare nebulized and particle formulations.

Twelve healthy nonsmoking subjects took part in the study.[61] Three study regimens on different days involved replicate doses of PulmoSphere tobramycin to assess reproducibility of delivery. Six gelatine capsules were administered on each of 3 days. Each capsule contained 13.5 mg of PulmoSphere tobramycin powder (total of 81 mg of tobramycin). The powder was inhaled at a targeted peak inhaled flow rate of 70 L/min from a simple passive unit-dose DPI (Turbospin®, PH&T S.p.A., Milan, Italy). The total delivery time was about 2 min. On another day, 300 mg of tobramycin (TOBI) in 5 mL of diluent was delivered by Pari LC Plus® nebulizer coupled to a Pari Master® (both Pari GmbH, Starnberg, Germany) compressor with a nebulization time of 15 min.

The formulations were radiolabeled with ^{99m}Tc, and appropriate *in vitro* testing was undertaken to ensure that the radiolabel was a valid marker for the drug across all size bands. Two-dimensional scintigraphic imaging of the lungs, oropharynx, and apparatus was performed immediately after completion of dosing. The fractionation of the dose for each delivery system is shown in Figure 12.7.

Mean lung depositions were 34.3 and 5.0% of the nominal doses for PulmoSphere particles and for the Pari nebulizer, respectively. These figures corresponded to means of 27.8 and 15.0 mg of tobramycin, respectively. The replicate measures of lung deposition for PulmoSpheres showed inter- and intrasubject coefficients of variation of less than 20%. The DPI delivered tobramycin PulmoSphere powder efficiently, with only about 10% of the nominal dose being retained in either the capsule or the device. Plasma concentrations of PulmoSphere tobramycin measured up to 24 h postdose were approximately double those of tobramycin given by nebulizer (mean maximum plasma concentrations, 0.6 µg/mL for PulmoSphere particles and 0.28 µg/mL for nebulizer), and these data correlated well with the lung deposition data.

This proof-of-concept study demonstrated the ability of a PulmoSphere particle formulation to deposit at least as much tobramycin in the lungs as a nebulizer, but starting with only about one quarter of the nominal dose, and in a small fraction of the delivery time. It was considered that these differences should have important implications for the cost-effectiveness of inhaled tobramycin therapy and for improving patient compliance with treatment.

12.3.2 SPECT Imaging for Assessing Delivery of a New Pulmonary Formulation of Flunisolide

Inhaled corticosteroids are now accepted as first-line therapy for asthma in many countries.[62] The phasing out of chlorofluorocarbon (CFC) propellants for environmental reasons has meant that companies wishing to continue marketing pressurized metered dose inhaler (pMDI) products have had to seek alternative propellant formulations, comprising hydrofluoroalkane (HFA) 134a or 227.[63] While developing these new formulations, some companies have sought to deliver drug more efficiently to the peripheral airways of the lungs, recognizing that the alveoli and bronchial smooth muscle contain high concentrations of glucocorticosteroid receptors.[64]

A novel HFA formulation of the corticosteroid flunisolide (Aerospan®) has been developed by Forest Laboratories Inc. (New York, NY) to replace its already marketed CFC formulation (Aerobid®). We undertook a two-dimensional scintigraphic study[65] to compare total and regional lung depositions of flunisolide delivered by CFC pMDI (ex-valve (metered) dose, 294 µg) and by HFA pMDI (ex-valve (metered)

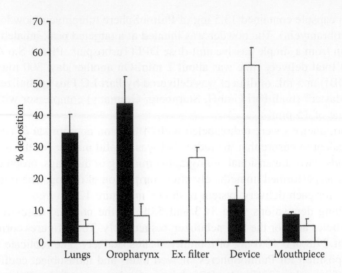

Figure 12.7 Percentage distribution of tobramycin dose delivered either as PulmoSphere particles or from a jet nebulizer. The results are expressed as a percentage of the powder capsule dose for the PulmoSphere particle formulation and as a percentage of the volume fill for the nebulizer. ■, PulmoSphere; □, nebulizer. (Data from Newhouse, M.T. et al., *Chest*, 124, 360, 2003.)

dose, 145 µg). The CFC formulation was a suspension of micronized particles with a mass median aerodynamic diameter (MMAD) of 3.8 µm, while the HFA formulation was a solution with an MMAD of 1.2 µm. Radiolabeling validation testing was undertaken successfully for each product. Mean (SD) whole-lung depositions from two-dimensional scintigraphy were 40.4 (5.5)% and 17.0 (10.4)% of the ex-valve dose for HFA and CFC formulations, respectively. However, the regional lung deposition pattern, expressed as a peripheral zone-to-central zone deposition ratio was the same for each product (mean values, 1.3 vs. 1.4).

The finding of the same regional lung distribution for CFC and HFA products was surprising, since the smaller-size HFA formulation aerosol would have been expected to penetrate more deeply into the lungs. It was considered that the finding could have resulted from the complex three-dimensional structure of the lungs, which was being viewed in only two dimensions, and that the ratio of peripheral zone to central zone deposition in two dimensions could be relatively insensitive to differences in regional depositions between products.[66] Therefore, the study was repeated,[67] but this time using SPECT imaging to assess regional lung deposition patterns. After inhalation, a SPECT imaging sequence was undertaken consisting of 32 pairs of images with a double-headed camera (ADAC Forte®, Philips Medical Systems, Best, Netherlands), as the camera heads rotated through 180°. The complete imaging sequence took approximately 8 min. Corrections to the data were made to allow for clearance of the radiolabel out of the lungs during the imaging process. The images were used to reconstruct the three-dimensional lung distribution for CFC–flunisolide and HFA–flunisolide, and the data from a transverse section through the lungs at the level of the hilum were analyzed. The data were presented as the ratio of deposition in an outer lung zone to that in an inner lung zone.

Now the data showed a significantly higher outer zone/inner zone deposition ratio for HFA–flunisolide than for CFC–flunisolide (mean values, 2.70 vs. 1.85).

Taken overall, the data showed that HFA–flunisolide was targeted more effectively to the lung periphery than CFC–flunisolide, and demonstrated the utility of using SPECT imaging in a situation where the assessment of regional deposition patterns within the lungs was a major study objective.

12.3.3 Delivery of a Nasal Insulin Formulation Assessed by Gamma Scintigraphy

Patients with diabetes who require regular therapy with insulin normally need to take this by injection. However, injections are inconvenient and painful, factors that can reduce compliance with treatment. A novel intranasal formulation of insulin was developed (Novo Nordisk A/S, Copenhagen, Denmark), and a two-dimensional scintigraphic study was undertaken to assess deposition in (and clearance from) the nasal cavity, changes in blood glucose, and whether or not any of the intranasal dose had reached the lungs. The issue of possible pulmonary deposition had been raised by a regulatory authority, and it was vital to address this question in order to help allay concerns about pulmonary accumulation of the formulation during long-term use of the product. Radionuclide imaging is ideal for assessing whether any lung deposition occurs, information that is probably impossible to obtain by any other noninvasive method.

Twelve healthy subjects were studied,[68] and there were four treatment regimens, representing a range of dose volumes (80 to 160 µL) and breathing maneuvers (gentle vs. vigorous sniffing). The dose was delivered from a nasal pump spray device, and the formulation was radiolabeled by the addition of ^{99m}Tc–human serum albumin (HSA). Volunteers ate a carbohydrate-rich meal immediately before dosing, in order to avoid the risk of hypoglycemia. The initial deposition pattern in the nasal cavity was assessed by an IGE Maxi® (IGE Medical Systems, Slough, U.K.) γ-camera, and then the clearance from the nose was followed by sequential imaging over 4 h. Blood glucose measurements were undertaken before dosing, and then at intervals up to 4 h postdose using an ExacTech® (MediSense (U.K.), Ltd., Abingdon, U.K.) meter.

The study showed that the entire dose was deposited in the nasal cavity, with no deposition in the lungs in any subject for any regimen. The formulation showed the expected two-phase clearance from the nasal cavity, with the fast phase representing mucociliary clearance from the area of the turbinates and the slow phase representing clearance from the nonciliated regions in the anterior part of the nasal cavity. Differences in nasal clearance between the regimens were minor. The data confirmed theoretical predictions, since pump spray devices generally comprise a spray of droplets greater than 10 µm in diameter,[69] which are too large to penetrate significantly through the nasal passages to enter the lungs.[70]

12.3.4 Proof-of-Concept Study to Assess Performance of an Enteric-Coated Tablet Formulation Using Gamma Scintigraphy

The oral route is preferred for most drugs because of its convenience, but the usefulness of nonsteroidal anti-inflammatory drugs (NSAIDs) is limited by gastric side effects. Enteric-coated tablets can overcome this limitation, since they are designed to remain intact in the stomach and then release their contents in the intestines. Gamma scintigraphy can be used to prove whether or not a new enteric-coated tablet preparation behaves according to its intended rationale. Furthermore, by relating scintigraphic data to plasma concentrations of drug obtained in a pharmacoscintigraphic study, it is possible to relate the biodistribution of the delivery system to drug absorption.

A novel enteric-coated formulation of the NSAID Naproxen® (Syntex Puerto Rico, Inc.) was investigated.[71] Each tablet contained 500 mg of Naproxen and was radiolabeled by the neutron-activation method. This involved incorporating 2 mg of samarium oxide (comprising isotopically enriched ^{152}Sm) into the tablet during its manufacture. Tablets were then irradiated in a nuclear reactor for 4 min at a neutron flux of 10^{12} neutrons /cm^2/sec, which converted the stable isotope ^{152}Sm into ^{153}Sm. Tests were carried out to demonstrate that the neutron activation procedure did not alter either the release characteristics of the formulation or the stability of the drug. The study was a randomized crossover comparison in seven healthy male subjects, both with (fed) and without (fasted) a light breakfast. Two enteric-coated tablets were given together on each study day, and the gastrointestinal transit of the ^{153}Sm-labeled tablets (total, 1 MBq ^{153}Sm) was tracked by sequential two-dimensional imaging of the stomach and intestines over 24 h. A drink of water containing ^{99m}Tc-DTPA was given to outline the gastrointestinal tract, and hence to aid with anatomical localization of the enteric-coated tablets.

Sequential images showed that there was no loss of tablet integrity in the stomach, and that all tablets disintegrated in the small intestine. In the fasting state, tablets disintegrated at a mean of 87 min (range, 11 to 134 min) postgastric emptying, compared with 94 min (range, 27 to 140 min) in the fed state (Table 12.2). Appearance of Naproxen in serum samples coincided with the observed tablet disintegration times, and maximum Naproxen concentrations in plasma were similar in fed and fasted states.

Table 12.2 Mean (Range) Times for Gastric Residence, Disintegration Time after Dosing, and Disintegration Time after Stomach Emptying for Enteric-Coated Naproxen Tablets Given in the Fed and Fasted States

	Fed	Fasted
Gastric residence (min)	110	47
	(67–187)	(6–162)
Disintegration time postdose (min)	204	134
	(130–247)	(78–263)
Disintegration time post-gastric emptying (min)	94	87
	(27–140)	(11–134)

Source: Wilding, I.R. et al., Pharm. Res., 9, 1436, 1992.

In summary, the study showed that the enteric-coated Naproxen tablets behaved as predicted, and in accordance with their intended rationale, allowing the new formulation to be developed and promoted with confidence.

REFERENCES

1. Maisey, M.N., Britton, K.E., and Gilday, B.L., *Clinical Nuclear Medicine*, 2nd ed., Chapman & Hall, London, 1991.
2. Parker, R.P., Smith, P.H.S., and Taylor, D.M., *Basic Science of Nuclear Medicine*, Churchill-Livingstone, New York, 1984.
3. Perkins, A.C., *Nuclear Medicine: Science and Safety*, John Libbey and Company, London, 1995.
4. Wagner, H.J., Hal Anger: nuclear medicine's quiet genius, *J. Nucl. Med.*, 44, 26, 2003.
5. Fleming, J.S., A history of the gamma camera: looking back to Anger, *Scope*, 6, 16, 1997.
6. Anger, H.O., Scintillation camera with multi-channel collimators, *J. Nucl. Med.*, 5, 151, 1964.
7. Pitcairn, G.R. et al., Radionuclide imaging for assessing pulmonary drug delivery: SPECT imaging and a novel radiolabelling method, *Drug Delivery Syst. Sci.*, 3, 5, 2003.
8. Davis, S.S. et al., Gamma scintigraphy in the evaluation of pharmaceutical dosage forms, *Eur. J. Nucl. Med.*, 19, 971, 1992.
9. Meseguer, G., Gurny, R., and Buri, P., *In vivo* evaluation of dosage forms: application of gamma scintigraphy to non-enteral routes of administration, *J. Drug Targeting*, 2, 269, 1994.
10. Wilson, C.G., Application of gamma scintigraphy to modern dosage form design, *Eur. J. Pharm. Sci.*, 2, 47, 1994.
11. Digenis, G.A. and Sandefer, E.P., Acceleration of pharmaceutical research and development with application of gamma scintigraphy, *European Pharmaceutical Contractor*, September, 22, 1999.
12. Wilding, I.R., Coupe, A.J., and Davis, S.S., The role of gamma scintigraphy in oral drug delivery, *Adv. Drug Del. Rev.*, 46, 103, 2001.
13. Newman, S.P. et al., Radionuclide imaging technologies and their use in evaluating asthma drug deposition in the lungs, *Adv. Drug Del. Rev.*, 55, 851, 2003.
14. Newman, S.P. and Illum, L., Radionuclide imaging studies in the assessment of nasal drug delivery in humans, *Am. J. Drug Delivery*, 2, 101, 2004.
15. Wilson, C.G., Assessing ocular drug delivery with lachrimal scintigraphy, *Pharm. Sci. Technol. Today*, 2, 321, 1999.
16. Washington, N. et al., A gamma scintigraphic study of gastric coating by Expidet, tablet and liquid formulations, *Int. J. Pharm.*, 57, 17, 1989.
17. Brown, J., Haines, S., and Wilding, I.R., Colonic spread of three rectally administered mesalazine (Pentasa) dosage forms in healthy volunteers as assessed by gamma scintigraphy, *Alimnet. Pharmacol. Ther.*, 11, 685, 1997.
18. Brown, J. et al., Spreading and retention of vaginal formulations in post-menopausal women as assessed by gamma scintigraphy, *Pharm. Res.*, 14, 1073, 1997.
19. Davis, S.S. and Illum, L., Colloidal carriers and drug targeting, *Acta Pharm. Technol.*, 32, 4, 1986.

20. Jones, T., New opportunities in molecular imaging using PET, *Drug Inf. J.*, 31, 991, 1997.
21. Wilding, I.R., Scintigraphic evaluation of colonic delivery systems, *STP Pharm. Sci.*, 5, 13, 1995.
22. Digenis, G.A. and Sandefer, E., Gamma scintigraphy and neutron activation techniques in the *in vivo* assessment of orally administered dosage forms, *Crit. Rev. Ther. Drug Carrier Syst.*, 7, 309, 1991.
23. Pitcairn, G.R. et al., TechneCoat: a novel method for radiolabelling dry powder formulations in radionuclide imaging studies, in *Respiratory Drug Delivery VIII*, Dalby, R.N. et al., Eds., Davis Horwood, Raleigh, NC, 2002, p. 553.
24. Burch, W.M., Sullivan, P.J., and McLaren, C.J., Technegas: a new ventilation agent for lung scanning, *Nucl. Med. Commun.*, 7, 865, 1986.
25. Conway, J.H. et al., Three-dimensional description of the deposition of inhaled terbutaline sulphate administered via Turbuhaler, in *Respiratory Drug Delivery VII*, Dalby, R.N. et al., Eds., Serentec Press, Raleigh, NC, 2000, p. 607.
26. Perkins, A. and Frier, M., Nuclear medicine imaging and drug delivery, *Nucl. Med. Commun.*, 21, 415, 2000.
27. Dolovich, M., Hahmias, C., and Coates, G., Unleashing the PET: 3D imaging of the lung, in *Respiratory Drug Delivery VII*, Dalby, R.N. et al., Eds., Serentec Press, Raleigh, NC, 2000, p. 215.
28. Berridge, M.S., Lee, Z., and Heald, D.L., Regional distribution and kinetics of inhaled pharmaceuticals, *Curr. Pharm. Des.*, 6, 1631, 2000.
29. Pozzi, F. et al., The TIME CLOCK system: a new oral dosage form for fast and complete release of drug after a predetermined time lag, *J. Cont. Rel.*, 31, 99, 1994.
30. Dashe, C.K. et al., The distribution of nebulised isoproterenol and its effect on regional ventilation and perfusion, *Am. Rev. Respir. Dis.*, 110, 293, 1974.
31. Walker, P.S. et al., An advanced and detailed *in vitro* validation procedure for the radiolabelling of carrier-free terbutaline sulphate dry powder, *J. Aerosol Med.*, 14, 227, 2001.
32. Warren, S. et al., Gamma scintigraphic evaluation of a novel budesonide dry powder inhaler using a validated radiolabeling technique, *J. Aerosol Med.*, 15, 15, 2002.
33. Hallworth, G.W., Particle size analysis of therapeutic aerosols, in *Aerosols in Medicine: Principles, Diagnosis and Therapy*, Morén, F. et al., Eds., Elsevier, Amsterdam, 1993, p. 351.
34. Snell, N.J.C. and Ganderton, D., Assessing lung deposition of inhaled medications, *Respir. Med.*, 93, 123, 1999.
35. Wilding, I.R., Coupe, A.J., and Davis, S.S., The role of gamma scintigraphy in oral drug delivery, *Adv. Drug Del. Rev.*, 7, 87, 1991.
36. Pitcairn, G.R. and Newman, S.P., Tissue attenuation corrections in gamma scintigraphy, *J. Aerosol Med.*, 3, 187, 1997.
37. Lee, Z. et al., The effect of scatter and attenuation on aerosol deposition as determined by gamma scintigraphy, *J. Aerosol Med.*, 14, 167, 2001.
38. Macey, D.J. and Marshall, R., Absolute quantitation of radiotracer uptake in the lungs using a gamma camera, *J. Nucl. Med.*, 23, 731, 1982.
39. Pitcairn, G.R. et al., An improved method of quantifying aerosol deposition from scintigraphic images, in *Proceedings of Drug Delivery to the Lungs XIII*, The Aerosol Society, Portishead, Bristol, 2002, p. 31.
40. Everard, M.L. and Dolovich, M.B., *In vivo* measurement of lung dose, in *Drug Delivery to the Lung*, Bisgaard, H., O'Callaghan, C., and Smaldone, G.C., Eds., Marcel Dekker, New York, 2002, p. 173.

41. Warren, S. and Taylor, G., Quality control aspects of pharmaceutical gamma scintigraphy studies, *European Pharmaceutical Contractor*, March 2004.
42. Bondesson, E. et al., Planar gamma scintigraphy: points to consider when quantifying pulmonary dry powder aerosol deposition, *Int. J. Pharm.*, 258, 227, 2003.
43. Perkins, A.C., Mann, C., and Wilson, C.G., Three-dimensional visualisation of the large bowel: a potential tool for assessing targeted drug delivery and colonic pathology, *Eur. J. Nucl. Med.*, 22, 1035, 1995.
44. Berridge, M.S. et al., Biodistribution and kinetics of nasal C-11 triamcinolone acetonide, *J. Nucl. Med.*, 39, 1972, 1998.
45. Dolovich, M.B., Measuring total and regional lung deposition using inhaled radiotracers, *J. Aerosol Med.*, 14 (Suppl. 1), S35, 2001.
46. Fleming, J.S. and Conway, J.H., Three-dimensional imaging of aerosol deposition, *J. Aerosol Med.*, 14, 147, 2001.
47. Pitcairn, G.R. et al., Lung penetration profiles: a new method for analyzing regional lung deposition data in scintigraphic studies, in *Respiratory Drug Delivery VIII*, Dalby, R.N. et al., Eds., Davis Horwood, Raleigh, NC, 2002, p. 549.
48. Pitcairn, G.R. et al., Radionuclide imaging for assessing pulmonary drug delivery: new methodologies for quantifying whole lung and regional lung deposition, *Int. J. Pharm. Med.*, 17, 11, 2003.
49. Perring, S. et al., A new method of quantification of the pulmonary regional distribution of aerosols using combined CT and SPECT and its application to nedocromil sodium administered by metered dose inhaler, *Br. J. Radiol.*, 67, 46, 1994.
50. Pitcairn, G.R. et al., Development of a standard method for quantifying regional lung deposition from SPECT and relating the data to airway anatomy, in *Respiratory Drug Delivery IX*, Dalby, R.N. et al., Eds., Davis Healthcare International, River Grove, IL, 2004, p. 621.
51. Fleming, J.S., Measuring drug deposition by airway generation in humans, in *Respiratory Drug Delivery IX*, Dalby, R.N. et al., Eds., Davis Healthcare International, River Grove, IL, 2004, p. 187.
52. Fleming, J.S. et al., Evaluation of the accuracy and precision of lung aerosol deposition measurements from single-photon emission computed tomography using simulation, *J. Aerosol Med.*, 13, 187, 2000.
53. Fleming, J.S. et al., Comparison of methods for deriving aerosol deposition by aerosol generation from three-dimensional radionuclide imaging, *J. Aerosol Sci.*, 31, 1251, 2000.
54. Pitcairn GR, Reader S, Pavia D. Deposition of corticosteroid aerosol in the human lung by Respimat soft mist inhaler compared to deposition by metered dose inhaler or by Turbuhaler dry powder inhaler. J. Aerosol Med 2005; 18: 264–272.
55. Finlay, W.H. et al., Solving a major *in vitro-in vivo* correlation problem: impactor induction ports, in *Respiratory Drug Delivery IX*, Dalby, R.N. et al., Eds., Davis Healthcare International, River Grove, IL, 2004, p. 203.
56. Newman, S.P., Pitcairn, G.R., and Dalby, R.N., Drug delivery to the nasal cavity: *in vitro* and *in vivo* assessment, *Crit. Rev. Ther. Drug Delivery Syst.*, 21, 21, 2004.
57. Suman, J.D. et al., Validity of *in vitro* tests on aqueous spray pumps as surrogates for nasal deposition, *Pharm. Res.*, 19, 1, 2002.
58. Newman, S.P., Wilding, I.R., and Hirst, P.H., Human lung deposition data: the bridge between *in vitro* and clinical evaluations for inhaled drug products?, *Int. J. Pharm.*, 208, 49, 2000.
59. Ramsey, B.W. et al., Intermittent administration of inhaled tobramycin in patients with cystic fibrosis, *N. Engl. J. Med.*, 340, 23, 1999.

60. Tarara, T.E., Weers, J., and Dellamary, L., Engineered powders for inhalation, in *Respiratory Drug Delivery VII*, Dalby, R.N. et al., Eds., Serentec Press, Raleigh, NC, 2000, p. 413.
61. Newhouse, M.T. et al., Inhalation of a dry powder tobramycin PulmoSphere formulation in healthy volunteers, *Chest*, 124, 360, 2003.
62. Barnes, P.J., Pedersen, S., and Busse, W.W., Efficacy and safety of inhaled corticosteroids: new developments, *Am. J. Respir. Crit. Care Med.*, 157, S1, 1998.
63. Partridge, M.R. et al., Chlorofluorocarbon-free inhalers: are we ready for the change?, *Eur. Respir. J.*, 11, 1006, 1998.
64. Lipworth, B.J., Targets for inhaled treatment, *Respir. Med.*, 94 (Suppl. D), S13, 2000.
65. Richards, J.C. et al., Deposition and pharmacokinetics of flunisolide delivered from pressurized inhalers containing non-CFC and CFC propellants, *J. Aerosol Med.*, 14, 197, 2001.
66. Phipps, P.R. et al., Comparisons of planar and tomographic gamma scintigraphy to measure the penetration index of inhaled aerosols, *Am. Rev. Respir. Dis.*, 139, 1516, 1989.
67. Newman, S.P. et al., Using gamma scintigraphy and single photon emission computed tomography to assess the pulmonary deposition of a new inhaled formulation of flunisolide, in *Proceedings of Drug Delivery to the Lungs XIII*, The Aerosol Society, Portishead, Bristol, 2002, p. 87.
68. Newman, S.P. et al., The distribution of an intranasal insulin formulation in healthy volunteers. Effect of different administration techniques, *J. Pharm. Pharmacol.*, 46, 657, 1994.
69. Petri, W., Schmiedel, R., and Sandow, J., Development of a metered-dose nebulizer for intranasal peptide administration, in *Transnasal Systemic Medications*, Chien, Y.W., Ed., Elsevier Science Publishers, Amsterdam, 1985, p. 161.
70. Heyder, J. et al., Deposition of particles in the human respiratory tract in the size range 0.005 to 15 μm, *J. Aerosol Sci.*, 17, 811, 1986.
71. Wilding, I.R. et al., *In vivo* evaluation of enteric-coated naproxen tablets using gamma scintigraphy, *Pharm. Res.*, 9, 1436, 1992.

Prefix	Symbol	Power of 10
Yotta	Y	10^{24}
Zetta	Z	10^{21}
Exa	E	10^{18}
Peta	P	10^{15}
Tera	T	10^{12}
Giga	G	10^{9}
Mega	M	10^{6}
Kilo	K	10^{3}
Milli	m	10^{-3}
Micro	μ	10^{-6}
Nano	n	10^{-9}
Pico	p	10^{-12}
Femto	f	10^{-15}
Atto	a	10^{-18}
Zepto	z	10^{-21}
Yocto	y	10^{-24}

Index

A

Accelerator mass spectrometry, 11, 29, 56, 233–249
  absolute bioavailability, 244–245
  data handling, 240–241
  defined, 233
  drug development, 243–247
  drug metabolism studies, 56
  as enabling technology, 243
  experimental populations, 244–245
  future developments, 247
  instrumentation, 235–237
  isotopes, 237–238
  metabolism, 56
  microdosing, 245–247
  precision of, 241–242
  radioactivity, 11, 29
  sample preparation, 238–239
  sensitivity, 241–242
  tandem accelerator, derivation of term, 236
Active guard detectors, 196–197
Administration of Radioactive Substances Advisory Committee, 14
Administration of radioactivity, 13–14
Alpha decay, 19
AMS. *See* Accelerator mass spectrometry
Approval of drug, 4
ARSAC. *See* Administration of Radioactive Substances Advisory Committee
Atoms, 18
Auger electrons, 21
Autoradiolysis, radioactivity, 35–37

B

Background reduction, 195–202
  instrument design, 196
  liquid scintillation counting, 195–202
    active guard detectors, 196–197
    instrument design, 196
    pulse amplitude comparison, 199
    pulse height analysis, 197
    pulse shape analysis, 197–199
    time-resolved liquid scintillation counting, 199–201
    TR-LSC guard detectors, 201
Beta decay, 19–20
Bile, sample preparation for liquid scintillation counting, 223–224
Bile duct cannulation, 63
Bioanalysis, 65–66
Biological tissues, sample preparation for liquid scintillation counting, 226–229
Biomedical accelerator mass spectrometry, 233–249
  absolute bioavailability, 244–245
  data handling, 240–241
  defined, 233
  drug development, 243–247
  as enabling technology, 243
  experimental populations, 244–245
  future developments, 247
  instrumentation, 235–237
  isotopes, 237–238
  microdosing, 245–247
  precision of, 241–242
  sample preparation, 238–239